THE HEALTH CARE SYSTEM

ISSN 1543-2556

THE HEALTH CARE SYSTEM

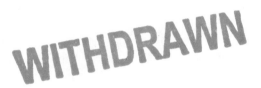

Barbara Wexler

INFORMATION PLUS® REFERENCE SERIES
Formerly Published by Information Plus, Wylie, Texas

GALE
CENGAGE Learning·

Detroit • New York • San Francisco • New Haven, Conn • Waterville, Maine • London

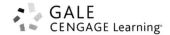

The Health Care System

Barbara Wexler

Kepos Media, Inc.: Paula Kepos and Janice Jorgensen, Series Editors

Project Editors: Kathleen J. Edgar, Elizabeth Manar, Kimberley McGrath

Rights Acquisition and Management: Leitha Etheridge-Sims

Composition: Evi Abou-El-Seoud, Mary Beth Trimper

Manufacturing: Rita Wimberley

For product information and technology assistance, contact us at
Gale Customer Support, 1-800-877-4253.
For permission to use material from this text or product,
submit all requests online at **www.cengage.com/permissions.**
Further permissions questions can be e-mailed to
permissionrequest@cengage.com

Cover photograph: © Anetta/Shutterstock.com.

Gale
27500 Drake Rd.
Farmington Hills, MI 48331-3535

ISBN-13: 978-0-7876-5103-9 (set)   ISBN-10: 0-7876-5103-6 (set)
ISBN-13: 978-1-4144-8145-6   ISBN-10: 1-4144-8145-4

ISSN 1543-2556

This title is also available as an e-book.
ISBN-13: 978-1-5730-2285-9 (set)
ISBN-10: 1-5730-2285-3 (set)
Contact your Gale sales representative for ordering information.

Printed in the United States of America
2 3 4 5 6   18 17 16 15 14

TABLE OF CONTENTS

PREFACE

The Health Care System is part of the *Information Plus Reference Series*. The purpose of each volume of the series is to present the latest facts on a topic of pressing concern in modern American life. These topics include the most controversial and studied social issues of the 21st century: abortion, capital punishment, care for the elderly, child abuse, crime, energy, the environment, gambling, immigration, minorities, national security, social welfare, women, youth, and many more. Even though this series is written especially for high school and undergraduate students, it is an excellent resource for anyone in need of factual information on current affairs.

By presenting the facts, it is the intention of Gale, Cengage Learning to provide its readers with everything they need to reach an informed opinion on current issues. To that end, there is a particular emphasis in this series on the presentation of scientific studies, surveys, and statistics. These data are generally presented in the form of tables, charts, and other graphics placed within the text of each book. Every graphic is directly referred to and carefully explained in the text. The source of each graphic is presented within the graphic itself. The data used in these graphics are drawn from the most reputable and reliable sources, such as from the various branches of the U.S. government and from private organizations and associations. Every effort has been made to secure the most recent information available. Readers should bear in mind that many major studies take years to conduct and that additional years often pass before the data from these studies are made available to the public. Therefore, in many cases the most recent information available in 2013 is dated from 2010 or 2011. Older statistics are sometimes presented as well, if they are landmark studies or of particular interest and no more-recent information exists.

Although statistics are a major focus of the *Information Plus Reference Series*, they are by no means its only content. Each book also presents the widely held positions and important ideas that shape how the book's subject is discussed in the United States. These positions are explained in detail and, where possible, in the words of their proponents. Some of the other material to be found in these books includes historical background, descriptions of major events related to the subject, relevant laws and court cases, and examples of how these issues play out in American life. Some books also feature primary documents or have pro and con debate sections that provide the words and opinions of prominent Americans on both sides of a controversial topic. All material is presented in an evenhanded and unbiased manner; readers will never be encouraged to accept one view of an issue over another.

HOW TO USE THIS BOOK

The U.S. health care system is a multifaceted establishment consisting of health care providers, patients, and treatment facilities, just to name a few components. This book examines the state of the nation's health care system, the education and training of health care providers, and the various types of health care institutions. The landmark health care reform legislation, efforts to control the cost of health care, prevalence of insurance, mental health care, and a comparison of health care throughout the world are also covered.

The Health Care System consists of nine chapters and three appendixes. Each chapter is devoted to a particular aspect of the health care system in the United States. For a summary of the information that is covered in each chapter, please see the synopses that are provided in the Table of Contents. Chapters generally begin with an overview of the basic facts and background information on the chapter's topic, then proceed to examine subtopics of particular interest. For example, Chapter 8: Change, Challenges, and Innovation in Health Care Delivery begins by describing changes in the U.S. health care system including new types of practitioners, the passage of the Patient Protection and Affordable Care Act and the Health Care and Education Reconciliation Act in 2010, and the use of information technology. Next, the chapter considers initiatives aimed at improving the safety and quality of health care delivery. This is followed by a discussion of the use of clinical practice guidelines to standardize care and treatment. The chapter details how communication and information management technologies, including telemedicine, online patient-physician consultations, and robotics, may be used to improve access to care and the outcomes of care. It concludes with a discussion of innovation, the diffusion of new technology, and how to present data about comparative costs and quality to consumers to better enable them to make informed health care purchases. Readers can find their way through a chapter by looking for the section and subsection headings, which are clearly set off from the text. They can also refer to the book's extensive Index if they already know what they are looking for.

Statistical Information

The tables and figures featured throughout *The Health Care System* will be of particular use to readers in learning about this issue. These tables and figures represent an extensive collection of the most recent and important statistics on the health care system, as well as related issues—for example, graphics cover the rate of supply and demand for registered nurses, the number of emergency department visits, the national health expenditure amounts, the percentage of people without health insurance, and public opinion on whether the health care reform law will help or hurt the U.S. economy. Gale, Cengage Learning believes that making this information available to readers is the most important way to fulfill the goal of this book: to help readers understand the issues and controversies surrounding the health care system in the United States and reach their own conclusions.

Each table or figure has a unique identifier appearing above it, for ease of identification and reference. Titles for the tables and figures explain their purpose. At the end of each table or figure, the original source of the data is provided.

To help readers understand these often complicated statistics, all tables and figures are explained in the text. References in the text direct readers to the relevant statistics. Furthermore, the contents of all tables and figures are fully indexed. Please see the opening section of the Index at the back of this volume for a description of how to find tables and figures within it.

Appendixes

Besides the main body text and images, *The Health Care System* has three appendixes. The first is the Important Names and Addresses directory. Here, readers will find contact information for a number of government and private organizations that can provide further information on aspects of the health care system. The second appendix is the Resources section, which can also assist readers in conducting their own research. In this section, the author and editors of *The Health Care System* describe some of the sources that were most useful during the compilation of this book. The final appendix is the Index. It has been greatly expanded from previous editions and should make it even easier to find specific topics in this book.

ADVISORY BOARD CONTRIBUTIONS

The staff of Information Plus would like to extend its heartfelt appreciation to the Information Plus Advisory Board. This dedicated group of media professionals provides feedback on the series on an ongoing basis. Their comments allow the editorial staff who work on the project to make the series better and more user-friendly. The staff's top priority is to produce the highest-quality and most useful books possible, and the Information Plus Advisory Board's contributions to this process are invaluable.

The members of the Information Plus Advisory Board are:

- Kathleen R. Bonn, Librarian, Newbury Park High School, Newbury Park, California

- Madelyn Garner, Librarian, San Jacinto College, North Campus, Houston, Texas

- Anne Oxenrider, Media Specialist, Dundee High School, Dundee, Michigan

- Charles R. Rodgers, Director of Libraries, Pasco-Hernando Community College, Dade City, Florida

- James N. Zitzelsberger, Library Media Department Chairman, Oshkosh West High School, Oshkosh, Wisconsin

COMMENTS AND SUGGESTIONS

The editors of the *Information Plus Reference Series* welcome your feedback on *The Health Care System*. Please direct all correspondence to:

Editors
Information Plus Reference Series
27500 Drake Rd.
Farmington Hills, MI 48331-3535

CHAPTER 1
THE U.S. HEALTH CARE SYSTEM

When asked to describe the U.S. health care system, most Americans would probably offer a description of just a single facet of a huge, complex interaction of people, institutions, and technology. Like snapshots, each account offers an image, frozen in time, of one of the many health care providers and the settings in which medical care is delivered. Examples of these include:

- Physician offices: for many Americans, health care may be described as the interaction between a primary care physician and a patient to address minor and urgent medical problems, such as colds, allergies, or back pain. A primary care physician (usually a general practitioner, family practitioner, internist, or pediatrician) is the frontline caregiver—the first practitioner to evaluate and treat the patient. Routine physical examinations, prevention management actions such as immunization and health screening to detect disease, and treatment of acute and chronic diseases commonly take place in physicians' offices.

- Medical clinics: these settings provide primary care services comparable to those provided in physicians' offices and may be organized to deliver specialized support such as prenatal care for expectant mothers, well-baby care for infants, or treatment for specific medical conditions such as hypertension (high blood pressure), diabetes, or asthma.

- Hospitals: these institutions contain laboratories, imaging centers (also known as radiology departments, where x-rays and other imaging studies are performed), and other equipment for diagnosis and treatment, as well as emergency departments, operating rooms, and highly specialized personnel.

Medical care is also provided through many other venues, including outpatient surgical centers, school health programs, pharmacies, worksite clinics, and voluntary health agencies such as Planned Parenthood, the American Red Cross, and the American Lung Association.

IS THE U.S. HEALTH CARE SYSTEM AILING?

Even though medical care in the United States is often considered to be the best available, some observers feel the system that delivers it is fragmented and in serious disarray. This section offers some of the many opinions about the challenges of the present health care system and how to improve it. For example, in "A Grim Diagnosis for Our Ailing Health Care System" (*Washington Post*, November 27, 2011), Robert J. Samuelson describes the nation's health care system as "fragmented and overspecialized" and opines that it "delivers the worst of both worlds: pay more, get less."

Joe Flower believes that the United States can deliver better health care for half the cost. In *Healthcare beyond Reform: Doing It Right for Half the Cost* (2012), he contends that the current U.S. health care system is in crisis because it is driven by the aims, methods, and preferences of health care providers and payers instead of by the needs of health care consumers. Flower argues that the U.S. health care system must eliminate a significant percentage of the medical procedures that are currently performed and replace expensive procedures with less costly procedures by detecting health problems earlier.

Flower proposes a number of measures to improve quality and reduce costs, including:

- Institute employer- and government-sponsored prevention and wellness programs so that chronic diseases are identified and managed earlier.

- Focus the efforts of teams of health professionals on people with chronic illnesses to reduce the need for higher-cost care. Even though this strategy is labor-intensive, it produces a high rate of return on the investment.

- Change how providers are compensated. Instead of paying physicians, hospitals, and other providers for individual medical procedures, they should be compensated by case rates and outcome-based payments that place them at financial risk. When providers are paid to keep patients healthy, costs will decline.

- Encourage the widespread use of health care teams and other proven measures to improve the efficiency of patient care.

- Target the highest-cost patients with interventions to reduce the costs that are associated with their care.

- Reduce the cost of variability by directing patients to the highest value providers—those that provide the same services and procedures with comparable outcomes for the lowest cost.

- Reduce the unnecessary costs that are associated with end-of-life care.

Primary care physicians also find fault with the health care system. In "Too Little? Too Much? Primary Care Physicians' Views on US Health Care: A Brief Report" (*Archives of Internal Medicine*, vol. 171, no. 17, September 26, 2011), Brenda E. Sirovich, Steven Woloshin, and Lisa M. Schwartz report the findings of a survey of primary care physicians. Nearly half of the physicians surveyed feel that their patients receive too much medical care, and more than 25% report that they themselves deliver too much care, largely by practicing "defensive medicine" to guard against malpractice suits. They are also concerned about overly aggressive practice among midlevel primary care providers (nurse practitioners and physician assistants) and physician subspecialists. Sirovich, Woloshin, and Schwartz assert that "physicians believe there is substantial unnecessary care that could be reduced, particularly by increasing time with patients, reforming the malpractice system, and reducing financial incentives to do more."

David De Ferranti and Julio Frenk observe in "Toward Universal Health Coverage" (*New York Times*, April 5, 2012) that the 25 wealthiest nations in the world, except the United States, have some form of universal health coverage. Even though health care legislation championed by the Obama administration had already expanded coverage by mid-2012, De Ferranti and Frenk aver that mandating large and midsized employers to provide coverage still left many people—the self-employed, people employed by small businesses, the unemployed, and retired people—without coverage.

The previously described ideas are just a few of the wide variety of ways in which people have proposed improvements to the existing health care system in the United States. Besides individual ideas, large-scale reforms have been proposed by presidential administrations, such as by the Clinton administration during the early 1990s. More recently, sweeping health care reform legislation was signed into law by President Barack Obama (1961–) in 2010. The Patient Protection and Affordable Care Act

(PPACA) contains numerous health-related provisions that began taking effect in 2010 and that will be phased in through 2014. Key provisions aim to extend coverage to millions of uninsured Americans, institute measures to contain and control health care costs and improve system efficiency, and eliminate denial of health care coverage based on preexisting conditions.

Reforming the U.S. Health Care System

Derek Bok of Harvard University observes in "The Great Health Care Debate of 1993–94" (1998, http://www.upenn.edu/pnc/ptbok.html) that while in 1993 it appeared that President Bill Clinton (1946–) might successfully enact sweeping reform of the health care system, by September 1994 the legislation his administration had championed was dead. Bok attributes the demise of the legislation to divisive special interest groups and to inadequate efforts to educate the public, which resulted in confusion and misunderstanding of the provisions of the legislation and opposition to it. Bok asserts that because many Americans mistakenly assumed that eliminating excess health care costs generated by fraud and waste would not free up enough money to provide coverage for all of the uninsured, they opposed the Clinton initiative, which they deemed too costly. Bok also recounts that even as public sentiment appeared to be opposed to the Clinton plan, a poll asking respondents to evaluate various health plans without disclosing their sponsors found that 76% of respondents favored the Clinton initiative.

Health care reform was a key issue during the 2008 presidential election. Shortly after taking office, President Obama announced his intention to make his campaign resolve—to fix health care by expanding coverage of the uninsured and helping Americans afford coverage and care—a reality. After a year of bitter partisan (adhering to one party) conflict, the PPACA was signed by President Obama and became law on March 23, 2010. A few days later this act was amended by the Health Care and Education Reconciliation Act, which became law on March 30, 2010.

Together, the PPACA and the Health Care and Education Reconciliation Act (which are now commonly known as the ACA) aim to expand coverage, contain health care costs, and improve the health care delivery system. More specifically, the ACA requires most U.S. citizens and legal residents to have health insurance and promises the creation of health insurance exchanges and other mechanisms to enable people with low incomes and small businesses to purchase insurance coverage. Beginning in 2014, all employers with more than 50 employees will be required to offer coverage; failing to do so will result in penalties. The ACA expands Medicaid (a state and federal health insurance program for low-income people) and the Children's Health Insurance Program to ensure that these public programs cover eligible people.

It also strengthens Medicare (a federal health insurance program for people aged 65 years and older and people with disabilities) prescription drug benefits. Furthermore, it eliminates lifetime and annual limits on coverage.

Opposition to the ACA mounted as soon as it was passed with federal judges ruling along party lines—those appointed by Democrats upheld the law and those appointed by Republicans deemed portions of the law, most notably the mandate requiring individuals to purchase health insurance, unconstitutional. For example, Michael Cooper observes in "Conservatives Sowed Idea of Health Care Mandate, Only to Spurn It Later" (*New York Times*, February 14, 2012) that even though the mandate was initially favored by conservatives, in 2012 it was "Republicans and conservatives who oppose the individual mandate, arguing that it is unconstitutional, while Democrats, who were long resistant to it, are its biggest defenders." In "Health Care Ruling, Vast Implications for Medicaid" (*New York Times*, June 15, 2012), Robert Pear indicates that more than half the states also challenged the constitutionality of the ACA requirement to expand Medicaid. The U.S. Supreme Court was called on to determine the constitutionality of the ACA and industry observers speculated that the court might overturn part or all of the complicated landmark legislation.

On June 28, 2012, in *National Federation of Independent Business v. Sebelius, Secretary of Health and Human Services* (No. 11-393), the Supreme Court voted 5–4 to uphold the ACA, with Chief Justice John G. Roberts (1955–) casting the deciding vote to affirm the health care reform legislation. Writing for the majority opinion, Roberts explained that requiring individuals who choose to forgo health insurance to pay a penalty is not unlike a tax. Because taxation is constitutional, it was not necessary for the court to prohibit it or even opine about its merit. However, the court did limit the ACA's requirements that the states expand Medicaid coverage, rejecting the plan to deny federal payments to states that failed to increase this coverage.

While supporters of the ACA celebrated the Supreme Court decision, its detractors, many of whom were Republican, vowed to continue their efforts to repeal it. John Parkinson explains in "House Gears up to Repeal Obamacare (Again)" (ABCnews.com, July 10, 2012) that even though there were insufficient votes in the U.S. Senate to repeal the ACA in July 2012, the U.S. House of Representatives had voted 32 times to "defund, dismantle and repeal" it and that it would continue to oppose the legislation despite the dwindling odds of successful repeal.

THE COMPONENTS OF THE HEALTH CARE SYSTEM

The health care system consists of all personal medical care services—prevention, diagnosis, treatment, and rehabilitation (services to restore function and independence)—plus the institutions and personnel that provide these services and the government, public, and private organizations and agencies that finance service delivery.

The health care system may be viewed as a complex consisting of three interrelated components: health care consumers (people in need of health care services), health care providers (people who deliver health care services—the professionals and practitioners), and the institutions and organizations of the health care system (the public and private agencies that organize, plan, regulate, finance, and coordinate services) that provide the systematic arrangements for delivering health care. The institutional component includes hospitals, clinics, and home-health agencies; the insurance companies and programs that pay for services (such as Blue Cross/Blue Shield), managed care plans (such as health maintenance organizations), and preferred provider organizations; and entitlement programs such as Medicare and Medicaid. Other health care institutions are the professional schools that train students for careers in medical, public health, dental, and allied health professions, such as nursing and laboratory technology. Also included are agencies and associations that research and monitor the quality of health care services; license and accreditation providers and institutions; local, state, and national professional societies; and the companies that produce medical technology, equipment, and pharmaceuticals.

Much of the interaction among the three components of the health care system occurs directly between individual health care consumers and providers. Other interactions are indirect and impersonal such as immunization programs or screenings to detect disease, which are performed by public health agencies for whole populations. All health care delivery relies on interactions among the three components. The ability to benefit from health care depends on an individual's or group's ability to gain entry to the health care system. The process of gaining entry to the health care system is referred to as access, and many factors can affect access to health care. This chapter provides an overview of how Americans access the health care system.

ACCESS TO THE HEALTH CARE SYSTEM

In the 21st century access to health care services is a key measure of the overall health and prosperity of a nation or a population, but access and availability were not always linked to good health status. In fact, many medical historians assert that until the beginning of the 20th century, a visit with a physician was as likely to be harmful as it was helpful. Only since the early 20th century has medical care been considered to be a positive influence on health and longevity.

There are three aspects of accessibility: consumer access, comprehensive availability of services, and supply of services adequate to meet community demand. Quality health care services must be accessible to health care consumers when and where they are needed. The health care provider must have access to a full range of facilities, equipment, drugs, and services provided by other practitioners. The institutional component of health care delivery—the hospitals, clinics, and payers—must have timely access to information to enable them to plan an adequate supply of appropriate services for their communities.

Consumer Access to Care

Access to health care services is influenced by a variety of factors. Characteristics of health care consumers strongly affect when, where, and how they access services. Differences in age, educational attainment, economic status, race, ethnicity, cultural heritage, and geographic location determine when consumers seek health care services, where they go to receive them, their expectations of treatment, and the extent to which they wish to participate in decisions about their own medical care.

People have different reasons for seeking access to health care services. Their personal beliefs about health and illness, motivations to obtain care, expectations of the care they will receive, and knowledge about how and where to receive care vary. For an individual to have access to quality care, there must be appropriately defined points of entry into the health care system. For many consumers, a primary care physician is their portal to the health care system. Besides evaluating and addressing the patient's immediate health care need, the primary care physician also directs the consumer to other providers of care such as physician specialists or mental health professionals.

Some consumers access the health care system by seeking care from a clinic or hospital outpatient department, where teams of health professionals are available at one location. Others gain entry by way of a public health nurse, school nurse, social worker, or pharmacist, who refers them to an appropriate source, site, or health care practitioner.

Comprehensive Availability of Health Care Services

Historically, the physician was the exclusive provider of all medical services. Until the 20th century the family doctor served as physician, surgeon, pharmacist, therapist, adviser, and dentist. He carried all the tools of his trade in a small bag and could easily offer state-of-the-art medical care in the patient's home, because hospitals had little more to offer in the way of equipment or facilities. In the 21st century it is neither practical nor desirable to ask one practitioner to serve in all these roles. It would be impossible for one professional to perform the full range of health care services, from primary prevention of disease and diagnosis to treatment and rehabilitation. Modern physicians and other health care practitioners must have access to a comprehensive array of trained personnel, facilities, and equipment so that they can, in turn, make them accessible to their patients.

Even though many medical problems are effectively treated in a single office visit with a physician, even simple diagnosis and treatment relies on a variety of ancillary (supplementary) services and personnel. To make the diagnosis, the physician may order an imaging study such as an x-ray or ultrasound that is performed by a radiology technician and interpreted by a radiologist (physician specialist in imaging techniques). Laboratory tests may be performed by technicians and analyzed by pathologists (physicians who specialize in microscopic analysis and diagnosis). More complicated medical problems involve teams of surgeons and high-tech surgical suites that are equipped with robotic assistants and rehabilitation programs in which physical and occupational therapists assist patients to regain function and independence.

Some health care services are more effectively, efficiently, and economically provided to groups rather than to individuals. Immunization to prevent communicable diseases and screening to detect diseases in their earliest and most treatable stages are examples of preventive services best performed as cooperative efforts of voluntary health organizations, medical and other professional societies, hospitals, and public health departments.

Access Requires Enough Health Care Services to Meet Community Needs

For all members of a community to have access to the full range of health care services, careful planning is required to ensure both the adequate supply and distribution of needed services. To evaluate community needs and effectively allocate health care resources, communities must gather demographic data and information about the social and economic characteristics of the population. They must also monitor the spread of disease and the frequency of specific medical conditions over time. All these population data must be considered in relation to available resources, including health care personnel; the distribution of facilities, equipment, and human resources (the available health care workforce); and advances in medicine and technology.

For example, a predicted shortage of nurses may prompt increased spending on nursing education; reviews of nurses' salary, benefits, and working conditions; and the cultivation of nonnursing personnel to perform specific responsibilities that were previously assigned to nurses. Similarly, when ongoing surveillance anticipates an especially virulent influenza (flu) season, public health officials, agencies, and practitioners intensify efforts to provide timely immunization to vulnerable populations such as older adults. Government agencies such as the Centers for Disease Control and Prevention (CDC), the National Institutes of Health, state and local health departments, professional societies, voluntary health agencies, and universities work together to research, analyze, and forecast health care needs. Their recommendations allow health care planners, policy makers, and legislators to allocate resources so that supply keeps pace with demand and to ensure that new services and strategies are developed to address existing and emerging health care concerns.

A REGULAR SOURCE OF HEALTH CARE IMPROVES ACCESS

According to the CDC, the determination of whether an individual has a regular source (i.e., a regular provider or site) of health care is a powerful predictor of access to health care services. Generally, people without regular sources have less access or access to fewer services, including key preventive medical services such as prenatal care, routine immunization, and health screening. Many factors have been found that contribute to keeping individuals from having regular sources of medical care, with income level being the best predictor of unmet medical needs or problems gaining access to health care services.

Patricia M. Barnes et al. of the National Center for Health Statistics (NCHS) analyze the 2011 National Health Interview Survey (NHIS), an annual nationwide survey of about 55,000 people in the United States, in *Early Release of Selected Estimates Based on Data from the January–September 2011 National Health Interview Survey* (March 2012, http://www.cdc.gov/nchs/data/nhis/earlyrelease/earlyrelease201203.pdf). The researchers find that between 1997 and September 2011 the percentage of people of all ages with a usual source of medical care did

not substantially vary—ranging from a high of 87.9% in 2003 to a low of 85.4% in 2010. (See Figure 1.1.)

Still, between 1998 and September 2011 the percentage of people who needed medical care but did not obtain it because of financial barriers to access increased each year. The annual percentage of people who experienced this lack of access to medical care rose from 4.2% in 1998 to nearly 7% in 2010 and 2011. (See Figure 1.2.)

Barnes et al. reveal that people aged 18 to 24 years were the least likely to have a regular source of care, but the likelihood of having a regular source of medical care increased among people aged 25 years and older. (See Figure 1.3.) Children under the age of 18 years were more likely than adults aged 18 to 64 years to have a usual place to go for medical care. Among adults (aged 18 to 64 years), women were more likely than men to have a usual place to seek medical care. Barnes et al. indicate that not having a regular health care provider is a greater predictor of delay in seeking care than insurance status. Health care consumers with a regular physician or a source of health care services are less likely to use the hospital emergency department to obtain routine nonemergency medical care and are less likely to be hospitalized for preventable illnesses.

In *Health Care Access and Utilization among Young Adults Aged 19–25: Early Release of Estimates from the National Health Interview Survey, January–September 2011* (May 2012, http://www.cdc.gov/nchs/data/nhis/earlyrelease/Young_Adults_Health_Access_052012.pdf), Whitney K. Kirzinger, Robin A. Cohen, and Renee M. Gindi of the NCHS reiterate that health insurance

FIGURE 1.1

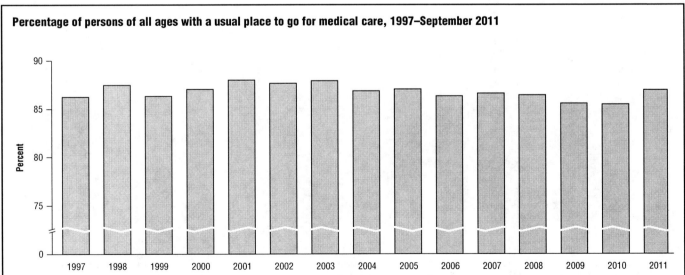

Percentage of persons of all ages with a usual place to go for medical care, 1997–September 2011

Notes: Data are based on household interviews of a sample of the civilian noninstitutionalized population. The usual place to go for medical care does not include a hospital emergency room. The analyses excluded persons with an unknown usual place to go for medical care (about 1.5% of respondents each year).

SOURCE: P. M. Barnes, B. W. Ward, and J. S. Schiller, "Figure 2.1. Percent of Persons of All Ages with a Usual Place to Go for Medical Care: United States, 1997–September 2011," in *Early Release of Selected Estimates Based on Data from the January–September 2011 National Health Interview Survey*, National Center for Health Statistics, March 2012, http://www.cdc.gov/nchs/data/nhis/earlyrelease/201203_02.pdf (accessed June 11, 2012)

FIGURE 1.2

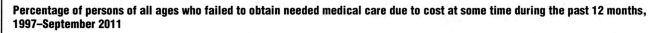

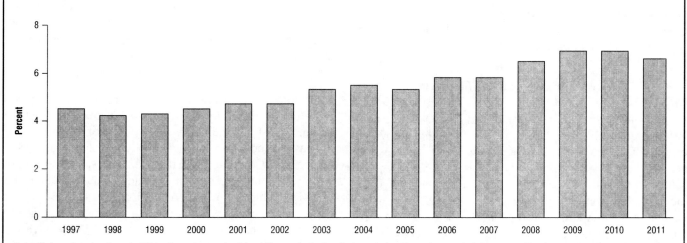

Percentage of persons of all ages who failed to obtain needed medical care due to cost at some time during the past 12 months, 1997–September 2011

Notes: Data are based on household interviews of a sample of the civilian noninstitutionalized population. The analyses excluded persons with unknown responses to the question on failure to obtain needed medical care due to cost (about 0.2% of respondents each year).

SOURCE: P. M. Barnes, B. W. Ward, and J. S. Schiller, "Figure 3.1. Percentage of Persons of All Ages Who Failed to Obtain Needed Medical Care Due to Cost at Some Time during the Past 12 Months: United States, 1997–September 2011," in *Early Release of Selected Estimates Based on Data from the January–September 2011 National Health Interview Survey*, National Center for Health Statistics, March 2012, http://www.cdc.gov/nchs/data/nhis/earlyrelease/201203_03.pdf (accessed June 11, 2012)

FIGURE 1.3

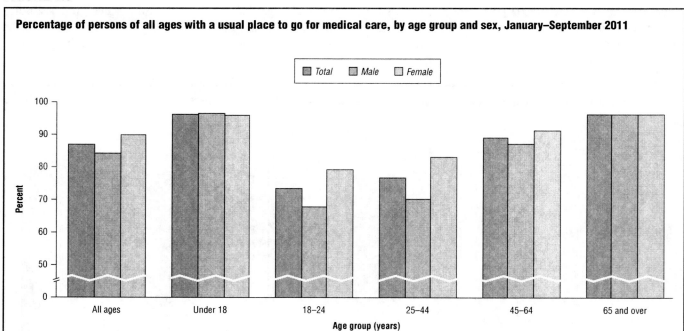

Percentage of persons of all ages with a usual place to go for medical care, by age group and sex, January–September 2011

Notes: Data are based on household interviews of a sample of the civilian noninstitutionalized population. The usual place to go for medical care does not include a hospital emergency room. The analyses excluded 0.3% of persons with an unknown usual place to go for medical care.

SOURCE: P. M. Barnes, B. W. Ward, and J. S. Schiller, "Figure 2.2. Percentage of Persons of All Ages with a Usual Place to Go for Medical Care, by Age Group and Sex: United States, January–September 2011," in *Early Release of Selected Estimates Based on Data from the January–September 2011 National Health Interview Survey*, National Center for Health Statistics, March 2012, http://www.cdc.gov/nchs/data/nhis/earlyrelease/201203_02.pdf (accessed June 11, 2012)

FIGURE 1.4

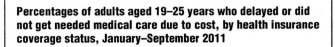

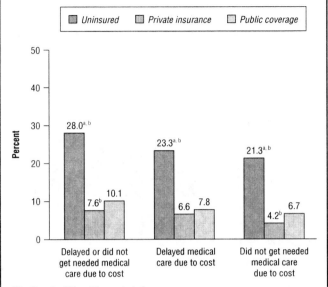

Percentages of adults aged 19–25 years who delayed or did not get needed medical care due to cost, by health insurance coverage status, January–September 2011

[a]Significantly different from private insurance.
[b]Significantly different from public coverage.
Notes: Estimates for 2011 are based on data collected from January through September. Data are based on household interviews of a sample of the civilian noninstitutionalized population.

SOURCE: Whitney K. Kirzinger, Robin A. Cohen, and Renee M. Gindi, "Figure 5. Percentages of Adults Aged 19–25 Years Who Delayed or Did Not Get Needed Medical Care Due to Cost, by Health Insurance Coverage Status: United States, January–September 2011," in *Health Care Access and Utilization among Young Adults Aged 19–25: Early Release of Estimates from the National Health Interview Survey, January–September 2011*, National Center for Health Statistics, May 2012, http://www.cdc.gov/nchs/data/nhis/earlyrelease/Young_Adults_Health_Access_052012.pdf (accessed June 12, 2012)

status is a key determinant of access to medical care. The researchers report that young adults (aged 19 to 25 years) without insurance (28%) were three and half times more likely to delay or forgo needed medical care because of cost than those with private insurance (7.6%). (See Figure 1.4.) Approximately 21.3% of uninsured young adults did not obtain needed medical care, compared with just 4.2% of those with private insurance and 6.7% with public coverage.

The National Association of Community Health Centers (NACHC) is a nonprofit organization that represents the interests of federally supported and other federally qualified health centers and serves as an information source about health care for poor and medically underserved populations in the United States. The NACHC reports in *Access Endangered: Profiles of the Medically Disenfranchised* (August 2011, http://www.nachc.org/client//NAC_AccessEndangered_FINAL_Lo.pdf) that in 2011, 60 million Americans of all income levels, race, and ethnicity were "medically disenfranchised" (at risk

of inadequate access to basic medical services and "without a regular and continuous source of primary care"). The NACHC asserts that besides the uninsured and low-income populations, which are disproportionately affected, people lack access for a variety of reasons such as scarcity of health care resources, geographically inaccessible services, and health care that is culturally sensitive.

Race and Ethnicity Continue to Affect Access to Health Care

According to Barnes et al., Hispanic adults continue to be less likely to have a regular source for medical care than non-Hispanic white and non-Hispanic African-American adults. After adjusting for age and gender, 78% of Hispanics had a usual source of medical care, compared with 89.1% of non-Hispanic whites and 85.3% of non-Hispanic African-Americans. (See Figure 1.5.) Hispanics and non-Hispanic African-Americans are more likely than non-Hispanic whites to suffer financial barriers to access. After adjusting for age and gender, 7.8% of Hispanics and 8.2% of non-Hispanic African-Americans were unable to obtain needed medical care because of financial barriers, compared with 6% of non-Hispanic whites. (See Figure 1.6.) Health educators speculate that language barriers and the lack of information about the availability of health care services may serve to widen this gap.

FIGURE 1.5

Age- and sex-adjusted percentage of persons of all ages with a usual place to go for medical care, by race/ethnicity, January–September 2011

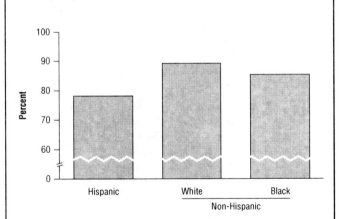

Notes: Data are based on household interviews of a sample of the civilian noninstitutionalized population. The usual place to go for medical care does not include a hospital emergency room. The analyses excluded 0.3% of persons with an unknown usual place to go for medical care. Estimates are age-sex-adjusted using the projected 2000 U.S. population as the standard population and using five age groups: under 18, 18–24, 25–44, 45–64, and 65 and over.

SOURCE: P. M. Barnes, B. W. Ward, and J. S. Schiller, "Figure 2.3. Age-sex-adjusted Percentage of Persons of All Ages with a Usual Place to Go for Medical Care, by Race/Ethnicity: United States, January–September 2011," in *Early Release of Selected Estimates Based on Data from the January–September 2011 National Health Interview Survey*, National Center for Health Statistics, March 2012, http://www.cdc.gov/nchs/data/nhis/earlyrelease/201203_02.pdf (accessed June 11, 2012)

FIGURE 1.6

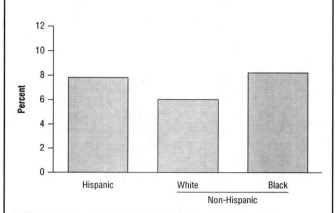

Age- and sex-adjusted percentage of persons of all ages who failed to obtain needed medical care due to cost at some time during the past 12 months, by race/ethnicity, January–September 2011

Notes: Data are based on household interviews of a sample of the civilian noninstitutionalized population. The analyses excluded 0.1% of persons with unknown responses to the question on failure to obtain needed medical care due to cost. Estimates are age-sex-adjusted using the projected 2000 U.S. population as the standard population and using three age groups: under 18, 18–64, and 65 and over.

SOURCE: P. M. Barnes, B. W. Ward, and J. S. Schiller, "Figure 3.3. Age-sex-adjusted Percentage of Persons of All Ages Who Failed to Obtain Needed Medical Care Due to Cost at Some Time during the Past 12 Months, by Race/Ethnicity: United States, January–September 2011," in *Early Release of Selected Estimates Based on Data from the January–September 2011 National Health Interview Survey*, National Center for Health Statistics, March 2012, http://www.cdc.gov/nchs/data/nhis/earlyrelease/201203_02.pdf (accessed June 11, 2012)

FIGURE 1.7

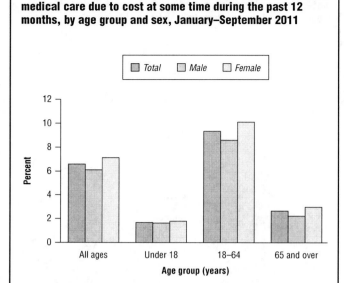

Percentage of persons of all ages who failed to obtain needed medical care due to cost at some time during the past 12 months, by age group and sex, January–September 2011

Notes: Data are based on household interviews of a sample of the civilian noninstitutionalized population. The analyses excluded 0.1% persons with unknown responses to the question on failure to obtain needed medical care due to cost.

SOURCE: P. M. Barnes, B. W. Ward, and J. S. Schiller, "Figure 3.2. Percentage of Persons of All Ages Who Failed to Obtain Needed Medical Care Due to Cost at Some Time during the Past 12 Months, by Age Group and Sex: United States, January–September 2011," in *Early Release of Selected Estimates Based on Data from the January–September 2011 National Health Interview Survey*, National Center for Health Statistics, March 2012, http://www.cdc.gov/nchs/data/nhis/earlyrelease/201203_02.pdf (accessed June 11, 2012)

Women Face Additional Obstacles

According to the Kaiser Family Foundation (KFF), in *Impact of Health Reform on Women's Access to Coverage and Care* (April 2012, http://www.kff.org/womenshealth/upload/7987-02.pdf), women fare worse than men in terms of access to health care services. The KFF notes that just 50% of women receive health coverage via employment, compared with 57% of men. Because women are more likely to be covered as a dependent on their spouse's plan, they are at greater risk of losing their coverage should they divorce or if their spouse becomes unemployed or dies.

Barnes at al. also document gender-based disparities in access. Women aged 18 to 64 years and those aged 65 years and older were more likely than men to have failed to obtain needed medical care because of financial barriers to access. (See Figure 1.7.)

The KFF observes that the ACA will serve to improve access to care and coverage for women by instituting insurance system reforms, lowering out-of-pocket costs, and mandating comprehensive benefits packages to meet the health service needs of women of all ages.

Children Need Better Access to Health Care, Too

Barbara Bloom, Robin A. Cohen, and Gulnar Freeman of the NCHS analyzed data from the 2010 NHIS to look at selected health measures, including children's access to care, and compiled their findings in *Summary Health Statistics for U.S. Children: National Health Interview Survey, 2010* (December 2011, http://www.cdc.gov/nchs/data/series/sr_10/sr10_250.pdf). Among other factors, the researchers' analysis focuses on the unmet health care needs of children under the age of 18 years, poverty status, insurance coverage, and usual place of medical care.

Bloom, Cohen, and Freeman note that in 2010, 5% of children in the United States did not have a regular source of medical care. Non-Hispanic African-American children (95%) and non-Hispanic white children (97%) were more likely to have a regular source of care, compared with Hispanic children (91%). The researchers also reveal a relationship between not having a usual source of medical care and family structure, family income, poverty status, and health insurance coverage. The likelihood of lacking a regular source of care was higher among poor and near-poor families of all races and ethnic groups. (See Table 1.1.)

TABLE 1.1

Frequency and location of usual place of health care for children under age 18, by selected characteristics, 2010

Selected characteristic	All children under age 18 years	Has usual place of health care[a] No	Yes	Clinic	Location of usual place of health care[b] Doctor's office	Emergency room	Hospital outpatient	Some other place	Doesn't go to one place most often
					Number in thousands[c]				
Total[d] (crude)	74,626	3,640	70,940	16,815	52,617	402	661	223	177
Sex									
Male	38,135	1,869	36,241	8,511	27,012	210	333	*70	90
Female	36,491	1,771	34,699	8,304	25,605	192	328	154	*87
Age									
0–4 years	21,414	676	20,713	5,521	14,760	116	214	†	*33
5–11 years	28,666	1,313	27,332	6,038	20,839	129	191	*87	*40
12–17 years	24,546	1,651	22,895	5,255	17,017	157	256	*73	104
Race									
One race[e]	71,490	3,495	67,949	16,198	50,312	386	653	189	166
White	56,170	2,638	53,504	12,207	40,322	301	382	*146	106
Black or African American	11,030	555	10,466	2,861	7,239	82	217	*43	†
American Indian or Alaska Native	768	*65	703	*402	287	—	†	—	†
Asian	3,354	224	3,120	657	2,379	†	*44	—	*37
Native Hawaiian or other Pacific Islander	168	†	156	*70	*86	—	—	—	—
Two or more races[f]	3,136	146	2,991	617	2,305	†	†	†	†
Black or African American and white	1,373	*44	1,329	253	1,040	†	†	†	†
American Indian or Alaska Native and white	473	†	431	168	249	—	—	†	†
Hispanic or Latino origin[g] and race									
Hispanic or Latino	17,167	1,518	15,640	6,120	9,077	159	150	*60	70
Mexican or Mexican American	11,590	1,185	10,399	4,492	5,650	*94	80	†	*48
Not Hispanic or Latino	57,460	2,122	55,300	10,695	43,539	244	511	164	106
White, single race	40,766	1,283	39,466	6,676	32,200	147	254	*100	*51
Black or African American, single race	10,430	512	9,909	2,628	6,931	79	206	*43	†
Family structure[h]									
Mother and father	51,329	2,329	48,976	10,395	37,676	213	357	194	132
Mother, no father	18,026	1,011	17,011	5,076	11,494	143	203	†	*32
Father, no mother	2,835	142	2,680	629	1,968	†	*48	—	†
Neither mother nor father	2,436	157	2,273	714	1,478	†	†	—	†
Parent's education[i]									
Less than high school diploma	9,301	905	8,396	3,850	4,284	108	88	†	*26
High school diploma or GED[j]	14,750	966	13,780	3,943	9,509	112	105	*66	*20
More than high school	47,913	1,609	46,267	8,224	37,219	160	415	116	116
Family income[k]									
Less than $35,000	24,323	1,714	22,600	8,123	13,741	212	328	*74	94
$35,000 or more	47,072	1,708	45,337	8,043	36,579	189	309	136	*77
$35,000–$49,999	9,438	615	8,807	2,439	6,118	129	63	†	†
$50,000–$74,999	12,473	592	11,881	2,428	9,219	†	*131	*57	†
$75,000–$99,999	8,919	216	8,701	1,299	7,299	†	*61	†	†
$100,000 or more	16,241	286	15,948	1,877	13,942	†	*55	†	†
Poverty status[l]									
Poor	15,701	1,064	14,637	5,670	8,517	115	231	†	*48
Near poor	15,562	1,083	14,470	4,283	9,765	178	131	*52	*57
Not poor	38,768	1,155	37,601	5,786	31,374	69	193	*103	*72
Health insurance coverage[m]									
Private	40,015	1,028	38,966	5,406	33,280	*65	118	*65	*32
Medicaid or other public	26,404	972	25,428	8,904	15,900	163	353	†	*57
Other	2,140	*67	2,068	706	1,187	†	*128	†	—
Uninsured	5,877	1,543	4,323	1,749	2,153	155	*58	*114	85
Place of residence[n]									
Large MSA	40,071	1,991	38,044	8,016	29,077	290	415	*87	119
Small MSA	23,245	1,153	22,082	5,253	16,425	*92	188	*72	*47
Not in MSA	11,310	496	10,814	3,546	7,114	*20	†	†	†
Region									
Northeast	11,610	249	11,361	1,656	9,484	*30	148	†	†
Midwest	17,664	617	17,036	4,980	11,719	*106	138	†	†
South	26,791	1,550	25,225	4,816	19,854	165	203	*79	103
West	18,561	1,225	17,317	5,363	11,560	101	173	*66	*54

TABLE 1.1

Frequency and location of usual place of health care for children under age 18, by selected characteristics, 2010 [CONTINUED]

Selected characteristic	All children under age 18 years	Has usual place of health care[a]			Location of usual place of health care[b]				
		No	Yes	Clinic	Doctor's office	Emergency room	Hospital outpatient	Some other place	Doesn't go to one place most often
Current health status					Number in thousands[c]				
Excellent or very good	61,019	2,796	58,185	12,999	44,154	269	418	194	132
Good	11,915	751	11,161	3,364	7,391	112	206	†	*45
Fair or poor	1,692	*93	1,594	451	1,072	†	†	†	—

*Estimates preceded by an asterisk have a relative standard error greater than 30% and less than or equal to 50% and should be used with caution as they do not meet standards of reliability or precision.
†Estimates with a relative standard error greater than 50% are indicated with a dagger, but data are not shown.
—Quantity zero.
[a]Based on the question, "Is there a place that [child's name] USUALLY goes when [he/she] is sick or you need advice about [his/her] health?"
[b]Based on the question, "What kind of place is it/What kind of place does [child's name] go to most often-clinic or health center, doctor's office or HMO, hospital emergency room, hospital outpatient department or some other place?"
[c]Unknowns for the columns are not included in the frequencies, but they are included in the "All children under age 18 years" column.
[d]Includes other races not shown separately and children with unknown family structure, parent's education, family income, poverty status, health insurance, or current health status. Additionally, numbers within selected characteristics may not add to totals because of rounding.
[e]In accordance with the 1997 standards for federal data on race and Hispanic or Latino origin, the category "One race" refers to persons who indicated only a single race group. Persons who indicated a single race other than the groups shown are included in the total for "One race" but are not shown separately due to small sample sizes. Therefore, the frequencies for the category "One race" will be greater than the sum of the frequencies for the specific groups shown separately. Persons of Hispanic or Latino origin may be of any race or combination of races.
[f]Refers to all persons who indicated more than one race group. Only two combinations of multiple race groups are shown due to small sample sizes for other combinations. Therefore, the frequencies for the category "Two or more races" will be greater than the sum of the frequencies for the specific combinations shown separately.
[g]Persons of Hispanic or Latino origin may be of any race or combination of races. Similarly, the category "Not Hispanic or Latino" refers to all persons who are not of Hispanic or Latino origin, regardless of race.
[h]Refers to parents living in the household. "Mother and father" can include biological, adoptive, step, in-law, or foster relationships. Legal guardians are classified in "Neither mother nor father."
[i]Refers to the education level of the parent with the higher level of education, regardless of that parent's age.
[j]GED is General Educational Development high school equivalency diploma.
[k]The categories "Less than $35,000" and "$35,000 or more" include both persons reporting dollar amounts and persons reporting only that their incomes were within one of these two categories. The indented categories include only those persons who reported dollar amounts. Because of the different income questions used in 2007, income estimates may not be comparable with those from earlier years.
[l]Based on family income and family size using the U.S. Census Bureau's poverty thresholds for the previous calendar year. "Poor" persons are defined as below the poverty threshold. "Near poor" persons have incomes of 100% to less than 200% of the poverty threshold. "Not poor" persons have incomes that are 200% of the poverty threshold or greater. Because of the different income questions used in 2007, poverty ratio estimates may not be comparable with those from earlier years.
[m]Classification of health insurance coverage is based on a hierarchy of mutually exclusive categories. Persons with more than one type of health insurance were assigned to the first appropriate category in the hierarchy. Persons under age 65 years and those aged 65 years and over were classified separately due to the predominance of Medicare coverage in the older population. The category "Private" includes persons who had any type of private coverage either alone or in combination with other coverage. For example, for persons aged 65 years and over, "Private" includes persons with only private or private in combination with Medicare. The category "Uninsured" includes persons who had no coverage as well as those who had only Indian Health Service coverage or had only a private plan that paid for one type of service such as accidents or dental care.
[n]MSA is metropolitan statistical area. Large MSAs have a population size of 1 million or more; small MSAs have a population size of less than 1 million. "Not in MSA" consists of persons not living in a metropolitan statistical area.
Note: Estimates are based on household interviews of a sample of the civilian noninstitutionalized population.

SOURCE: Barbara Bloom, Robin Cohen, and Gulnur Freeman, "Table 11. Frequencies of Having a Usual Place of Health Care and Frequency Distributions of Location of Usual Place of Health Care for Children with a Usual Place of Health Care for Children under Age 18 Years, by Selected Characteristics: United States, 2010," in *Summary Health Statistics for U.S. Children: National Health Interview Survey, 2010*, 2011, http://www.cdc.gov/nchs/data/series/sr_10/sr10_250.pdf (accessed June 12, 2012)

Having health insurance and the type of health insurance also predicted whether a child had a regular source of care. In 2010 children with no health insurance (1.5 million out of a total of 3.6 million children aged 18 years and younger, or 42%) were less likely to have a usual place for health care than children with private health insurance (1 million out of 3.6 million, or 28%). (See Table 1.1.)

Bloom, Cohen, and Freeman also find that in 2010 more than twice as many children with private health insurance (33.3 million) received health care in a physician's office than children with Medicaid or other public health insurance (15.9 million). (See Table 1.1.) Children without health insurance were more likely to receive routine health care in an emergency department than were children with private health insurance.

In 2010, 7.8% of U.S. children had no health insurance coverage. (See Table 1.2.) Of those children who were uninsured, 11.8% lived in families with incomes of less than $35,000 per year and another 11.8% lived in families with an income of $35,000 to $49,999, compared with 2.1% of children in households with incomes of $100,000 or more. Children from poor and near-poor families were more likely to be uninsured, have unmet medical needs, and delayed care because of costs more frequently than children from families that were not poor. Health professionals are especially concerned about delayed or missed medical visits for children because well-child visits provide an opportunity for early detection of developmental problems and timely treatment of illnesses and ensure that children receive the recommended schedule of immunizations.

The Health Care System

TABLE 1.2

Age-adjusted percentages of selected measures of health care access for children under age 18, by selected characteristics, 2010

Selected characteristic	All children under age 18 years	Selected measures of health care access					
		Uninsured for health care[a]	Unmet medical need[b]	Delayed care due to cost[c]	Uninsured for health care[a]	Unmet medical need[b]	Delayed care due to cost[c]
		Number in thousands[d]			Percenet[e]		
Total[f] (age-adjusted)	74,625	5,791	1,581	2,938	7.8	2.1	4.0
Total[f] (crude)	74,625	5,791	1,581	2,938	7.8	2.1	3.9
Sex							
Male	38,134	3,037	849	1,506	8.0	2.2	4.0
Female	36,491	2,754	732	1,432	7.6	2.0	4.0
Age[g]							
0–4 years	21,485	1,324	325	659	6.2	1.5	3.1
5–11 years	28,972	2,102	602	1,164	7.3	2.1	4.0
12–17 years	24,168	2,364	654	1,115	9.8	2.7	4.6
Race							
One race[h]	71,622	5,591	1,528	2,802	7.9	2.1	3.9
White	56,223	4,391	1,172	2,274	7.9	2.1	4.1
Black or African American	11,085	698	294	391	6.4	2.7	3.6
American Indian or Alaska Native	772	†	†	†	*27.0		
Asian	3,374	271	41	76	8.2	1.2	2.2
Native Hawaiian or Other Pacific Islander	168	†	†	†			
Two or more races[i]	3,003	199	53	136	7.0	1.9	4.8
Black or African American and white	1,306	95	*29	78	8.0	*2.1	6.2
American Indian or Alaska Native and white	497	*44	†	†	*8.7		
Hispanic or Latino origin[j] and race							
Hispanic or Latino	17,166	2,221	444	787	13.5	2.7	4.7
Mexican or Mexican American	11,629	1,704	329	562	15.2	2.9	5.0
Not Hispanic or Latino	57,459	3,570	1,136	2,151	6.2	2.0	3.7
White, single race	40,804	2,340	749	1,543	5.7	1.8	3.8
Black or African American, single race	10,480	663	285	374	6.4	2.7	3.6
Family structure[k]							
Mother and father	51,483	3,744	957	1,873	7.4	1.9	3.7
Mother, no father	17,915	1,426	488	862	8.0	2.7	4.8
Father, no mother	2,745	317	89	118	11.2	2.8	4.0
Neither mother nor father	2,482	303	*47	86	11.7	*1.8	3.4
Parent's education[l]							
Less than high school diploma	9,348	1,383	243	351	15.3	2.7	3.9
High school diploma or GED[m]	14,745	1,649	409	630	11.4	2.8	4.4
More than high school	47,454	2,385	880	1,870	5.1	1.9	4.0
Family income[n]							
Less than $35,000	23,698	2,688	641	1,058	11.8	2.8	4.6
$35,000 or more	45,422	2,709	874	1,743	6.0	1.9	3.8
$35,000–$49,999	9,210	1,065	327	595	11.8	3.6	6.5
$50,000–$74,999	12,151	963	315	611	8.0	2.6	5.1
$75,000–$99,999	8,492	354	117	241	4.2	1.4	2.8
$100,000 or more	15,570	327	116	295	2.1	0.7	1.9
Poverty status[o]							
Poor	15,355	1,576	342	540	10.7	2.3	3.7
Near poor	15,119	1,914	564	999	13.0	3.8	6.7
Not poor	37,335	1,723	552	1,181	4.6	1.5	3.2
Health insurance coverage[p]							
Private	40,184	—	419	1,175		1.0	2.9
Medicaid or other public	26,156	—	374	557		1.5	2.3
Other	2,131	—	†	†			
Uninsured	5,791	5,791	764	1,172	100.0	13.2	20.3
Place of residence[q]							
Large MSA	40,084	3,035	929	1,697	7.6	2.3	4.3
Small MSA	23,248	1,788	451	909	7.8	2.0	3.9
Not in MSA	11,293	968	201	332	8.7	1.8	3.0
Region							
Northeast	11,620	509	148	314	4.4	1.3	2.7
Midwest	17,472	859	253	535	5.0	1.5	3.1
South	26,939	2,591	691	1,225	9.8	2.6	4.6
West	18,594	1,831	488	863	9.9	2.7	4.7

TABLE 1.2

Age-adjusted percentages of selected measures of health care access for children under age 18, by selected characteristics, 2010
[CONTINUED]

		Selected measures of health care access					
Selected characteristic	All children under age 18 years	Uninsured for health care[a]	Unmet medical need[b]	Delayed care due to cost[c]	Uninsured for health care[a]	Unmet medical need[b]	Delayed care due to cost[c]
Current health status		Number in thousands[d]				Percenet[e]	
Excellent or very good	61,275	4,538	1,074	2,115	7.5	1.8	3.5
Good	11,822	1,147	426	701	9.7	3.6	5.9
Fair or poor	1,504	105	81	122	6.8	5.3	7.9

[†]Estimates with a relative standard error greater than 50% are indicated with a dagger, but data are not shown.

[*]Estimates preceded by an asterisk have a relative standard error greater than 30% and less than or equal to 50% and should be used with caution as they do not meet standards of reliability or precision.

—Quantity zero.

[a]Based on the following question in the family core section of the survey: "[Are you/Is anyone] covered by health insurance or some other kind of health care plan?"

[b]Based on the following question in the family core section of the survey: "DURING THE PAST 12 MONTHS, was there any time when [you/someone in the family] needed medical care, but did not get it because [you/the family] couldn't afford it?"

[c]Based on the following question in the family core section of the survey: "DURING THE PAST 12 MONTHS, [have/has] [you/anyone in the family] delayed seeking medical care because of worry about the cost?"

[d]Unknowns for the columns are not included in the frequencies, but they are included in the "All children under age 18 years" column.

[e]Unknowns for the column variables are not included in the denominators when calculating percentages.

[f]Includes other races not shown separately and children with unknown family structure, parent's education, family income, poverty status, health insurance, or current health status. Additionally, numbers within selected characteristics may not add to totals because of rounding.

[g]Estimates for age groups are not age adjusted.

[h]In accordance with the 1997 standards for federal data on race and Hispanic or Latino origin, the category "One race" refers to persons who indicated only a single race group. Persons who indicated a single race other than the groups shown are included in the total for "One race" but are not shown separately due to small sample sizes. Therefore, the frequencies for the category "One race" will be greater than the sum of the frequencies for the specific groups shown separately. Persons of Hispanic or Latino origin may be of any race or combination of races.

[i]Refers to all persons who indicated more than one race group. Only two combinations of multiple race groups are shown due to small sample sizes for other combinations. Therefore, the frequencies for the category "Two or more races" will be greater than the sum of the frequencies for the specific combinations shown separately.

[j]Persons of Hispanic or Latino origin may be of any race or combination of races. Similarly, the category "Not Hispanic or Latino" refers to all persons who are not of Hispanic or Latino origin, regardless of race. The tables in this report use the current (1997) Office of Management and Budget race and Hispanic origin terms.

[k]Refers to parents living in the household. "Mother and father" can include biological, adoptive, step, in-law, or foster relationships. Legal guardians are classified in "Neither mother nor father."

[l]Refers to the education level of the parent with the higher level of education, regardless of that parent's age.

[m]GED is General Educational Development high school equivalency diploma.

[n]The categories "Less than $35,000" and "$35,000 or more" include both persons reporting dollar amounts and persons reporting only that their incomes were within one of these two categories. The indented categories include only those persons who reported dollar amounts. Because of the different income questions used in 2007, income estimates may not be comparable with those from earlier years.

[o]Based on family income and family size using the U.S. Census Bureau's poverty thresholds for the previous calendar year. "Poor" persons are defined as below the poverty threshold. "Near poor" persons have incomes of 100% to less than 200% of the poverty threshold. "Not poor" persons have incomes that are 200% of the poverty threshold or greater. Because of the different income questions used in 2007, poverty ratio estimates may not be comparable with those from earlier years. Because of the different income questions used in 2007, poverty ratio estimates may not be comparable with those from earlier years.

[p]Classification of health insurance coverage is based on a hierarchy of mutually exclusive categories. Persons with more than one type of health insurance were assigned to the first appropriate category in the hierarchy. Persons under age 65 years and those aged 65 years and over were classified separately due to the predominance of Medicare coverage in the older population. The category "Private" includes persons who had any type of private coverage either alone or in combination with other coverage. For example, for persons aged 65 years and over, "Private" includes persons with only private or private in combination with Medicare. The category "Uninsured" includes persons who had no coverage as well as those who had only Indian Health Service coverage or had only a private plan that paid for one type of service such as accidents or dental care.

[q]MSA is metropolitan statistical area. Large MSAs have a population size of 1 million or more; small MSAs have a population size of less than 1 million. "Not in MSA" consists of persons not living in a metropolitan statistical area.

Notes: Estimates are based on household interviews of a sample of the civilian noninstitutionalized population.

SOURCE: Barbara Bloom, Robin Cohen, and Gulnur Freeman, "Table 15. Frequencies and Age-Adjusted Percentages (with Standard Errors) of Selected Measures of Health Care Access for Children under 18 Years of Age, by Selected Characteristics: United States, 2010," in *Summary Health Statistics for U.S. Children: National Health Interview Survey, 2010*, 2011, http://www.cdc.gov/nchs/data/series/sr_10/sr10_250.pdf (accessed June 12, 2012)

According to Bloom, Cohen, and Freeman, there was significant geographic variation in insurance status, which was strongly linked to children's access to health care services. Approximately 10% of children in the South and West were uninsured in 2010—twice as many as were uninsured in the Midwest (5%) and the Northeast (4.4%). (See Table 1.2.)

How to Reduce Disparities in Access to Care

Health care researchers believe many factors contribute to differences in access, including cultural perceptions and beliefs about health and illness, patient preferences, availability of services, and provider bias. They recommend special efforts to inform and educate minority health care consumers and to increase understanding and sensitivity among practitioners and other providers of care. Besides factual information, minority consumers must overcome the belief that they are at a disadvantage because of their race or ethnicity. Along with action to dispel barriers to access, educating practitioners, policy makers, and consumers can help reduce the perception of disadvantage.

For decades, health care researchers have documented sharp differences in the ability of ethnic and racial groups to access medical services. The federal government has repeatedly called for an end to these disparities. Even though some observers believe universal health insurance coverage is an important first step in eliminating disparities, there is widespread concern that the challenge is more complicated and calls for additional analysis and action.

FIGURE 1.8

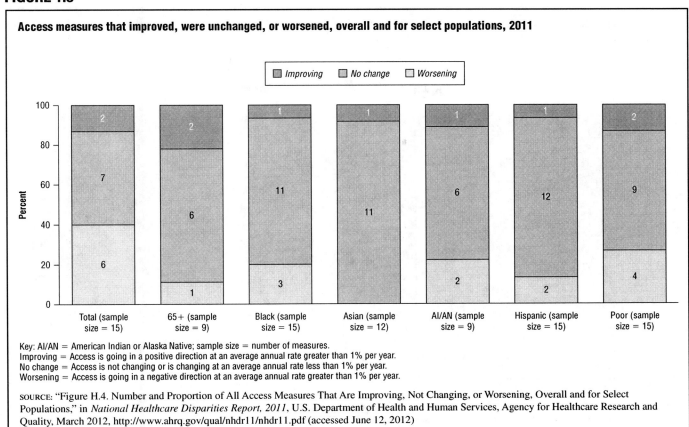

Access measures that improved, were unchanged, or worsened, overall and for select populations, 2011

Key: AI/AN = American Indian or Alaska Native; sample size = number of measures.
Improving = Access is going in a positive direction at an average annual rate greater than 1% per year.
No change = Access is not changing or is changing at an average annual rate less than 1% per year.
Worsening = Access is going in a negative direction at an average annual rate greater than 1% per year.

SOURCE: "Figure H.4. Number and Proportion of All Access Measures That Are Improving, Not Changing, or Worsening, Overall and for Select Populations," in *National Healthcare Disparities Report, 2011*, U.S. Department of Health and Human Services, Agency for Healthcare Research and Quality, March 2012, http://www.ahrq.gov/qual/nhdr11/nhdr11.pdf (accessed June 12, 2012)

In "The Affordable Care Act's Coverage Expansions Will Reduce Differences in Uninsurance Rates by Race and Ethnicity" (*Health Affairs*, vol. 31, no. 5, May 2012), Lisa Clemans-Cope et al. estimate that full implementation of the ACA could reduce the 8% differential in health insurance coverage between African-Americans and whites by more than half and reduce the 19% differential between Hispanics and whites by about a quarter. The researchers also anticipate gains in access and outcomes (how people fare following treatment), opining, "If uninsurance is reduced to the extent projected in this analysis, sizable reductions in long-standing racial and ethnic differentials in access to health care and health status are likely to follow."

Because the U.S. Supreme Court ruling on the ACA will likely limit Medicaid expansion, the Congressional Budget Office forecasts in *Estimates for the Insurance Coverage Provisions of the Affordable Care Act Updated for the Recent Supreme Court Decision* (July 2012, http://www.cbo.gov/sites/default/files/cbofiles/attachments/43472-07-24-2012-CoverageEstimates.pdf) that once the legislation is fully implemented an estimated 30 million people will gain coverage under the ACA—about 3 million fewer people than previously anticipated. In "Court's Ruling May Blunt Reach of the Health Law" (*New York Times*, July 24, 2012), Robert Pear explains that while it is not yet known how many states will choose not to expand their Medicaid programs, the Congressional Budget Office estimates that 6 million fewer people will be covered by Medicaid; however, half of them will likely be able to obtain private health care coverage from insurance exchanges.

AHRQ Report Documents Disparities in Access

In July 2003 the Agency for Healthcare Research and Quality (AHRQ) released its first *National Healthcare Disparities Report* (http://www.ahrq.gov/qual/nhdr03/nhdr2003.pdf), a report requested by Congress that documented racial health disparities including access to care. Among other things, the report cited the finding that African-Americans and low-income Americans have higher mortality rates for cancer than the general population because they are less likely to receive screening tests for certain forms of the disease and other preventive services. Even though the report asserted that differential access may lead to disparities in quality and observed that opportunities to provide preventive care are often missed, it conceded that knowledge about why disparities exist is limited.

The AHRQ report generated fiery debate in the health care community and among legislators and painted a rather bleak view of disparities. The report called for detailed data to support quality improvement initiatives and observed that "community-based participatory research has numerous examples of communities working

FIGURE 1.9

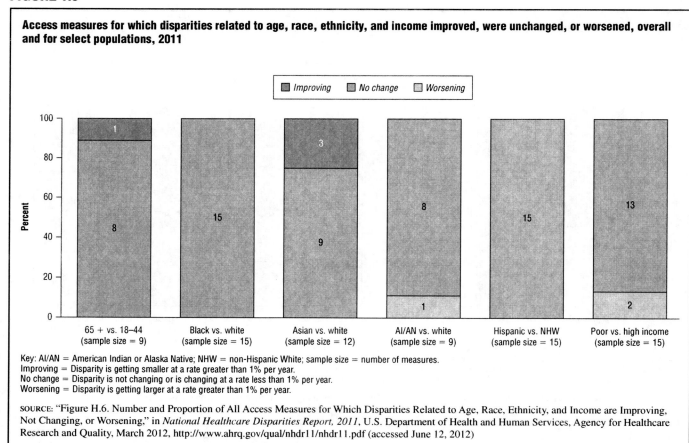

Access measures for which disparities related to age, race, ethnicity, and income improved, were unchanged, or worsened, overall and for select populations, 2011

Key: AI/AN = American Indian or Alaska Native; NHW = non-Hispanic White; sample size = number of measures.
Improving = Disparity is getting smaller at a rate greater than 1% per year.
No change = Disparity is not changing or is changing at a rate less than 1% per year.
Worsening = Disparity is getting larger at a rate greater than 1% per year.

SOURCE: "Figure H.6. Number and Proportion of All Access Measures for Which Disparities Related to Age, Race, Ethnicity, and Income are Improving, Not Changing, or Worsening," in *National Healthcare Disparities Report, 2011*, U.S. Department of Health and Human Services, Agency for Healthcare Research and Quality, March 2012, http://www.ahrq.gov/qual/nhdr11/nhdr11.pdf (accessed June 12, 2012)

to improve quality overall, while reducing healthcare disparities for vulnerable populations."

Highlights from the *National Healthcare Disparities Report 2011*

In *National Healthcare Disparities Report 2011* (March 2012, http://www.ahrq.gov/qual/nhdr11/nhdr11.pdf), the AHRQ tracks the measures of access to care that the first report, *National Healthcare Disparities Report*, identified in 2003. These measures include factors that facilitated access, such as having a primary care provider, and factors that were barriers to access, such as having no health insurance. The AHRQ's principal findings about access are:

- Access is not improving. Across the measures of health care access that were analyzed, about half showed no improvement and 40% worsened. Figure 1.8 shows the number and proportion of access measures that improved, were unchanged, or worsened.

- Racial and ethnic minorities and poor people continue to encounter disproportionate barriers to care. For about one-third of all access measures analyzed, African-Americans had worse access to care than whites and Hispanics had worse access to care than non-Hispanic whites across about two-thirds of the measures.

Figure 1.9 shows that almost no disparities related to age, race, ethnicity, and income improved.

- Socioeconomic status accounts for differences in access—poor people had worse access to care than high-income people on 89% of measures.

HEALTH CARE REFORM PROMISES TO IMPROVE ACCESS

The 2010 enactment of the PPACA promised to help the United States make great strides toward expanding coverage and access to health care for many more Americans. The landmark legislation has been hailed as the most sweeping social legislation since the enactment of Social Security in 1935 and Medicare and Medicaid in 1965. The act is intended to improve access to care by extending health care coverage to millions of uninsured Americans and by preventing health insurance companies from denying coverage to people with preexisting medical conditions or dropping them when they develop costly medical problems.

The months leading up to this historic moment were tense, so much so that the future of the PPACA remained in jeopardy until Congress passed it. The Senate approved its version of the health care reform bill, the Patient Protection and Affordable Care Act, in December

FIGURE 1.10

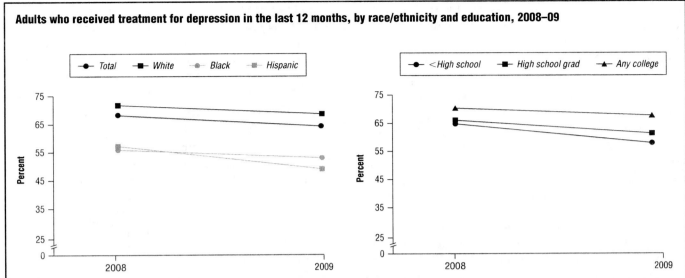

Adults who received treatment for depression in the last 12 months, by race/ethnicity and education, 2008–09

SOURCE: "Figure 2.31. Adults with a Major Depressive Episode in the Last 12 Months Who Received Treatment for Depression in the Last 12 Months, by Race/Ethnicity and Education, 2008–2009," in *National Healthcare Disparities Report, 2011*, U.S. Department of Health and Human Services, Agency for Healthcare Research and Quality, March 2012, http://www.ahrq.gov/qual/nhdr11/nhdr11.pdf (accessed June 12, 2012)

2009 in a 60–39 vote that adhered to party lines. Every Republican senator opposed the bill even though it was much more conservative than the corresponding bill, the Service Members Home Ownership Tax Act, in the House of Representatives. The House bill contained a public insurance option—a government-run health insurance company—and stronger sanctions for employers who failed to provide insurance for their workers. The Senate bill replaced the public insurance option with the creation of insurance exchanges (regulated marketplaces where insurance companies can compete to gain the business of individuals and small companies purchasing health insurance). The intent of these exchanges is to guarantee that insurance offerings are both comprehensive in terms of coverage and competitively priced.

Because there were no Republican supporters of the legislation, House Democrats worked feverishly to secure the 216 votes necessary to pass the bill. Last-minute accommodations were made to secure the votes, most notably by inserting language that ensured that the long-standing ban on using federal funds for abortion would not be overturned. Because it was a budget bill, it could be approved under reconciliation, a process that requires a majority to pass and is not subject to filibuster (the use of obstructive tactics to prevent adoption of a measure favored by the majority).

The Health Care and Education Reconciliation Act, which was intended to enable the PPACA to be amended, was introduced by Representative John M. Spratt Jr. (1942–; D-SC) on March 17, 2010, and the House passed the bill on March 21. The Senate amended the bill and passed its amended version on March 25. Fifty-six Dem-

ocrats voted in favor of the bill and a bipartisan (two-party) group of 43 senators voted against it. The amended bill was then returned to the House, where it was passed on March 30 in a vote of 220 in favor and 207 not in favor.

Even after it was signed into law, the PPACA remained controversial. In 2012 the U.S. Supreme Court considered the constitutionality of the law that aims to extend insurance coverage to most Americans. Much of the fiery debate about the law centered on the individual mandate—the provision that requires most Americans to have insurance by 2014 or pay a penalty should they forgo health insurance coverage.

ACCESS TO MENTAL HEALTH CARE

Besides the range of barriers to access faced by all Americans trying to access the health care system, people seeking mental health care face unique challenges, not the least of which is that they are even less able than people in good mental health to successfully navigate the fragmented mental health service delivery system. Furthermore, because people with serious mental illness frequently suffer from unemployment and disability, they are likely to join the ranks of the impoverished, uninsured, and homeless, which only compounds access problems. Finally, the social stigmas (deeply held negative attitudes) that promote discrimination against people with mental illness are a powerful deterrent to seeking care.

The social stigmas attached to being labeled "crazy" prevent some sufferers of mental illness from seeking and obtaining needed care. Myths about mental illness persist, especially the mistaken beliefs that mental illness is a sign of moral weakness or that an affected individual can simply choose to "wish or will away" the symptoms of mental illness. People with mental illness cannot just "pull themselves together" and will themselves well. Without treatment, symptoms can worsen and persist for months or even years.

People with mental illness experience other types of social stigmas as well. They may face discrimination in the workplace, in school, and in finding housing. Thwarted in their efforts to maintain independence, people suffering from mental illness may become trapped in a cycle characterized by feelings of worthlessness and hopelessness and may be further isolated from the social and community supports and treatments most able to help them recover.

Disparities in Access to Mental Health Care

The principal barriers to access of mental health care are the cost of mental health services, the lack of sufficient insurance for these services, the fragmented organization of these services, the mistrust of providers, and the social stigmas toward mental illness. These obstacles may act as deterrents for all Americans, but for racial and ethnic minorities they are compounded by language barriers, ethnic and cultural compatibility of practitioners, and geographic availability of services.

The AHRQ finds in *National Healthcare Disparities Report 2011* that when compared with whites and people with a high school education or higher, minorities and people with less than a high school education have less access to care and are less likely to receive needed services. For example, according to the AHRQ, African-Americans and Hispanics were less likely than whites to receive treatment for depression in 2009. Similarly, people with less than a high school education were less likely than people with a high school education or higher to receive treatment. (See Figure 1.10.)

IS ACCESS A RIGHT OR A PRIVILEGE?

The AHRQ and other health care researchers and policy makers observe that having health insurance does not necessarily ensure access to medical care. They contend that many other factors, including cost-containment measures put in place by private and public payers, have reduced access to care. Nonetheless, reduced access affects vulnerable populations—the poor, people with mental illness and other disabilities, and immigrants—more than others.

Health care is a resource that is rationed. The United States is the only developed country in the world that does not have a government-funded universal or national program of health insurance. As a result, Americans with greater incomes and assets are more likely than low-income families to have health insurance and have greater access to health care services. It is for this reason that the 2010 health care reform legislation is regarded by some as groundbreaking. Supporters of this legislation anticipate that as previously uninsured people obtain insurance, access will be greatly improved.

The National Economic and Social Right Initiative (NESRI) asserts that health care is a public good, not a commodity. In "Human Right to Health" (2012, http://www.nesri.org/programs/health), the NESRI states that "the human right to health guarantees a system of health protection for all. . . . NESRI supports groups that seek to mobilize people to stand up for their right to health care and motivate policymakers to make health care a public good, with costs and benefits shared equitably. We have a right to get the health care we need, and a responsibility to ensure that everyone else can do the same."

Various groups and organizations support the premise that health care is a fundamental human right, rather than a privilege. These organizations include Physicians for a National Health Program, the AARP, National Health Care for the Homeless, Inc., and the Friends Committee on National Legislation, a Quaker public interest lobby.

Others disagree with the notion that access to health care is a fundamental right. For example, Richard M. Salsman argues in "Memo to the Supreme Court: Health Care Is Not a Right" (*Forbes*, April 3, 2012) that "health care is not a right. It's a valuable service provided by intelligent, hard-working professionals with years of painstaking education and training, people who, like other Americans, deserve equal protection under the law, people who, like other Americans, have a right to their own life, liberty, property and the pursuit of their own happiness." Salsman believes that because people pay for health care, as they do for other goods and services, it is a privilege. Furthermore, he opposes the 2010 health care reform legislation, contending that mandating health coverage and requiring hospitals to treat patients who cannot pay violate both personal rights and the U.S. Constitution.

Concurring with Salsman, many groups and organizations assert that health care is not a fundamental right. These include Americans for Free Choice in Medicine, the Atlas Society, the United States Conference of Catholic Bishops, and the Heritage Foundation.

CHAPTER 2
HEALTH CARE PRACTITIONERS

The art of medicine consists of amusing the patient while nature cures the disease.

—Voltaire

One of the first duties of the physician is to educate the masses not to take medicine.

—William Osler, *Sir William Osler: Aphorisms, from His Bedside Teachings and Writings* (1950)

PHYSICIANS

Physicians routinely perform medical examinations, provide preventive medicine services, diagnose illness, treat patients suffering from injury or disease, and offer counsel about how to achieve and maintain good health. There are two types of physicians trained in traditional Western medicine: the Doctor of Medicine (MD) is schooled in allopathic medicine and the Doctor of Osteopathy (DO) learns osteopathy. Allopathy is the philosophy and system of curing disease by producing conditions that are incompatible with disease, such as prescribing antibiotics to combat bacterial infection. The philosophy of osteopathy is different; it is based on recognition of the body's capacity for self-healing, and it emphasizes structural and manipulative therapies such as postural education, manual treatment of the musculoskeletal system (osteopathic physicians are trained in hands-on diagnosis and treatment), and preventive medicine. Osteopathy is also considered a holistic practice because it considers the whole person, rather than simply the diseased organ or system.

In modern medical practice, the philosophical differences may not be obvious to most health care consumers because MDs and DOs use many comparable methods of treatment, including prescribing medication and performing surgery. In fact, the American Osteopathic Association (2012, https://www.osteopathic.org/inside-aoa/about/Pages/default.aspx), the national medical professional society that represents more than 100,000 DOs and DO students, admits that many people who seek care from osteopathic physicians may be entirely unaware of their physician's training, which emphasizes holistic interventions or special skills such as manipulative techniques. Like MDs, DOs complete four years of medical school and postgraduate residency training; may specialize in areas such as surgery, psychiatry, or obstetrics; and must pass state licensing examinations to practice.

Medical School, Postgraduate Training, and Qualifications

Modern medicine requires considerable skill and extensive training. The road to gaining admission to medical school and becoming a physician is long, difficult, and intensely competitive. Medical school applicants must earn excellent college grades, achieve high scores on entrance exams, and demonstrate emotional maturity and motivation to be admitted to medical school. Once admitted, medical students spend the first two years primarily in laboratories and classrooms learning basic medical sciences such as anatomy (detailed understanding of body structure), physiology (biological processes and vital functions), and biochemistry. They also learn how to take medical histories, perform complete physical examinations, and recognize symptoms of diseases. During their third and fourth years, the medical students work under supervision at teaching hospitals and clinics. By completing clerkships—spending time in different specialties such as internal medicine, obstetrics and gynecology, pediatrics, psychiatry, and surgery—they acquire the necessary skills and gain experience to diagnose and treat a wide variety of illnesses.

Following medical school, new physicians must complete a year of internship, also referred to as postgraduate year one, that emphasizes either general medical practice or one specific specialty and provides clinical experience in various hospital services (e.g., inpatient care, outpatient clinics, emergency departments, and operating rooms). In the past, many physicians entered practice after this first year of postgraduate training. However, in the present era of specialization most physicians choose to continue in residency training, which lasts an additional three to six years, depending on the specialty. Those who choose a subspecialty such as cardiology, infectious diseases, oncology, or plastic surgery must spend additional years in residency and may then choose to complete fellowship training. Immediately after residency, they are eligible to take an examination to earn board certification in their chosen specialty. Fellowship training involves a year or two of laboratory and clinical research work as well as opportunities to gain additional clinical and patient care expertise.

Medical School Applicants

According to the Association of American Medical Colleges (AAMC), in "U.S. Medical School Applicants and Students 1982–1983 to 2011–2012" (2012, https://www.aamc.org/download/153708/data/charts1982to2012.pdf), the number of students entering medical school for the 2011–12 academic year rose to 19,230, which was a 16.6% increase from the 2002–03 academic year. The students were selected from a pool of 43,919 applicants.

Conventional and Newer Medical Specialties

Rapid advances in science and medicine and changing needs have resulted in a variety of new medical and surgical specialties, subspecialties, and concentrations. For example, geriatrics, the medical subspecialty concerned with the prevention and treatment of diseases in older adults, has developed in response to growth in this population. The term *geriatrics* is derived from the Greek *geras* (old age) and *iatrikos* (physician). Geriatricians are physicians trained in primary care, such as internal medicine or family practice, who receive further training and become eligible for certification as specialists in the medical care of older adults. In "Frequently Asked Questions" (June 2012, http://www.americangeriatrics.org/files/documents/Adv_Resources/gwps_faqs.pdf), the American Geriatrics Society (AGS) reports that as of March 2011 there were 7,162 board-certified geriatricians and 1,751 board-certified geriatric psychiatrists in the United States. It also observes that the United States needs more geriatricians to care for its growing population of older adults. In 2011 there was one geriatrician for every 2,620 adults aged 75 years and older. In 2030 the AGS estimates that there will be one geriatrician for every 3,798 older adults.

Another relatively new medical specialty has resulted in physician intensivists. Intensivists, as the name indicates, are trained to staff hospital intensive care units (ICUs, which are sometimes known as critical care units), where the most critically ill patients are cared for using a comprehensive array of state-of-the-art technology and equipment. This specialty arose in response to both the increasing complexity of care provided in ICUs and the demonstrated benefits of immediate availability of highly trained physicians to care for critically ill patients. The Health Resources and Services Administration (HRSA) notes in *The Critical Care Workforce: A Study of the Supply and Demand for Critical Care Physicians* (July 2006, http://bhpr.hrsa.gov/healthworkforce/reports/studycriticalcarephys.pdf) that "demand for intensivists will continue to exceed available supply through the year 2020 if current supply and demand trends continue." Assuming optimal utilization, the HRSA predicts a shortfall of 1,500 intensivists in 2020. (See Figure 2.1.) According to David J. Wallace et al., in "Nighttime Intensivist Staffing and Mortality among Critically Ill Patients" (*New England Journal of Medicine*, vol. 366, no. 22, May 31, 2012), hospitals are increasingly staffed by intensivists 24 hours per day, rather than simply during daytime hours, to improve the care of ICU patients. The researchers analyzed nighttime intensivist staffing and how well patients fare in the ICU. Their analysis finds a reduction in ICU deaths with nighttime intensivists staffing. Wallace et al. speculate that nighttime intensivists may institute more timely resuscitation of unstable patients, initiate effective medical therapies earlier, and manage complex therapies more efficiently. Their availability may also serve to reduce medical errors.

The fastest-growing new specialty is hospitalists—physicians who are hospital based as opposed to office

FIGURE 2.1

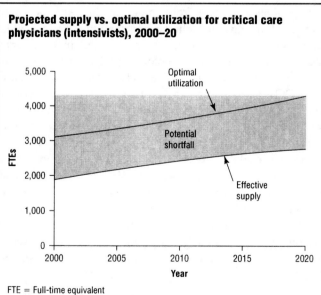

Projected supply vs. optimal utilization for critical care physicians (intensivists), 2000–20

FTE = Full-time equivalent

SOURCE: Elizabeth M. Duke, "Exhibit 15. Projected Supply vs. Optimal Utilization for Intensivists, 2000–2020," in *Report to Congress—The Critical Care Workforce: A Study of the Supply and Demand for Critical Care Physicians*, U.S. Department of Health and Human Services, Health Resources and Services Administration, May 2006, http://bhpr.hrsa.gov/healthworkforce/reports/studycriticalcarephys.pdf (accessed June 13, 2012)

based and who provide a variety of services from caring for hospitalized patients who do not have personal physicians to explaining complex medical procedures to patients and families and coordinating many aspects of inpatient care. Robert M. Wachter and Derek Bell report in "Renaissance of Hospital Generalists" (*BMJ*, vol. 344, no. 10, February 2012) that there were more than 30,000 hospitalists in the United States in 2012 and that their ranks are expected to grow in coming years. The researchers attribute the rise in hospitalists to evidence that the use of hospitalists improved outcomes and to hospitalists' willingness to champion safety and quality improvement programs. Financial considerations also promoted hospitalist growth. Wachter and Bell observe that "hospitals benefited from savings in cost and length of stay generated by hospitalists and were therefore willing to provide financial support for hospitalist programmes."

More traditional medical specialties include:

- Anesthesiologist—administers anesthesia (partial or complete loss of sensation) and monitors patients in surgery

- Cardiologist—diagnoses and treats diseases of the heart and blood vessels

- Dermatologist—trained to diagnose and treat diseases of the skin, hair, and nails

- Family practitioner—delivers primary care to people of all ages and, when necessary, refers patients to other physician specialists

- Gastroenterologist—specializes in digestive system disorders

- Internist—provides diagnosis and nonsurgical treatment of a broad array of illnesses affecting adults

- Neurologist—specializes in the nervous system and provides diagnosis and treatment of brain, spinal cord, and nerve disorders

- Obstetrician-gynecologist—provides health care for women and their reproductive systems, as well as care for mothers and babies before, during, and immediately following delivery

- Oncologist—dedicated to the diagnosis and treatment of cancer

- Otolaryngologist—skilled in the medical and surgical treatment of ear, nose, and throat disorders and related structures of the face, head, and neck

- Pathologist—uses skills in microscopic chemical analysis and diagnostics to detect disease in body tissues and fluids

- Psychiatrist—specializes in the prevention, diagnosis, and treatment of mental health and emotional disorders

- Pulmonologist—specializes in diseases of the lungs and respiratory system

- Urologist—provides diagnosis as well as medical and surgical treatment of the urinary tract in both men and women as well as male reproductive health services

HIGH COSTS, LONG HOURS, AND LOW WAGES. According to Laura McMullen, in "10 Least Expensive Public Medical Schools for In-State Students" (*U.S. News & World Report*, May 1, 2012), the tuition and fees for the 2011–12 academic year at public medical schools were $28,812 and the tuition and fees at private medical schools were $45,870. The AAMC (2012, https://services.aamc.org/tsfreports/select.cfm?year_of_study=2012) reports that public medical school tuition and fees increased by an average of 7.7% for in-state residents and by 6.3% for nonresidents from the previous academic year. Similarly, private medical school tuition and fees increased by 4.3% for in-state residents and by 4.6% for nonresidents.

In "10 Medical Schools That Lead to the Most Debt" (*U.S. News & World Report*, May 22, 2012), Kelsey Sheehy indicates that the average 2010 medical school graduate had an educational debt of $145,020. Even though a physician's earning power is considerable, and many students are able to repay their educational debt during their first years of practice, some observers believe the extent of medical students' indebtedness may unduly influence their career choices. They may train for higher-paying specialties and subspecialties rather than follow their natural interests or opt to practice in underrepresented specialties or underserved geographic areas. The high cost of medical education is also believed to limit the number of minority applicants to medical school.

Historically, medical training has been difficult and involved long hours. Working long hours without adequate rest has been found to increase the occurrence of preventable medical errors and thereby adversely affect patient safety. Since July 1, 2011, the Accreditation Council for Graduate Medical Education (ACGME) restricts the duty hours of the more than 100,000 U.S. residents. The ACGME Common Program Requirements (http://www.acgme.org/acWebsite/home/Common_Program_Requirements_07012011.pdf) stipulate that:

- Residents' "duty hours must be limited to 80 hours per week, averaged over a four-week period"

- "Residents must be scheduled for a minimum of one day free of duty every week"

- First-year residents (interns) must not work more than 16 hours and "should have 10 hours, and must have eight hours, free of duty between scheduled duty periods"

- Second-year residents and above "may be scheduled to a maximum of 24 hours of continuous duty in the hospital"

- "Programs must encourage residents to use alertness management strategies in the context of patient care responsibilities. Strategic napping, especially after 16 hours of continuous duty and between the hours of 10:00 p.m. and 8:00 a.m., is strongly suggested."

In "Residents' Response to Duty-Hour Regulations—A Follow-up National Survey" (*New England Journal of Medicine*, vol. 366, no. 35, June 14, 2012), Brian C. Drolet, Derrick A. Christopher, and Staci A. Fischer report the results of a survey of residents one year after the ACGME requirements went into effect. Even though the regulations were intended to improve residents' quality of life, only interns (61.8%) reported a positive change. In contrast, senior residents said their quality of life had worsened (49.7%) and, overall, residents claimed their work schedules were worse (43%). The researchers note that "50.1% of residents said that the amount of rest they obtained was unchanged, and 58.9% said the total number hours they worked was unchanged."

The Number of Physicians in Practice Is Increasing

In 2009, of the 972,376 physicians in the United States, 307,586 (31.6%) were primary care physicians. (See Table 2.1.) Primary care physicians are the front line of the health care system—the first health professionals most people see for medical problems or routine care. Family practitioners, internists, pediatricians, obstetrician/gynecologists, and general practitioners are considered to be primary care physicians. Primary care physicians tend to see the same patients regularly and develop relationships with patients over time as they offer preventive services, scheduled visits, follow-up, and urgent medical care. When necessary, they refer patients for consultation with, and care from, physician specialists.

In 2009, 560,381 physicians maintained office-based practices, 189,185 were in hospital-based practices, and 109,065 were residents and interns. (See Table 2.2.) Besides the growing number of graduates of U.S. medical

TABLE 2.1

Doctors in primary care, by specialty, selected years 1949–2009

Specialty	1949[a]	1960[a]	1970	1980	1990	1995	2000	2008	2009
					Number				
Total doctors of medicine[b]	201,277	260,484	334,028	467,679	615,421	720,325	813,770	954,224	972,376
Active doctors of medicine[c]	191,577	247,257	310,845	414,916	547,310	625,443	692,368	784,199	792,805
General primary care specialists	113,222	125,359	134,354	170,705	213,514	241,329	274,653	305,264	307,586
General practice/family medicine	95,980	88,023	57,948	60,049	70,480	75,976	86,312	93,761	94,671
Internal medicine	12,453	26,209	39,924	58,462	76,295	88,240	101,353	115,314	116,148
Obstetrics/gynecology	—	—	18,532	24,612	30,220	33,519	35,922	38,272	38,573
Pediatrics	4,789	11,127	17,950	27,582	36,519	43,594	51,066	57,917	58,194
Primary care subspecialists	—	—	3,161	16,642	30,911	39,659	52,294	71,794	74,000
Family medicine	—	—	—	—	—	236	483	1,193	1,303
Internal medicine	—	—	1,948	13,069	22,054	26,928	34,831	47,779	49,324
Obstetrics/gynecology	—	—	344	1,693	3,477	4,133	4,319	4,363	4,282
Pediatrics	—	—	869	1,880	5,380	8,362	12,661	18,459	19,091
				Percent of active doctors of medicine					
General primary care specialist	59.1	50.7	43.2	41.1	39.0	38.6	39.7	38.9	38.8
General practice/family medicine	50.1	35.6	18.6	14.5	12.9	12.1	12.5	12.0	11.9
Internal medicine	6.5	10.6	12.8	14.1	13.9	14.1	14.6	14.7	14.7
Obstetrics/gynecology	—	—	6.0	5.9	5.5	5.4	5.2	4.9	4.9
Pediatrics	2.5	4.5	5.8	6.6	6.7	7.0	7.4	7.4	7.3
Primary care subspecialists	—	—	1.0	4.0	5.6	6.3	7.6	9.2	9.3
Family medicine	—	—	0.0	0.0	0.0	0.0	0.1	0.2	0.2
Internal medicine	—	—	0.6	3.1	4.0	4.3	5.0	6.1	6.2
Obstetrics/gynecology	—	—	0.1	0.4	0.6	0.7	0.6	0.6	0.5
Pediatrics	—	—	0.3	0.5	1.0	1.3	1.8	2.4	2.4

—Data not available.

0.0 Percentage greater than zero but less than 0.05.

[a]Estimated by the Bureau of Health Professions, Health Resources Administration. Active doctors of medicine (MDs) include those with address unknown and primary specialty not classified.

[b]Includes MDs engaged in federal and nonfederal patient care (office-based or hospital-based) and other professional activities.

[c]Starting with 1970 data, MDs who are inactive, have unknown address, or primary specialty not classified are excluded.

Notes: Data are as of December 31 except for 1990–1994 data, which are as of January 1, and 1949 data, which are as of midyear. Outlying areas include Puerto Rico, the U.S. Virgin Islands, and the Pacific islands of Canton, Caroline, Guam, Mariana, Marshall, American Samoa, and Wake. Data have been revised and differ from previous editions of *Health, United States*.

SOURCE: "Table 111. Doctors of Medicine in Primary Care, by Specialty: United States and Outlying U.S. Areas, Selected Years 1949–2009," in *Health, United States, 2011: With Special Feature on Socioeconomic Status and Health*, U.S. Department of Health and Human Services, Centers for Disease Control and Prevention, National Center for Health Statistics, May 2012, http://www.cdc.gov/nchs/data/hus/hus11.pdf (accessed June 14, 2012). Data from the American Medical Association (AMA).

TABLE 2.2

Medical doctors by activity and place of medical education, selected years 1975–2009

Place of medical education and activity	1975	1985	1995	2000	2005	2007	2008	2009
				Number of doctors of medicine				
Total doctors of medicine	393,742	552,716	720,325	813,770	902,053	941,304	954,224	972,376
Active doctors of medicine[a]	340,280	497,140	625,443	692,368	762,438	776,554	784,199	792,805
Place of medical education								
U.S. medical graduates	—	392,007	481,137	527,931	571,798	580,336	586,421	591,835
International medical graduates[b]	—	105,133	144,306	164,437	190,640	196,218	197,778	200,970
Activity								
Patient care[c, d]	287,837	431,527	564,074	631,431	718,473	732,234	740,867	749,566
Office-based practice	213,334	329,041	427,275	490,398	563,225	562,897	556,818	560,381
General and family practice	46,347	53,862	59,932	67,534	74,999	75,952	75,443	76,514
Cardiovascular diseases	5,046	9,054	13,739	16,300	17,519	17,504	17,352	17,443
Dermatology	3,442	5,325	6,959	7,969	8,795	9,036	9,066	9,192
Gastroenterology	1,696	4,135	7,300	8,515	9,742	10,042	10,119	10,293
Internal medicine	28,188	52,712	72,612	88,699	107,028	108,552	107,943	109,305
Pediatrics	12,687	22,392	33,890	42,215	51,854	52,095	51,719	52,420
Pulmonary diseases	1,166	3,035	4,964	6,095	7,321	7,490	7,535	7,677
General surgery	19,710	24,708	24,086	24,475	26,079	25,434	24,640	24,536
Obstetrics and gynecology	15,613	23,525	29,111	31,726	34,659	34,405	33,968	34,092
Ophthalmology	8,795	12,212	14,596	15,598	16,580	15,852	15,656	15,731
Orthopedic surgery	8,148	13,033	17,136	17,367	19,115	19,299	19,110	19,205
Otolaryngology	4,297	5,751	7,139	7,581	8,206	8,177	8,034	8,025
Plastic surgery	1,706	3,299	4,612	5,308	6,011	6,100	6,093	6,110
Urological surgery	5,025	7,081	7,991	8,460	8,955	8,796	8,656	8,678
Anesthesiology	8,970	15,285	23,770	27,624	31,887	31,617	31,389	31,294
Diagnostic radiology	1,978	7,735	12,751	14,622	17,618	17,327	17,197	17,100
Emergency medicine	—	—	11,700	14,541	20,173	20,036	19,965	19,978
Neurology	1,862	4,691	7,623	8,559	10,400	10,476	10,386	10,433
Pathology, anatomical/clinical	4,195	6,877	9,031	10,267	11,747	11,191	10,738	10,554
Psychiatry	12,173	18,521	23,334	24,955	27,638	27,492	26,521	26,235
Radiology	6,970	7,355	5,994	6,674	7,049	6,913	6,809	6,837
Other specialty	15,320	28,453	29,005	35,314	39,850	39,111	38,479	38,729
Hospital-based practice	74,503	102,486	136,799	141,033	155,248	169,337	184,049	189,185
Residents and interns[e]	53,527	72,159	93,650	95,125	95,391	98,688	108,073	109,065
Full-time hospital staff	20,976	30,327	43,149	45,908	59,857	70,649	75,976	80,120
Other professional activity[f]	24,252	44,046	40,290	41,556	43,965	44,320	43,332	43,239
Inactive	21,449	38,646	72,326	75,168	99,823	111,551	119,239	121,704
Not classified	26,145	13,950	20,579	45,136	39,304	52,740	50,347	57,427
Unknown address	5,868	2,980	1,977	1,098	488	459	439	440

—Data not available.

[a]Doctors of medicine who are inactive, have unknown address, or primary specialty not classified are excluded.
[b]International medical graduates received their medical education in schools outside the United States and Canada.
[c]Specialty information is based on the physician's self-designated primary area of practice. Categories include generalists and specialists.
[d]Starting with 2003 data, estimates include federal and nonfederal doctors of medicine. Prior to 2003, estimates were for nonfederal doctors of medicine only.
[e]Starting with 1990 data, clinical fellows are included in this category. In prior years, clinical fellows were included in the other professional activity category.
[f]Includes medical teaching, administration, research, and other. Prior to 1990, this category also included clinical fellows.
Notes: Data for doctors of medicine are as of December 31, except for 1990–1994 data, which are as of January 1. Outlying areas include Puerto Rico, the U.S. Virgin Islands, and the Pacific islands of Canton, Caroline, Guam, Mariana, Marshall, American Samoa, and Wake.

SOURCE: "Table 110. Doctors of Medicine, by Place of Medical Education and Activity: United States and Outlying U.S. Areas, Selected Years 1975–2009," in *Health, United States, 2011: With Special Feature on Socioeconomic Status and Health*, U.S. Department of Health and Human Services, Centers for Disease Control and Prevention, National Center for Health Statistics, May 2012, http://www.cdc.gov/nchs/data/hus/hus11.pdf (accessed June 14, 2012). Data from the American Medical Association (AMA).

schools, the ranks of international medical graduates grew by 3,192, from 197,778 in 2008 to 200,970 in 2009.

The number of active physicians devoted to patient care, as opposed to research, administration, or other roles, varied by geographic region and by state, from highs of 65 physicians per 10,000 civilian population in the District of Columbia and 39.6 per 10,000 civilian population in Massachusetts in 2009 to lows of 17.4 and 17.3 physicians per 10,000 civilian population in Idaho and Mississippi, respectively. (See Table 2.3.)

Physician Working Conditions and Earnings

Many physicians work long, irregular hours. The Bureau of Labor Statistics (BLS; July 11, 2011, http://www.bls.gov/k12/help06.htm) reports that in 2008 three out of 10 full-time physicians worked 60 hours or more per week performing patient care and administrative duties such as office management. According to the BLS (March 29, 2012, http://www.bls.gov/ooh/Health care/Physicians-and-surgeons.htm), physicians and surgeons worked at 691,000 jobs in 2010. Physicians in

TABLE 2.3

Active physicians and physicians in patient care, by state, selected years 1975–2009

State	Active physicians[a,b]						Physicians in patient care[a,b,c]					
	1975	1985	1995	2000[d]	2008	2009	1975	1985	1995	2000	2008	2009
	Number per 10,000 civilian population											
United States	**15.3**	**20.7**	**24.2**	**25.8**	**27.7**	**27.4**	**13.5**	**18.0**	**21.3**	**22.7**	**25.7**	**25.4**
Alabama	9.2	14.2	18.4	19.8	21.6	21.5	8.6	13.1	17.0	18.2	20.6	20.5
Alaska	8.4	13.0	15.7	18.5	24.2	24.2	7.8	12.1	14.2	16.3	22.5	22.6
Arizona	16.7	20.2	21.4	20.9	22.3	22.6	14.1	17.1	18.2	17.6	20.6	21.0
Arkansas	9.1	13.8	17.3	18.8	20.4	20.4	8.5	12.8	16.0	17.3	19.4	19.4
California	18.8	23.7	23.7	23.8	26.2	26.4	17.3	21.5	21.7	21.6	24.4	24.6
Colorado	17.3	20.7	23.7	24.0	26.6	26.8	15.0	17.7	20.6	20.9	24.7	25.0
Connecticut	19.8	27.6	32.8	33.7	36.6	36.8	17.7	24.3	29.5	30.3	33.5	33.9
Delaware	14.3	19.7	23.4	24.7	26.4	26.2	12.7	17.1	19.7	21.0	24.7	24.5
District of Columbia	39.6	55.3	63.6	62.5	74.9	73.8	34.6	45.6	53.6	54.5	65.9	65.0
Florida	15.2	20.2	22.9	24.1	25.8	26.0	13.4	17.8	20.3	21.2	24.2	24.4
Georgia	11.5	16.2	19.7	20.4	21.4	21.3	10.6	14.7	18.0	18.6	20.1	19.9
Hawaii	16.2	21.5	24.8	26.4	31.8	31.8	14.7	19.8	22.8	24.0	29.6	29.7
Idaho	9.5	12.1	13.9	15.8	17.9	18.4	8.9	11.4	13.1	14.4	17.0	17.4
Illinois	14.5	20.5	24.8	26.1	27.8	28.0	13.1	18.2	22.1	23.1	25.8	26.1
Indiana	10.6	14.7	18.4	20.0	22.2	22.3	9.6	13.2	16.6	18.0	21.0	21.0
Iowa	11.4	15.6	19.2	19.8	21.5	21.6	9.4	12.4	15.1	15.5	19.5	19.7
Kansas	12.8	17.3	20.8	21.8	23.8	24.1	11.2	15.1	18.0	18.8	22.0	22.4
Kentucky	10.9	15.1	19.2	20.6	23.1	23.3	10.1	13.9	18.0	19.1	21.7	22.0
Louisiana	11.4	17.3	21.7	23.8	25.3	25.4	10.5	16.1	20.3	22.4	24.2	24.3
Maine	12.8	18.7	22.3	26.8	31.1	31.6	10.7	15.6	18.2	21.7	28.2	28.7
Maryland	18.6	30.4	34.1	35.4	40.2	40.1	16.5	24.9	29.9	31.1	35.3	35.4
Massachusetts	20.8	30.2	37.5	38.6	43.6	43.4	18.3	25.4	33.2	34.4	39.7	39.6
Michigan	15.4	20.8	24.8	26.3	28.5	29.2	12.0	16.0	19.0	20.2	25.5	26.0
Minnesota	14.9	20.5	23.4	24.9	28.8	28.9	13.7	18.5	21.5	23.0	27.0	27.2
Mississippi	8.4	11.8	13.9	16.6	18.2	18.2	8.0	11.1	13.0	15.2	17.3	17.3
Missouri	15.0	20.5	23.9	24.7	26.2	26.1	11.6	16.3	19.7	20.2	24.1	24.1
Montana	10.6	14.0	18.4	20.4	23.0	23.0	10.1	13.2	17.1	18.8	21.9	21.9
Nebraska	12.1	15.7	19.8	21.7	24.7	24.9	10.9	14.4	18.3	20.1	23.1	23.5
Nevada	11.9	16.0	16.7	18.0	19.7	19.8	10.9	14.5	14.6	15.9	18.5	18.6
New Hampshire	14.3	18.1	21.5	23.8	28.6	29.3	13.1	16.7	19.8	21.7	26.9	27.6
New Jersey	16.2	23.4	29.3	31.1	32.9	33.0	14.0	19.8	24.9	26.2	30.0	30.1
New Mexico	12.2	17.0	20.2	20.9	23.9	23.9	10.1	14.7	18.0	18.5	22.3	22.2
New York	22.7	29.0	35.3	36.2	37.8	37.9	20.2	25.2	31.6	32.3	34.8	35.0
North Carolina	11.7	16.9	21.1	22.3	25.0	25.0	10.6	15.0	19.4	20.5	23.4	23.4
North Dakota	9.7	15.8	20.5	19.2	24.7	25.2	9.2	14.9	18.9	19.8	23.6	24.1
Ohio	14.1	19.9	23.8	25.4	28.2	28.5	12.2	16.8	20.0	21.3	25.9	26.2
Oklahoma	11.6	16.1	18.8	19.4	20.9	21.3	9.4	12.9	14.7	14.8	18.9	19.3
Oregon	15.6	19.7	21.6	22.9	27.8	28.0	13.8	17.6	19.5	20.5	26.1	26.4
Pennsylvania	16.6	23.6	30.1	31.6	33.1	33.1	13.9	19.2	24.6	25.4	29.6	29.6
Rhode Island	17.8	23.3	30.4	32.5	37.0	37.2	16.1	20.2	26.7	28.8	34.5	34.6
South Carolina	10.0	14.7	18.9	21.0	22.8	22.8	9.3	13.6	17.6	19.4	21.7	21.6
South Dakota	8.2	13.4	16.7	19.2	22.8	23.2	7.7	12.3	15.7	17.7	21.8	22.2
Tennessee	12.4	17.7	22.5	23.6	26.0	26.2	11.3	16.2	20.8	21.8	24.6	24.8
Texas	12.5	16.8	19.4	20.3	21.5	21.6	11.0	14.7	17.3	17.9	20.2	20.3
Utah	14.1	17.2	19.2	19.6	20.8	21.0	13.0	15.5	17.6	17.8	19.3	19.6
Vermont	18.2	23.8	26.9	32.0	36.0	35.9	15.5	20.3	24.2	28.8	33.3	33.3
Virginia	12.9	19.5	22.5	23.9	27.2	27.5	11.9	17.8	20.8	22.0	25.5	25.8
Washington	15.3	20.2	22.5	23.7	27.0	27.0	13.6	17.9	20.2	21.2	25.1	25.1
West Virginia	11.0	16.3	21.0	23.5	25.7	26.1	10.0	14.6	17.9	19.5	23.3	23.8
Wisconsin	12.5	17.7	21.5	23.1	26.2	26.5	11.4	15.9	19.6	20.9	24.6	24.9
Wyoming	9.5	12.9	15.3	17.3	19.9	19.9	8.9	12.0	13.9	15.7	18.7	18.8

[a]Includes active doctors of medicine (MDs) and active doctors of osteopathy (DOs).
[b]Starting with 2003 data, federal and nonfederal physicians are included. Data prior to 2003 included nonfederal physicians only.
[c]Prior to 2006, excludes DOs. Excludes physicians in medical teaching, administration, research, and other nonpatient care activities. Includes residents.
[d]Data for DOs are as of January 2001.
Notes: Data for MDs are as of December 31. Data for DOs are as of May 31, unless otherwise specified.

SOURCE: "Table 109. Active Physicians and Physicians in Patient Care, by State: United States, Selected Years 1975–2009," in *Health, United States, 2011: With Special Feature on Socioeconomic Status and Health*, U.S. Department of Health and Human Services, Centers for Disease Control and Prevention, National Center for Health Statistics, May 2012, http://www.cdc.gov/nchs/data/hus/hus11.pdf (accessed June 14, 2012). Data from the American Medical Association (AMA).

salaried positions, such as those employed by health maintenance organizations, usually have shorter and more regular hours and enjoy more flexible work schedules than those in private practice. Instead of working as

solo practitioners, growing numbers of physicians work in clinics or are partners in group practices or other integrated health care systems. Medical group practices allow physicians to have more flexible schedules, to

TABLE 2.4

Median annual compensation for selected medical specialties, 2010

Anesthesiology	$407,292
General surgery	343,958
Obstetrics/gynecology	281,190
Internal medicine	205,379
Psychiatry	200,694
Pediatrics/adolescent medicine	192,148
Family practice (without obstetrics)	189,402

SOURCE: "Median Annual Compensations for Selected Specialties in 2010," in *Occupational Outlook Handbook, 2012–13 Edition: Physicians and Surgeons*, Bureau of Labor Statistics, U.S. Department of Labor, March 29, 2012, http://www.bls.gov/ooh/Healthcare/Physicians-and-surgeons.htm#tab-5 (accessed June 14, 2012). Data from the Medical Group Management Association.

FIGURE 2.2

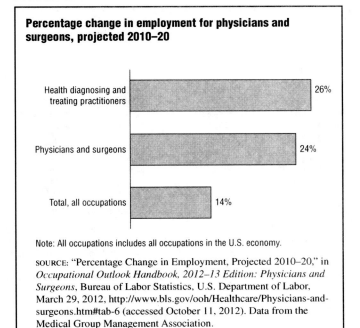

Percentage change in employment for physicians and surgeons, projected 2010–20

Note: All occupations includes all occupations in the U.S. economy.

SOURCE: "Percentage Change in Employment, Projected 2010–20," in *Occupational Outlook Handbook, 2012–13 Edition: Physicians and Surgeons*, Bureau of Labor Statistics, U.S. Department of Labor, March 29, 2012, http://www.bls.gov/ooh/Healthcare/Physicians-and-surgeons.htm#tab-6 (accessed October 11, 2012). Data from the Medical Group Management Association.

realize purchasing economies of scale, to pool their money to finance expensive medical equipment, and to be better able to adapt to changes in health care delivery, financing, and reimbursement.

Physicians' earnings are among the highest of any profession. The BLS (March 27, 2012, http://www.bls.gov/oes/current/oes291069.htm) notes that the median annual compensation (the point at which half earn more and half earn less) for all physicians in 2011 was $184,650; however, many specialists earn more. In 2010 family practitioners received a total median annual compensation of $189,402 and pediatricians received a total median annual compensation of $192,148. In contrast, the median annual compensation for general surgeons was $343,958 and for anesthesiologists it was $407,292. (See Table 2.4.) Salaries vary widely and are based on a physician's specialty, the number of years in practice, the hours worked, and the geographic location.

The BLS expects that physician employment will increase by 24% between 2010 and 2020, outpacing many other occupations. (See Figure 2.2.) This increase is attributable to an aging population and continued demand for physician services.

Physician Visits

In 2009 Americans made more than 1 million physician office visits, and 30% (316,395) of these visits were made by people aged 45 to 64 years. (See Table 2.5.) More than half (55.9%) of all Americans' physician office visits were to primary care physicians. (See Table 2.6.) Women aged 18 to 44 years visited primary care physicians more often than men did. As expected, visits to specialty care physicians increased with advancing age. For example, 54.1% of visits to physician specialists were made by people aged 75 years and older, compared with 38.5% of visits by people aged 18 to 44 years.

Physician Satisfaction

Changes in the health care delivery system—particularly the shift from traditional fee-for-service practice (paid for each visit, procedure, or treatment that is delivered) to managed care, with its efforts to standardize medical practice, which reduces physicians' ability to manage their time, schedules, and professional relationships—have been named as factors contributing to physicians' dissatisfaction with their choice of career. Other changes, including decreasing reimbursement and an ever-increasing emphasis on documentation to satisfy government and private payers, as well as administrative requirements that infringe on the time physicians would rather spend caring for patients, have also increased physician dissatisfaction.

In *Physician Compensation Report 2012* (2012, http://www.medscape.com/features/slideshow/compensation/2012/public), Leslie Kane reports on a survey of 24,216 U.S. physicians representing 25 specialties that was conducted by Medscape in February 2012. The survey indicates that physician frustration and dissatisfaction increased from the previous year. In 2012 slightly more than half (54%) of the physicians said they would choose medicine again as a career, down from 69% in 2011. Only half (51%) of the physicians surveyed felt they are fairly compensated for their work, and less than half of the primary care physicians—25% of internists, 32% of family physicians, and 46% of pediatricians—would choose the same specialty. The physicians also expressed dissatisfaction with their practice settings; only 23% would choose the same practice setting in 2012, compared with 50% in 2011.

TABLE 2.5

Visits to physician offices by age, selected years 1995–2009

Age, sex, and race	All places*				Physician offices			
	1995	2000	2008	2009	1995	2000	2008	2009
Age				Number of visits in thousands				
Total	860,859	1,014,848	1,189,619	1,270,001	697,082	823,542	955,969	1,037,796
Under 18 years	194,644	212,165	225,531	239,590	150,351	163,459	171,744	183,999
18–44 years	285,184	315,774	328,438	341,209	219,065	243,011	243,979	257,890
45–64 years	188,320	255,894	341,595	374,775	159,531	216,783	284,110	316,395
45–54 years	104,891	142,233	169,674	190,701	88,266	119,474	137,776	158,120
55–64 years	83,429	113,661	171,921	184,074	71,264	97,309	146,335	158,275
65 years and over	192,712	231,014	294,054	314,428	168,135	200,289	256,135	279,514
65–74 years	102,605	116,505	144,878	153,884	90,544	102,447	127,125	137,452
75 years and over	90,106	114,510	149,177	160,544	77,591	97,842	129,010	142,062

*All places includes visits to physician offices and hospital outpatient and emergency departments.

SOURCE: Adapted from "Table 96. Visits to Physician Offices, Hospital Outpatient Departments, and Hospital Emergency Departments, by Age, Sex, and Race: United States, Selected Years 1995–2009," in *Health, United States, 2011: With Special Feature on Socioeconomic Status and Health*, U.S. Department of Health and Human Services, Centers for Disease Control and Prevention, National Center for Health Statistics, May 2012, http://www.cdc.gov/nchs/data/hus/hus11.pdf (accessed June 14, 2012)

The 2011 survey found that dermatologists were among the most satisfied, with an 80% overall satisfaction rate. In 2012 only 64% were satisfied. The most dissatisfied physicians were plastic surgeons (41% were satisfied overall), internists (44%), and endocrinologists (45%).

As might be expected, the 2012 survey finds that physician dissatisfaction was fueled by fear of declining income, increased regulation and documentation requirements, and the perceived need to practice defensive medicine to guard against malpractice suits.

REGISTERED NURSES

Registered nurses (RNs) are licensed by the state to care for the sick and to promote health. RNs supervise hospital care, administer medication and treatment as prescribed by physicians, monitor the progress of patients, and provide health education. Nurses work in a variety of settings, including hospitals, nursing homes, physicians' offices, clinics, and schools.

Education for Nurses

There are three types of education for RNs: associate's degree (two-year community college program), baccalaureate degree (four-year program), and postgraduate degree (master's and doctorate programs). The baccalaureate degree provides more knowledge of community health services, as well as the psychological and social aspects of caring for patients, than does the associate's degree. Those who complete the four-year baccalaureate degree and the other advanced degrees are generally better prepared to eventually attain administrative or management positions and may have greater opportunities for upward mobility in related disciplines such as research, teaching, and public health.

The BLS (March 29, 2012, http://www.bls.gov/ooh/Healthcare/Registered-nurses.htm) indicates that in 2010 there were nearly 2.8 million RNs and predicts that employment of RNs will grow 26% between 2010 and 2020, faster than it will for all occupations. (See Figure 2.3.)

NEED FOR NURSES EXCEEDS SUPPLY. Even though the number of RNs holding baccalaureate degrees increased sharply during the 1990s, there is still a shortage of nurses that is predicted to persist through 2020. Figure 2.3 shows employment projections for RNs between 2010 and 2020. Figure 2.4 shows that the gap between supply and demand for RNs is projected to widen through 2020. In "United States Registered Nurse Workforce Report Card and Shortage Forecast" (*American Journal of Medical Quality*, vol. 27, no. 3, May–June 2012), Stephen P. Juraschek et al. present a state-by-state analysis of the nursing workforce that forecasts a national RN deficit of 300,000 to 1 million RN jobs in 2020. The researchers assert that the aging U.S. population and growing demand for health services—the same factors that contribute to the growing need for geriatricians—are responsible for the shortage, and opine that it "will reach epic proportions in years when RN services are in highest demand."

Industry observers believe other factors have contributed to the shortage including expanding opportunities for women to pursue other careers, a sicker population of hospitalized patients requiring more labor-intensive care, and the public perception that nursing is a thankless, unglamorous job that requires grueling physical labor, long hours, and low pay. In "The Best Jobs of 2012" (*U.S. News & World Report*, February 2, 2012), Jada A. Graves ranks nursing as number one and explains that nursing salaries range from $44,190 to $95,130. Observers also note that the public, particularly high school students who are considering careers in health care, are unaware of the many new

TABLE 2.6

Visits to physician offices, by selected characteristics, selected years 1980–2009

Type of primary care generalist physician[a] — Percent of all physician office visits

Age, sex, and race	All primary care generalists				General and family practice				Internal medicine				Obstetrics and gynecology				Pediatrics				Specialty care physicians			
	1980	1990	2000	2009	1980	1990	2000	2009	1980	1990	2000	2009	1980	1990	2000	2009	1980	1990	2000	2009	1980	1990	2000	2009
Age																								
Total	**66.2**	**63.6**	**58.9**	**55.9**	**33.5**	**29.9**	**24.1**	**23.1**	**12.1**	**13.8**	**15.3**	**14.8**	**9.6**	**8.7**	**7.8**	**7.0**	**10.9**	**11.2**	**11.7**	**11.1**	**33.8**	**36.4**	**41.1**	**44.1**
Under 18 years	77.8	79.5	79.7	78.8	26.1	26.5	19.9	16.3	2.0	2.9	*	*	1.3	1.2	1.1	0.8	48.5	48.9	57.3	60.5	22.2	20.5	20.3	21.2
18–44 years	65.3	65.2	62.1	61.5	34.3	31.9	28.2	29.7	8.6	11.8	12.7	11.0	21.7	20.8	20.4	19.8	0.7	0.7	0.9	1.1	34.7	34.8	37.9	38.5
45–64 years	60.2	55.5	51.2	48.6	36.3	32.1	26.4	25.5	19.5	18.6	20.1	18.0	4.2	4.6	4.5	4.9	*	*	*	*	39.8	44.5	48.8	51.4
45–54 years	60.2	55.6	52.3	50.9	37.4	32.0	27.8	27.5	17.1	17.1	18.7	17.1	5.6	6.3	5.6	6.0	*	*	*	*	39.8	44.4	47.7	49.1
55–64 years	60.2	55.5	49.9	46.4	35.4	32.1	24.7	23.5	21.8	20.0	21.7	19.0	2.9	3.1	3.3	3.8	*	*	*	*	39.8	44.5	50.1	53.6
65 years and over	61.6	52.6	46.5	43.9	37.5	28.1	20.2	18.8	22.7	23.3	24.5	23.5	1.4	1.1	1.5	1.5	*	*	*	*	38.4	47.4	53.5	56.1
65–74 years	61.2	52.7	46.6	41.9	37.4	28.1	19.7	19.9	22.1	23.0	24.5	20.0	1.7	1.6	2.0	1.8	*	*	*	*	38.8	47.3	53.4	58.1
75 years and over	62.3	52.4	46.4	45.9	37.6	28.0	20.8	17.7	23.5	23.7	24.5	26.9	1.0	0.6	1.0	1.1	*	*	*	*	37.7	47.6	53.6	54.1
Sex and age																								
Male:																								
Under 18 years	77.3	78.1	77.7	77.6	25.6	24.1	18.3	15.2	2.0	3.0	*	*	—	—	—	—	49.4	50.7	58.0	61.2	22.7	21.9	22.3	22.4
18–44 years	50.8	51.8	51.5	52.4	38.0	35.9	34.2	36.6	11.5	15.0	14.4	14.1	—	—	—	—	1.0	0.7	1.7	1.8	49.2	48.2	48.5	47.6
45–64 years	55.6	50.6	49.4	45.2	34.4	31.0	28.7	26.4	20.5	19.2	19.8	18.7	—	—	—	—	*	*	*	*	44.4	49.4	50.6	54.8
65 years and over	58.2	51.2	43.1	38.6	35.6	27.7	19.3	18.3	22.3	23.3	23.8	20.1	—	—	—	—	*	*	*	*	41.8	48.8	56.9	61.4
Female:																								
Under 18 years	78.5	81.1	82.0	80.2	26.6	29.1	21.7	17.6	2.0	2.8	*	*	2.5	2.3	2.1	1.7	47.4	46.9	56.5	59.8	21.5	18.9	18.0	19.8
18–44 years	72.1	71.3	67.2	65.6	32.5	30.0	25.3	26.6	7.3	10.3	11.9	9.6	31.7	30.4	29.6	28.7	0.6	0.7	*	*	27.9	28.7	32.8	34.4
45–64 years	63.4	58.8	52.5	51.1	37.7	32.8	24.9	24.9	18.9	18.2	20.2	17.6	6.7	7.7	7.3	8.4	*	*	*	*	36.6	41.2	47.5	48.9
65 years and over	63.9	53.5	48.9	47.8	38.7	28.3	20.9	19.2	22.9	23.3	25.0	26.0	2.1	1.8	2.6	2.5	*	*	*	*	36.1	46.5	51.1	52.2
Race and age[b]																								
White:																								
Under 18 years	77.6	79.2	78.5	78.1	26.4	27.1	21.2	16.3	2.0	2.3	*	*	1.1	1.0	1.2	0.7	48.2	48.8	54.7	60.1	22.4	20.8	21.5	21.9
18–44 years	64.8	64.4	61.4	60.4	34.5	31.9	29.2	30.3	8.6	10.6	11.0	10.1	21.0	21.1	20.4	18.8	0.7	0.7	0.8	1.2	35.2	35.6	38.6	39.6
45–64 years	59.6	54.2	49.3	47.6	36.0	31.5	27.3	25.9	19.2	17.6	17.1	17.0	4.1	4.8	4.7	4.5	*	*	*	*	40.4	45.8	50.7	52.4
65 years and over	61.4	51.9	45.1	43.2	36.6	27.5	20.3	18.7	23.3	23.1	23.0	22.9	1.4	1.2	1.5	1.4	*	*	*	*	38.6	48.1	54.9	56.8
Black or African American:																								
Under 18 years	79.9	85.5	87.3	80.8	23.7	20.2	*	15.5	2.2	9.8	*	*	2.8	3.4	*	*	51.2	52.1	75.0	62.7	20.1	14.5	12.7	19.2
18–44 years	68.5	68.3	65.0	64.4	31.7	31.9	23.3	26.6	9.0	18.1	20.9	15.2	27.1	17.9	20.7	22.1	*	*	*	*	31.5	31.7	35.0	35.6
45–64 years	66.1	61.6	61.7	50.0	38.6	31.2	23.3	23.4	22.6	26.9	35.9	21.4	4.8	3.5	2.4	5.1	*	*	*	*	33.9	38.4	38.3	50.0
65 years and over	64.6	58.6	52.8	45.7	49.0	28.9	18.5	15.8	14.2	28.7	33.4	28.6	*	*	*	*	*	*	*	*	35.4	41.4	47.2	54.3

TABLE 2.6

Visits to physician offices, by selected characteristics, selected years 1980–2009 [CONTINUED]

*Estimates are considered unreliable.
—Category not applicable.

[a]Type of physician is based on physician's self-designated primary area of practice. Primary care generalist physicians are defined as practitioners in the fields of general and family practice, general internal medicine, general obstetrics and gynecology, and general pediatrics and exclude primary care specialists. Primary care generalists in general and family practice exclude primary care specialties, such as sports medicine and geriatrics. Primary care internal medicine physicians exclude internal medicine specialists, such as allergists, cardiologists, and endocrinologists. Primary care obstetrics and gynecology physicians exclude obstetrics and gynecology specialties, such as gynecological oncology, maternal and fetal medicine, obstetrics and gynecology critical care medicine, and reproductive endocrinology. Primary care pediatricians exclude pediatric specialists, such as adolescent medicine specialists, neonatologists, pediatric allergists, and pediatric cardiologists.

[b]Estimates by racial group should be used with caution because information on race was collected from medical records. In 2009, race data were missing and imputed for 24% of visits. Information on the race imputation process used in each data year is available in the public use file documentation. Starting with 1999 data, the instruction for the race item on the patient record form was changed so that more than one race could be recorded. In previous years only one racial category could be checked. Estimates for racial groups presented in this table are for visits where only one race was recorded. Because of the small number of responses with more than one racial group checked, estimates for visits with multiple races checked are unreliable and are not presented.

Notes: This table presents data on visits to physician offices and excludes visits to other sites, such as hospital outpatient and emergency departments. In 1980, the survey excluded Alaska and Hawaii. Data for all other years include all 50 states and the District of Columbia. Visits with specialty of physician unknown are excluded. Starting with *Health, United States, 2005*, data for 2001 and later years for physician offices use a revised weighting scheme. Data for additional years are available.

SOURCE: "Table 97. Visits to Primary Care Generalist and Specialist Physicians, by Selected Characteristics and Type of Physician: United States, Selected Years 1980–2009," in *Health, United States, 2011: With Special Feature on Socioeconomic Status and Health*, U.S. Department of Health and Human Services, Centers for Disease Control and Prevention, National Center for Health Statistics, May 2012, http://www.cdc.gov/nchs/data/hus/hus11.pdf (accessed June 14, 2012)

FIGURE 2.3

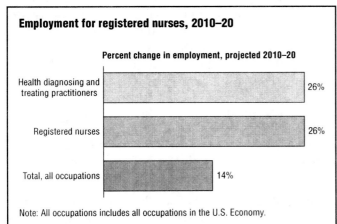

Employment for registered nurses, 2010–20

Percent change in employment, projected 2010–20

- Health diagnosing and treating practitioners — 26%
- Registered nurses — 26%
- Total, all occupations — 14%

Note: All occupations includes all occupations in the U.S. Economy.

SOURCE: "Registered Nurses: Percent Change in Employment, Projected 2010–2020," in *Occupational Outlook Handbook, 2012–13 Edition: Registered Nurses*, Bureau of Labor Statistics, U.S. Department of Labor, March 29, 2012, http://www.bls.gov/ooh/healthcare/print/registered-nurses.htm (accessed June 14, 2012)

FIGURE 2.4

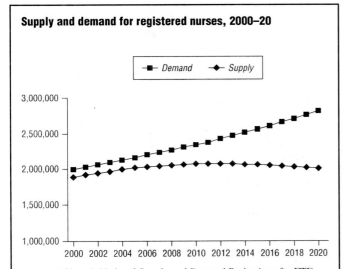

Supply and demand for registered nurses, 2000–20

- Demand
- Supply

SOURCE: "Chart 1. National Supply and Demand Projections for FTE Registered Nurses: 2000 to 2020," in *Projected Supply, Demand, and Shortages of Registered Nurses: 2000–2020*, U.S. Department of Health and Human Services, Health Resources and Services Administration, Bureau of Health Professions, National Center for Health Workforce Analysis, July 2002, http://www.ahcancal.org/research_data/staffing/Documents/Registered_Nurse_Supply_Demand.pdf (accessed June 14, 2012)

opportunities in nursing, such as advanced practice nursing, which offers additional independence and increased earning potential, and the technology-driven field of applied informatics (computer management of information).

ADVANCED PRACTICE NURSES AND PHYSICIAN ASSISTANTS

Much of the preventive medical care and treatment usually delivered by physicians may also be provided by midlevel practitioners—health professionals with less formal education and training than physicians. Advanced practice nurses make up a group that includes certified nurse midwives, nurse practitioners (NPs; RNs with advanced academic and clinical experience), and clinical nurse specialists (RNs with advanced nursing degrees who specialize in areas such as mental health, gerontology, cardiac or cancer care, or community or neonatal health). Physician assistants (PAs) are midlevel practitioners who work under the auspices, supervision, or direction of physicians. They conduct physical examinations, order and interpret laboratory and radiological studies, and prescribe medication. They even perform procedures (e.g., flexible sigmoidoscopy, biopsy, suturing, casting, and administering anesthesia) that were once performed exclusively by physicians.

The origins of each profession are key to understanding the differences between them. Nursing has the longer history, and nurses are recognized members of the health care team. For this reason, NPs were easily integrated into many practice settings.

PA is the newer of the two disciplines. PAs have been practicing in the United States since the early 1970s. The career originated as civilian employment for returning Vietnam War (1954–1975) veterans who had worked as medics. The veterans needed immediate employment and few had the educational prerequisites, time, or resources to pursue the training necessary to become physicians. At the same time, the United States was projecting a dire shortage of primary care physicians, especially in rural and inner-city practices. The use of NPs and PAs was seen as an ideal rapid response to the demand for additional medical services. They could be deployed quickly to serve remote communities or underserved populations for a fraction of the costs associated with physicians.

The numbers of NPs and PAs have increased dramatically since the beginning of the 1990s. Kevin M. Stange and Deborah A. Sampson find in *Nurse Practitioners and Physician Assistants in the United States: Current Patterns of Distribution and Recent Trends* (September 2010, http://thefutureofnursing.org/) that between 1995 and 2009 the number of NPs and PAs per primary care physician had more than doubled. As of 2010 the combined midlevel practitioner (NP-PA) workforce was already three-quarters the size of the physician workforce. The HRSA states in *The Registered Nurse Population: Findings from the 2008 National Sample Survey of Registered Nurses* (September 2010, http://bhpr.hrsa.gov/healthworkforce/rnsurveys/rnsurveyfinal.pdf) that in 2008 there were 250,527 advanced practice nurses—158,348 NPs, 59,242 clinical nurse specialists, 34,821 certified RN anesthetists, and 18,492 certified nurse midwives. According to the American Academy of Physician Assistants (AAPA), in "Quick Facts" (http://www.aapa.org/the_pa_profession/quick_facts/resources/item.aspx?id=3848), as of 2010 there were 84,066 nationally certified PAs.

Training, Certification, and Practice

Advanced practice nurses usually have considerable clinical nursing experience before completing certificate or master's degree NP programs. Key components of NP programs are instruction in nursing theory and practice and a period of direct supervision by a physician or NP. The American Academy of Nurse Practitioners explains in "State Practice Environment" (2012, http://www.aanp.org/ legislation-regulation/state-practice-environment) that NPs are a scope of practice that varies from state to state. For example, some states require state certification as well as national certification and some states permit independent practice for NPs (not requiring any physician involvement).

The Commission on Accreditation of Allied Health Education Programs accredits PA training programs. In "Becoming a PA" (2012, http://www.aapa.org/your _pa_career/becoming_a_pa.aspx), the AAPA notes that most students have an undergraduate degree and health care experience before they enter a PA training program, which lasts about 27 months. Graduates sit for a national certifying examination and, once certified, must earn 100 hours of continuing medical education every two years and pass a recertification exam every six years. PAs must also obtain a state license.

PA practice is always delegated by the physician and conducted with physician supervision. The extent and nature of physician supervision varies from state to state. For example, Connecticut permits a physician to supervise up to six PAs, whereas California limits a supervising physician to two. Even though PAs work interdependently with physicians, supervision is not necessarily direct and onsite; some PAs working in remote communities are supervised primarily by telephone.

Merion Matters reports in "Advances for NPs & PAs" (August 22, 2012, http://nurse-practitioners-and -physician-assistants.advanceweb.com/) that in 2011 the average annual income of PAs who were employed full time was $94,870 and the average NP working full time earned $90,583.

Distinctions between Midlevel Practitioners Blurring

Stacy Kess observes in "Nurse Practitioner vs. Physician Assistant" (*Washington Post*, January 9, 2011) that even though their training may be different, in terms of how patients view them and their day-to-day job responsibilities, NPs and PAs are essentially interchangeable. Both types of practitioners diagnose and treat illness, take medical histories, and perform physical examinations. They order diagnostic tests, prescribe medication, and assist in operating rooms and emergency departments.

In "Time to Expand NP Scope of Practice" (*Synapse*, May 3, 2012), Leah Sanchez calls for a standardized and expanded scope of practice for NPs. Sanchez offers examples of the variation in scope of practice— 22 states and the District of Columbia permit NPs to diagnose and treat patients without involvement of a physician, and 13 of those states allow NPs to prescribe without physician supervision. In Oregon an NP can prescribe narcotics and other drugs that are classified as controlled substances, whereas in Alabama an NP is not permitted to prescribe controlled substances. Sanchez asserts that "the current healthcare system needs an overhaul, starting with increasing access to care by allowing all NPs to work to the fullest extent of their advanced training."

Even though the roles of NPs have been gradually expanding over time, the Patient Protection and Affordable Care Act (PPACA) may accelerate broadening the responsibilities of NPs, because it will extend health insurance coverage to millions of previously uninsured Americans, which will create demand for services that cannot be met by physicians alone.

Several provisions of the PPACA expand the role of nurses by encouraging training and increasing compensation. These include:

- $50 million to clinics managed by nurses that provide care to low-income patients

- $50 million annually between 2012 and 2015 for hospitals to train nurses with advanced degrees to care for Medicare patients

- 10% bonuses from Medicare between 2011 and 2016 to primary care providers, including NPs, who work in physician-shortage areas

- An increase in Medicare reimbursement for certified nurse midwives, giving them the same compensation as physicians

DENTISTS

Dentists diagnose and treat problems of the teeth, gums, and mouth, take x-rays, apply protective plastic sealant to children's teeth, fill cavities, straighten teeth, and treat gum disease. The BLS (March 27, 2012, http:// www.bls.gov/ooh/Healthcare/Dentists.htm) reports that dentists held about 155,700 jobs in 2012.

Fluoridation of community water supplies and improved dental hygiene have dramatically improved the dental health of Americans. Dental caries (cavities) among all age groups have declined significantly. As a result, many dental services are shifting focus from young people to adults. In the 21st century many adults are choosing to have orthodontic services, such as straightening their teeth. In addition, the growing older adult population generally requires more complex dental procedures, such as endodontic (root canal) services, bridges, and dentures.

Many dentists own solo dental practices, where only one dentist operates in each office. Others are partners in a practice with other general dentists or dental specialists, and most manage a small staff, which may include dental hygienists and assistants. The BLS reports most dentists work full time and many work evenings and weekends to accommodate their patients.

Dental Specialists

In "Specialty Definitions" (2012, http://www.ada.org/495.aspx), the American Dental Association (ADA) identifies nine recognized specialties. Orthodontists, who straighten teeth, make up the largest group of specialists. The next largest group, oral and maxillofacial surgeons, operates on the mouth and jaw. The balance of the specialists concentrates in pediatric dentistry (dentistry for children), periodontics (treating the gums), prosthodontics (making dentures and artificial teeth), endodontics (root canals), public health dentistry (community dental health), and oral pathology (diseases of the mouth).

Training to Become a Dentist

Entry into dental schools requires two to four years of college-level predental education—most dental students have earned excellent grades and have at least a bachelor's degree when they enter dental school. Dentists should have good visual memory, excellent judgment about space and shape, a high degree of manual dexterity, and scientific ability. Development and maintenance of a successful private practice requires business acumen, the ability to manage and organize people and materials, and strong interpersonal skills.

Dental schools require applicants to take the Dental Admissions Test (DAT). During the admission process, schools consider scores earned on the DAT, applicants' grade-point averages, and information gleaned from recommendations and interviews. Dental school usually lasts four academic years. Students begin by studying the basic sciences, including anatomy, microbiology, biochemistry, and physiology. During the last two years students receive practical experience by treating patients, usually in dental clinics that are supervised by licensed dentists.

Visiting a Dentist

In 2010, 64.7% of Americans aged two years and older had visited a dentist at least once in the past year. (See Table 2.7.) Children aged two to 17 years (78.9%) were more likely to have visited a dentist than any other age group, and women aged 65 years and older (58.9%) were somewhat more likely to see a dentist than were men (56.2%). Among adults aged 18 to 64 years, the proportion of non-Hispanic whites (65.4%) visiting a dentist was considerably higher than the proportions of

non-Hispanic African-Americans (53.1%) and Hispanics (48.5%). People who were poor or near poor were much less likely to visit a dentist annually than those who were not poor. For example, among adults aged 18 to 64 years, 41% of people who were 100% below the poverty level had visited a dentist in the past year, compared with 77.5% of people who were 400% or more above the poverty level.

SEVERE SHORTAGES OF DENTISTS IN SOME AREAS. The United States boasts the highest concentration of dentists of any country in the world. Nonetheless, health care planners caution that the ranks of dentists will begin to decline in 2014, according to Margot Sanger-Katz, in "Nothing to Smile About" (*National Journal*, May 7, 2012). Sanger-Katz observes that the United States faces a shortage of dentists and that poor, rural regions are disproportionately affected. Large swaths of the country have few dentists. For example, in 2008 Georgia had just 4.4 dentists per 10,000 civilian population, compared with the District of Columbia, which boasted 10.7 dentists per 10,000 population. (See Table 2.8.)

ALLIED HEALTH CARE PROVIDERS

Many health care services are provided by an interdisciplinary team of health professionals. The complete health care team may include physicians, nurses, midlevel practitioners, and dentists; physical and occupational therapists; audiologists and speech-language pathologists; licensed practical nurses, nurses' aides, and home health aides; and pharmacists, optometrists, podiatrists, dental hygienists, social workers, registered dieticians, and others. Table 2.9 describes some of these allied health professions. Specific health care teams are assembled to meet the varying needs of patients. For example, the team involved in stroke rehabilitation might include a physician, a nurse, a speech-language pathologist, a social worker, and physical and occupational therapists.

Table 2.10 shows the growth in numbers of health care practitioners, allied health professionals, and health care support occupations such as assistants, aides, and massage therapists as well as their mean hourly wages during the first decade of the 21st century. For example, occupational therapists saw a 3% annual increase in wages between 2001 and 2010, whereas massage therapists realized a 10.8% increase during the same period. The only decreases were among dietetic technicians, dispensing opticians, recreational therapists, respiratory therapy technicians, medical transcriptionists, occupational therapy aides, and pharmacy aides.

Physical and Occupational Therapists

Physical therapists (PTs) are licensed practitioners who work with patients to preserve and restore function, improve capabilities and mobility, and regain independence

TABLE 2.7

Dental visits in the past year by selected characteristics, 1997–2010

Characteristic	2 years and over			2–17 years			18–64 years			65 years and over[a]		
	1997	2009	2010	1997	2009	2010	1997	2009	2010	1997	2009	2010
	Percent of persons with a dental visit in the past year[b]											
Total[c]	**65.1**	**65.4**	**64.7**	**72.7**	**78.4**	**78.9**	**64.1**	**62.0**	**61.1**	**54.8**	**59.6**	**57.7**
Sex												
Male	62.9	62.6	61.7	72.3	77.6	78.3	60.4	57.9	56.8	55.4	58.4	56.2
Female	67.1	68.0	67.5	73.0	79.3	79.6	67.7	65.9	65.4	54.4	60.5	58.9
Race[d]												
White only	66.4	66.3	65.6	74.0	79.1	79.2	65.7	63.1	62.4	56.8	61.8	59.3
Black or African American only	58.9	59.9	58.8	68.8	76.7	79.0	57.0	55.9	53.1	35.4	38.1	40.6
American Indian or Alaska Native only	55.1	53.1	57.4	66.8	68.5	73.2	49.9	47.3	49.8	*	44.2	72.2
Asian only	62.5	67.6	66.5	69.9	76.2	74.8	60.3	65.8	64.6	53.9	62.1	61.9
Native Hawaiian or other Pacific Islander only	—	*	*	—	*	*	—	*	*	—	*	*
2 or more races	—	63.5	65.2	—	80.0	77.9	—	50.0	54.7	—	58.5	48.1
Black or African American; white	—	67.1	72.5	—	78.7	78.4	—	45.3	62.1	—	*	*
American Indian or Alaska Native; white	—	56.0	54.7	—	76.5	70.0	—	47.9	49.0	—	58.3	54.5
Hispanic origin and race[d]												
Hispanic or Latino	54.0	56.0	56.5	61.0	73.0	74.8	50.8	48.1	48.5	47.8	47.9	42.1
Not Hispanic or Latino	66.4	67.1	66.2	74.7	80.0	80.1	65.7	64.5	63.4	55.2	60.5	59.0
White only	68.0	68.6	67.6	76.4	81.4	80.9	67.5	66.3	65.4	57.2	62.8	60.9
Black or African American only	58.8	59.8	58.7	68.8	76.7	79.2	56.9	55.9	53.1	35.3	38.4	40.5
Percent of poverty level[e]												
Below 100%	50.5	51.7	50.6	62.0	71.7	73.2	46.9	42.7	41.0	31.5	39.0	32.8
100%–199%	50.8	52.8	51.6	62.5	75.2	73.4	48.3	45.3	44.1	40.8	42.3	43.8
200%–399%	66.2	63.3	63.5	76.1	77.1	79.0	63.4	59.1	59.6	60.7	60.9	57.9
400% or more	78.9	79.5	79.3	85.7	87.8	88.0	77.7	77.9	77.5	74.7	77.5	77.2
Hispanic origin and race and percent of poverty level[d, e]												
Hispanic or Latino:												
Below 100%	45.7	51.7	50.8	55.9	71.7	74.3	39.2	37.6	34.7	33.6	42.7	32.4
100%–199%	47.2	51.7	50.8	53.8	72.4	71.1	43.5	41.4	40.2	47.9	37.5	39.5
200%–399%	61.2	57.1	59.1	70.5	73.8	76.5	57.5	51.3	54.1	57.0	54.4	46.0
400% or more	73.0	69.2	73.3	82.4	76.9	84.2	70.8	67.1	71.6	64.9	63.5	54.3
Not Hispanic or Latino:												
White only:												
Below 100%	51.7	51.3	49.3	64.4	69.6	69.1	50.6	46.3	44.4	32.0	42.2	36.4
100%–199%	52.4	52.7	52.7	66.1	76.2	75.3	50.4	46.4	47.2	42.2	44.4	45.4
200%–399%	67.5	64.7	64.7	77.1	79.1	79.6	65.0	60.7	61.4	61.9	62.4	59.8
400% or more	79.7	81.1	79.8	86.8	89.9	88.6	78.5	79.4	77.9	75.5	79.4	78.8
Black or African American only:												
Below 100%	52.8	52.6	52.0	66.1	74.0	78.0	46.2	42.1	39.7	27.7	28.8	20.9
100%–199%	48.7	53.0	50.0	61.2	79.2	75.9	46.3	45.1	41.5	26.9	26.9	33.6
200%–399%	63.3	61.6	61.2	75.0	74.4	81.2	60.7	59.5	57.2	41.5	46.7	45.3
400% or more	74.6	74.3	77.2	81.8	85.0	87.2	73.4	74.1	75.9	66.1	55.3	69.8

Notes: In 1997 the National Health Interview Survey questionnaire was redesigned.

*Estimates are considered unreliable.

—Data not available

[a]Based on the 1997–2010 National Health Interview Surveys, about 24%–30% of persons 65 years and over were edentulous (having lost all their natural teeth). In 1997–2010, about 69%–73% of older dentate persons, compared with 17%–21% of older edentate persons, had a dental visit in the past year.

[b]Respondents were asked "About how long has it been since you last saw or talked to a dentist?"

[c]Includes all other races not shown separately and unknown disability status.

[d]The race groups, white, black, American Indian or Alaska Native, Asian, Native Hawaiian or Other Pacific Islander, and 2 or more races, include persons of Hispanic and non-Hispanic origin. Persons of Hispanic origin may be of any race. Starting with 1999 data, race-specific estimates are tabulated according to the 1997 *Revisions to the Standards for the Classification of Federal Data on Race and Ethnicity* and are not strictly comparable with estimates for earlier years. The five single-race categories plus multiple-race categories shown in the table conform to the 1997 Standards. Starting with 1999 data, race-specific estimates are for persons who reported only one racial group; the category 2 or more races includes persons who reported more than one racial group. Prior to 1999, data were tabulated according to the 1977 Standards with four racial groups, and the Asian only category included Native Hawaiian or Other Pacific Islander. Estimates for single-race categories prior to 1999 included persons who reported one race or, if they reported more than one race, identified one race as best representing their race. Starting with 2003 data, race responses of other race and unspecified multiple race were treated as missing, and then race was imputed if these were the only race responses. Almost all persons with a race response of other race were of Hispanic origin.

[e]Percent of poverty level is based on family income and family size and composition using U.S. Census Bureau poverty thresholds. Missing family income data were imputed for 1997 and beyond.

[f]Any basic actions difficulty or complex activity limitation is defined as having one or more of the following limitations or difficulties: movement difficulty, emotional difficulty, sensory (seeing or hearing) difficulty, cognitive difficulty, self-care (activities of daily living or instrumental activities of daily living) limitation, social limitation, or work limitation. Starting with 2007 data, the hearing question, a component of the basic actions difficulty measure, was revised. Consequently, data prior to 2007 are not comparable with data for 2007 and beyond.

SOURCE: Adapted from "Table 98. Dental Visits in the Past Year, by Selected Characteristics: United States, Selected Years 1997–2010," in *Health, United States, 2011: With Special Feature on Socioeconomic Status and Health*, U.S. Department of Health and Human Services, Centers for Disease Control and Prevention, National Center for Health Statistics, May 2012, http://www.cdc.gov/nchs/data/hus/hus11.pdf (accessed June 14, 2012)

TABLE 2.8

Active dentists by state, selected years 1993–2008

State	1993	2000	2006	2007	2008	1993	2000	2006	2007	2008
			Number of dentists				Number of dentists per 10,000 civilian population			
United States	**155,087**	**166,383**	**179,594**	**181,725**	**181,774**	**6.1**	**6.1**	**6.0**	**6.0**	**6.0**
Alabama	1,779	1,912	2,032	2,032	2,032	4.3	4.3	4.4	4.4	4.4
Alaska	421	467	513	519	505	7.5	7.5	7.7	7.6	7.4
Arizona	2,032	2,322	3,107	3,225	3,302	5.3	4.5	5.0	5.1	5.1
Arkansas	1,001	1,080	1,146	1,162	1,125	4.2	4.0	4.1	4.1	3.9
California	20,909	22,963	26,887	27,654	27,922	6.8	6.8	7.4	7.6	7.6
Colorado	2,503	2,818	3,139	3,181	3,212	7.3	6.6	6.6	6.5	6.5
Connecticut	2,587	2,636	2,694	2,710	2,610	7.9	7.7	7.7	7.7	7.5
Delaware	331	357	395	403	403	4.8	4.6	4.6	4.7	4.6
District of Columbia	810	728	609	614	634	13.9	12.7	10.5	10.4	10.7
Florida	7,110	8,170	9,450	9,640	9,741	5.3	5.1	5.2	5.3	5.3
Georgia	3,251	3,611	4,167	4,295	4,260	4.9	4.4	4.5	4.5	4.4
Hawaii	976	992	1,046	1,043	1,039	8.8	8.2	8.1	8.1	8.1
Idaho	573	678	834	863	890	5.4	5.2	5.7	5.8	5.8
Illinois	7,978	8,205	8,249	8,268	8,192	6.9	6.6	6.4	6.4	6.3
Indiana	2,716	2,867	3,013	3,035	3,009	4.8	4.7	4.8	4.8	4.7
Iowa	1,545	1,564	1,583	1,610	1,600	5.5	5.3	5.3	5.4	5.3
Kansas	1,316	1,329	1,417	1,437	1,413	5.3	4.9	5.1	5.2	5.0
Kentucky	2,129	2,258	2,340	2,356	2,388	5.7	5.6	5.6	5.6	5.6
Louisiana	2,029	2,086	2,102	2,118	2,066	4.8	4.7	4.9	4.9	4.7
Maine	592	601	650	662	657	4.8	4.7	4.9	5.0	5.0
Maryland	3,753	3,986	4,132	4,212	4,138	7.7	7.5	7.4	7.5	7.3
Massachusetts	4,652	5,137	5,299	5,314	5,442	7.8	8.1	8.2	8.2	8.4
Michigan	5,884	5,913	6,141	6,126	6,060	6.2	5.9	6.1	6.1	6.1
Minnesota	2,913	2,960	3,137	3,196	3,174	6.5	6.0	6.1	6.1	6.1
Mississippi	1,040	1,115	1,173	1,190	1,160	4.0	3.9	4.0	4.1	3.9
Missouri	2,773	2,680	2,803	2,813	2,803	5.4	4.8	4.8	4.8	4.7
Montana	476	485	525	549	548	5.8	5.4	5.6	5.7	5.7
Nebraska	1,054	1,087	1,116	1,111	1,105	6.6	6.4	6.3	6.3	6.2
Nevada	570	763	1,185	1,285	1,330	4.3	3.8	4.7	5.0	5.1
New Hampshire	642	707	821	830	817	5.8	5.7	6.2	6.3	6.2
New Jersey	6,144	6,607	7,113	7,042	6,925	7.9	7.9	8.2	8.1	8.0
New Mexico	719	809	871	907	916	4.6	4.4	4.5	4.6	4.6
New York	14,395	15,159	15,110	15,184	14,980	8.0	8.0	7.8	7.9	7.7
North Carolina	2,968	3,394	4,031	4,108	4,183	4.4	4.2	4.6	4.5	4.5
North Dakota	315	300	323	326	329	5.0	4.7	5.1	5.1	5.1
Ohio	5,981	6,108	6,081	6,063	6,029	5.4	5.4	5.3	5.3	5.2
Oklahoma	1,584	1,683	1,774	1,804	1,805	5.0	4.9	5.0	5.0	5.0
Oregon	2,034	2,273	2,506	2,551	2,574	6.8	6.6	6.8	6.8	6.8
Pennsylvania	7,915	8,031	7,907	7,747	7,756	6.6	6.5	6.4	6.2	6.2
Rhode Island	581	589	596	569	573	5.8	5.6	5.6	5.4	5.5
South Carolina	1,601	1,803	2,006	2,026	2,065	4.5	4.5	4.6	4.6	4.6
South Dakota	347	359	387	397	406	4.9	4.8	4.9	5.0	5.0
Tennessee	2,748	2,993	3,031	3,076	3,015	5.5	5.3	5.0	5.0	4.9
Texas	8,860	9,873	10,758	10,981	10,936	5.1	4.7	4.6	4.6	4.5
Utah	1,162	1,398	1,671	1,713	1,743	6.4	6.3	6.6	6.5	6.4
Vermont	323	353	360	361	360	5.7	5.8	5.8	5.8	5.8
Virginia	3,686	4,036	4,489	4,563	4,640	5.9	5.7	5.9	5.9	6.0
Washington	3,271	3,860	4,510	4,528	4,579	6.4	6.5	7.1	7.0	7.0
West Virginia	816	828	854	847	844	4.5	4.6	4.7	4.7	4.7
Wisconsin	3,054	3,119	3,199	3,186	3,208	6.1	5.8	5.8	5.7	5.7
Wyoming	235	267	281	269	266	5.1	5.4	5.5	5.1	5.0

Notes: The data include professionally active dentists only. Professionally active dentist occupation categories include active practitioners (full- or part-time); dental school faculty or staff; armed forces dentists; government-employed dentists at the federal, state, or local levels; graduate students/interns and residents; and other health or dental organization staff members. U.S. totals include dentists with unknown state of practice not shown separately.

SOURCE: "Table 112. Active Dentists, by State: United States, Selected Years 1993–2008," in *Health, United States, 2011: With Special Feature on Socioeconomic Status and Health*, U.S. Department of Health and Human Services, Centers for Disease Control and Prevention, National Center for Health Statistics, May 2012, http://www.cdc.gov/nchs/data/hus/hus11.pdf (accessed June 14, 2012). Data from the American Dental Association and American Medical Association.

following an illness or injury. They also aim to prevent or limit disability and slow the progress of debilitating diseases. Treatment involves exercise to improve range of motion, balance, coordination, flexibility, strength, and endurance. PTs may also use electrical stimulation to promote healing, hot and cold packs to relieve pain and inflammation (swelling), and therapeutic massage.

According to the BLS (April 6, 2012, http://www.bls.gov/ooh/Healthcare/Physical-therapists.htm), PTs worked at 198,600 jobs in 2010, but some were part-time jobs and some PTs had two or more jobs at the same time. Approximately 65% of practicing PTs worked in hospitals and physicians' offices; the remaining PTs were employed in outpatient rehabilitation

TABLE 2.9

Allied health care providers

Dental hygienists provide services for maintaining oral health. Their primary duty is to clean teeth.

Emergency medical technicians (EMTs) provide immediate care to critically ill or injured people in emergency situations.

Home health aides provide nursing, household, and personal care services to patients who are homebound or disabled.

Licensed practical nurse (LPNs) are trained and licensed to provide basic nursing care under the supervision of registered nurses and doctors.

Medical records personnel analyze patient records and keep them up-to-date, complete, accurate, and confidential.

Medical technologists perform laboratory tests to help diagnose diseases and to aid in identifying their causes and extent.

Nurses' aides, orderlies, and attendants help nurses in hospitals, nursing homes, and other facilities.

Occupational therapists help disabled persons adapt to their disabilities. This may include helping a patient relearn basic living skills or modifying the environment.

Optometrists measure vision for corrective lenses and prescribe glasses.

Pharmacists are trained and licensed to make up and dispense drugs in accordance with a physician's prescription.

Physician assistants (PAs) work under a doctor's supervision. Their duties include performing routine physical exams, prescribing certain drugs, and providing medical counseling.

Physical therapists work with disabled patients to help restore function, strength, and mobility. PTs use exercise, heat, cold, water, and electricity to relieve pain and restore function.

Podiatrists diagnose and treat diseases, injuries, and abnormalities of the feet. They may use drugs and surgery to treat foot problems.

Psychologists are trained in human behavior and provide counseling and testing services related to mental health.

Radiation technicians take and develop x-ray photographs for medical purposes.

Registered dietitians (RDs) are licensed to use dietary principles to maintain health and treat disease.

Respiratory therapists treat breathing problems under a doctor's supervision and help in respiratory rehabilitation.

Social workers help patients to handle social problems such as finances, housing, and social and family problems that arise out of illness or disability.

Speech pathologists diagnose and treat disorders of speech and communication.

SOURCE: "Allied Health Care Providers," U.S. Department of Commerce, Washington, DC

clinics, nursing homes, and home health agencies. Even though most work in rehabilitation, PTs may specialize in areas such as sports medicine, pediatrics, or neurology. PTs often work as members of a health care team and may supervise PT assistants or aides. The BLS notes that the median annual wages for PTs were $76,310 in 2010.

The BLS indicates that PTs are required to earn a master's or doctorate degree from an accredited physical therapy program. To practice physical therapy, PTs must obtain state licensure, and even though the requirements vary by state, licensure generally requires graduation from an accredited physical therapy education program and passing a national examination. Many states also require continuing education as a condition of maintaining licensure.

Occupational therapists (OTs) focus on helping people relearn and improve their abilities to perform the "activities of daily living," meaning the tasks they perform during the course of their work and home life. Examples of activities of daily living that OTs help

patients regain are dressing, bathing, and meal preparation. For people with long-term or permanent disabilities, OTs may assist them to find new ways to accomplish their responsibilities on the job, sometimes by using adaptive equipment or by asking employers to accommodate workers with special needs such as people in wheelchairs. OTs use computer programs and simulations to help patients restore fine motor skills and practice reasoning, decision making, and problem solving.

A master's degree or higher in occupational therapy is the minimum educational requirement. The American Occupational Therapy Association states in "FAQ about the Entry-Level Master's and Doctoral Degrees for Occupational Therapist" (August 8, 2011, http://www.aota.org/Students/FAQDegrees.aspx) that "an entry-level degree for occupational therapists is the degree required to enter the profession and to be eligible to sit for the Occupational Therapist Registered…examination administered by the National Board for Certification in Occupational Therapy…. Occupational therapy requires that the entry-level degree be a postbaccalaureate degree." The BLS (June 26, 2012, http://www.bls.gov/ooh/Healthcare/Occupational-therapists.htm) reports that in 2010 OTs filled 108,800 jobs and that their median annual wages were $72,320.

The demand for PTs and OTs is expected to exceed the available supply through 2020, growing by 39% and 33%, respectively, between 2010 and 2020. Besides hospital and rehabilitation center jobs, it is anticipated that PTs and OTs will increasingly be involved in school program efforts to meet the needs of disabled and special education students.

Pharmacists

Pharmacists are involved in many more aspects of patient care than simply compounding and dispensing medication from behind the drugstore counter. According to the American Pharmacists Association, pharmacists provide pharmaceutical care that both improves patient adherence to prescribed drug treatment and reduces the frequency of drug therapy mishaps, which can have serious and even life-threatening consequences.

Studies citing the value of pharmacists in patient care describe pharmacists improving the rates of immunization against disease (pharmacists can provide immunization in all 50 states, the District of Columbia, and Puerto Rico), assisting patients to better control chronic diseases such as asthma and diabetes, reducing the frequency and severity of drug interactions and adverse reactions, and helping patients effectively manage pain and symptoms of disease, especially at the end of life. Pharmacists also offer public health education programs about prescription medication safety, prevention of poisoning, appropriate use of nonprescription (over-the-counter) drugs, and medical self-care.

TABLE 2.10

Health care workers and wages, selected years 2001–10

Occupation title	2001	2004	2008	2010	2001– 2010	2001	2004	2008	2010	2001– 2010
Health care practitioners and technical occupations	Employment[a]				AAPC[b]	Mean hourly wage[c]				AAPC[b]
Audiologists	11,040	9,810	12,480	12,860	1.7	$23.89	$26.47	$31.49	$33.58	3.9
Cardiovascular technologists and technicians	40,990	43,540	48,040	48,720	1.9	17.55	19.09	23.38	24.38	3.7
Dental hygienists	149,880	155,810	173,090	177,520	1.9	27.30	28.58	32.19	33.02	2.1
Diagnostic medical sonographers	32,990	41,280	48,920	53,010	5.4	23.08	25.78	30.12	31.20	3.4
Dietetic technicians	28,940	24,630	24,620	23,890	−2.1	11.23	11.89	13.26	13.86	2.4
Dietitians and nutritionists	43,200	46,530	53,630	53,510	2.4	19.74	21.46	24.75	26.13	3.2
Emergency medical technicians and paramedics	170,690	187,900	207,610	221,760	3.0	12.24	13.30	15.38	16.01	3.0
Licensed practical and licensed vocational nurses	683,790	702,740	730,500	730,290	0.7	15.14	16.75	19.28	19.88	3.1
Nuclear medicine technologists	17,360	17,520	21,200	21,600	2.5	24.65	29.43	32.44	33.20	3.4
Occupational therapists	77,080	83,560	94,800	100,300	3.0	25.10	27.19	32.65	35.28	3.9
Opticians, dispensing	63,120	62,350	59,470	62,200	−0.2	13.49	14.37	16.85	16.73	2.4
Pharmacists	223,630	222,960	266,410	268,030	2.0	35.02	40.56	50.13	52.59	4.6
Pharmacy technicians	207,140	255,290	324,110	333,500	5.4	10.82	11.87	13.70	14.10	3.0
Physical therapists	126,450	142,940	167,300	180,280	4.0	28.43	30.00	35.77	37.50	3.1
Physician assistants	56,200	59,470	71,950	81,420	4.2	30.00	33.07	39.24	41.89	3.8
Psychiatric technicians	59,750	59,010	54,800	72,650	2.2	12.94	13.43	15.48	15.15	1.8
Radiation therapists	13,460	14,470	14,850	16,590	2.4	25.71	29.05	36.28	37.64	4.3
Radiologic technologists and technicians	168,240	177,220	208,570	216,730	2.9	18.68	21.41	25.59	26.80	4.1
Recreational therapists	26,830	23,050	22,510	20,830	−2.8	14.92	16.48	19.20	19.92	3.3
Registered nurses	2,217,990	2,311,970	2,542,760	2,655,020	2.0	23.19	26.06	31.31	32.56	3.8
Respiratory therapists	82,930	91,350	103,870	109,270	3.1	19.17	21.24	25.55	26.54	3.7
Respiratory therapy technicians	28,700	24,190	16,210	13,570	−8.0	16.93	18.00	21.00	22.28	3.1
Speech-language pathologists	83,110	89,260	107,340	112,530	3.4	24.20	26.71	31.80	33.60	3.7
Health care support occupations										
Dental assistants	267,840	264,820	293,090	294,030	1.2	13.29	13.97	15.95	16.41	2.7
Home health aides	560,190	596,330	892,410	982,840	7.3	8.90	9.13	10.31	10.46	2.0
Massage therapists	26,440	32,200	51,250	60,040	10.8	15.93	17.63	19.16	19.12	2.3
Medical assistants	345,930	380,340	475,950	523,260	5.3	11.71	12.21	13.97	14.31	2.5
Medical equipment preparers	33,540	40,380	44,340	47,310	4.4	11.29	12.14	14.08	14.59	3.3
Medical transcriptionists	94,090	92,740	86,200	78,780	−2.2	12.99	14.01	15.84	16.12	2.7
Nursing aides, orderlies, and attendants	1,307,600	1,384,120	1,422,720	1,451,090	1.3	9.54	10.39	11.84	12.09	3.0
Occupational therapy aides	7,560	5,240	7,410	7,180	−0.6	11.70	12.51	14.22	14.95	3.1
Occupational therapy assistants	17,520	20,880	25,610	27,720	5.9	17.39	18.49	23.29	24.66	4.5
Pharmacy aides	58,130	47,720	53,190	49,580	−2.0	9.22	9.52	10.34	10.98	2.2
Physical therapist aides	35,250	41,910	44,410	45,900	3.4	10.45	11.14	11.91	12.02	1.8
Physical therapist assistants	47,810	57,420	61,820	65,960	4.1	17.18	18.14	22.26	23.95	4.2
Psychiatric aides	59,640	54,520	59,050	64,730	1.0	11.42	11.70	13.10	12.84	1.5

[a]Employment is the number of filled positions. This table includes both full-time and part-time wage and salary positions. Estimates do not include business establishments where persons are self-employed, owners and partners in unincorporated firms, household workers, or unpaid family workers and were rounded to the nearest 10.
[b]AAPC is average annual percent change.
[c]The mean hourly wage rate for an occupation is the total wages that all workers in the occupation earn in an hour divided by the total employment of the occupation.
Notes: This table excludes occupations such as dentists, physicians, and chiropractors, which have a large percentage of workers who are self-employed. Challenges in using Occupational Employment Statistics (OES) data as a time series include changes in the occupational, industrial, and geographical classification systems, changes in the way data are collected, changes in the survey reference period, and changes in mean wage estimation methodology, as well as permanent features of the methodology.

SOURCE: "Table 113. Health Care Employment and Wages, by Selected Occupations: United States, Selected Years 2001–2010," in *Health, United States, 2011: With Special Feature on Socioeconomic Status and Health*, U.S. Department of Health and Human Services, Centers for Disease Control and Prevention, National Center for Health Statistics, May 2012, http://www.cdc.gov/nchs/data/hus/hus11.pdf (accessed June 13, 2012)

Pharmacists must obtain a doctoral degree, called a Pharm.D., from an accredited school of pharmacy. Training leading to the Pharm.D. generally takes four years to complete and some Pharm.D. graduates obtain additional training. All states require a license to practice pharmacy and 44 states and the District of Columbia also require the Multistate Pharmacy Jurisprudence Exam, which tests pharmacy law. Some states also require additional exams and all require a stipulated number of hours of experience in a practice setting as a prerequisite for licensure.

The BLS (March 29, 2012, http://www.bls.gov/ooh/Healthcare/Pharmacists.htm) reports that pharmacists worked at 274,900 jobs in 2010. Approximately 62% worked in community pharmacies—either independently owned or part of a drugstore chain, grocery store, department store, or mass merchandiser. In 2010, 21% of pharmacists worked part time. Most full-time salaried pharmacists worked about 40 hours per week, and many self-employed pharmacists worked more than 50 hours per week. About 23% worked in hospitals in 2010. The median annual wages of pharmacists in 2010 were $111,570.

MENTAL HEALTH PROFESSIONALS

The mental health sector includes a range of professionals—psychiatrists, psychologists, psychiatric nurses, clinical social workers, and counselors—whose training, orientation, philosophy, and practice styles differ, even within a single discipline. For example, clinical psychologists may endorse and offer dramatically different forms of therapy—ranging from long-term psychoanalytic psychotherapy to short-term cognitive-behavioral therapy.

Psychiatrists

Psychiatrists are physicians who have completed residency training in the prevention, diagnosis, and treatment of mental illness, mental retardation, and substance abuse disorders. Because they are trained physicians, they are especially well equipped to care for people who have coexisting medical diseases and mental health problems and can prescribe medication including psychoactive drugs. Psychiatrists may also obtain additional training that prepares them to treat certain populations such as children and adolescents or older adults (this subspecialty is called geriatric psychiatry or geropsychiatry), or they may specialize in a specific treatment modality.

Psychologists

Research psychologists investigate the physical, cognitive, emotional, or social aspects of human behavior. They work in academic and private research centers and in business, nonprofit, and governmental organizations.

Clinical psychologists help mentally and emotionally disturbed clients better manage their symptoms and behaviors. Some work in rehabilitation, treating patients with spinal cord injuries, chronic pain or illness, stroke, arthritis, and neurologic conditions. Others help people cope during times of personal crisis, such as divorce or the death of a loved one. Psychologists are also called on to help communities recover from the trauma of natural or human-made disasters by working with, for example, people who have lost their homes to earthquakes, fires, or floods, or students who have witnessed school violence.

Clinical psychologists may specialize in health psychology, neuropsychology, or geropsychology. Health psychologists promote healthy lifestyles and behaviors and provide counseling such as smoking cessation, weight reduction, and stress management to assist people to reduce their health risks. Neuropsychologists often work in stroke rehabilitation and head injury programs, and geropsychologists work with older adults in institutional and community settings.

School psychologists identify, diagnose, and address students' learning and behavior problems. They work with teachers and school personnel to improve classroom management strategies and to design educational programs for students with disabilities or gifted and talented

students. They also work with parents to help improve parenting skills.

Industrial-organizational psychologists aim to improve productivity and the quality of life in the workplace. They screen prospective employees and conduct training and development, counseling, and organizational development and analysis. Industrial-organizational psychologists examine aspects of work life. They work in organizational consultation, market research, systems design, or other applied psychology fields. For example, industrial-organizational psychologists may be involved in efforts to understand and influence consumer-purchasing behaviors.

Social psychologists consider interpersonal relationships and interactions with the social environment and social experience. Many social psychologists specialize in particular aspects of social psychology, such as group behavior, leadership, aggression, attitudinal change, or social perception.

EDUCATION, TRAINING, LICENSURE, AND EARNINGS. Most psychologists hold a doctorate degree in psychology, which requires between five and seven years of graduate study. Clinical psychologists usually earn a Doctor of Philosophy or a Doctor of Psychology degree and complete an internship of at least a one-year duration. An educational specialist degree qualifies an individual to work as a school psychologist; however, most school psychologists complete a master's degree followed by a one-year internship. People with a master's degree in psychology may work as industrial-organizational psychologists or as psychological assistants, under the supervision of doctoral-level psychologists, and conduct research or psychological evaluations. Vocational and guidance counselors usually need two years of graduate education in counseling and one year of counseling experience. A master's degree in psychology requires at least two years of full-time graduate study. People with undergraduate degrees in psychology assist psychologists and other professionals in community mental health centers, vocational rehabilitation offices, and correctional programs.

Psychologists in clinical practice must be certified or licensed in all states and the District of Columbia. According to the BLS (March 29, 2012, http://www.bls.gov/ooh/Life-Physical-and-Social-Science/Psychologists.htm), the median annual wages for clinical, counseling, and school psychologists were $66,640 in 2010.

Psychiatric Nurses

Psychiatric nurses are required to have a degree in nursing, be licensed as an RN, and have additional experience in psychiatry. Advanced practice psychiatric nurses (RNs prepared at the master's level) may prescribe psychotropic medications and conduct individual, group, and family psychotherapy as well as perform crisis intervention and case management functions. Along with primary care physicians, they are often the first points of contact for people seeking mental health help.

The American Psychiatric Nurses Association (2012, http://www.apna.org/i4a/pages/index.cfm?pageid=3292) is the professional society that represents psychiatric nurses and examines the changing profile of the profession. The association explains that the pay scale for psychiatric nurses and psychiatric nurse practitioners "depends on many factors, such as level of education, years of experience, size of the agency or hospital, and geographic location." According to PayScale (September 5, 2012, http://www.payscale.com/research/US/Job=Psychiatric_Nurse_%28RN%29/Salary), a service that collects salary data, psychiatric nurses' salaries usually start at $38,482. PayScale (August 28, 2012, http://www.payscale.com/research/US/Job=Psychiatric_Nurse_Practitioner_%28NP%29/Salary) notes that advanced practice nurses' salaries start at $66,325.

Clinical Social Workers

Clinical social workers are the largest group of professionally trained mental health care providers in the United States. Clinical social workers offer psychotherapy or counseling and a range of diagnostic services in public agencies, clinics, and private practice. They assist people to improve their interpersonal relationships, solve personal and family problems, and advise them about how to function effectively in their communities.

According to the BLS (March 29, 2012, http://www.bls.gov/ooh/Community-and-Social-Service/Social-workers.htm), social workers held 650,500 positions in the United States in 2010. Of this total, 295,700 were child, family, and school social workers; 152,700 were health care social workers; and 126,100 were mental health and substance abuse social workers. The median annual wages of child, family, and school social workers were $40,210 in 2010. Health care social workers earned $47,230, and mental health and substance abuse social workers earned $38,600.

EDUCATION, CERTIFICATION, AND LICENSURE. A bachelor's degree in social work is usually the minimum requirement for employment as a social worker, and an advanced degree has become the standard for many positions. A master's degree in social work is necessary for positions in health and mental health settings and is typically required for certification for clinical work. Licensed clinical social workers hold a master's degree in social work along with additional clinical training. Supervisory, administrative, and staff training positions usually require an advanced degree, and university teaching positions and research appointments normally require a doctorate in social work.

All the states and the District of Columbia have licensing, certification, or registration requirements that delineate the scope of social work practice and the use of professional titles; however, standards for licensing vary by state. The National Association of Social Workers (2012, https://www.socialworkers.org/nasw/default.asp) represents 145,000 professional social workers and "works to enhance the professional growth and development of its members, to create and maintain professional standards, and to advance sound social policies."

Counselors

Counselors assist people with personal, family, educational, mental health, and job-related challenges and problems. Their roles and responsibilities depend on the clients they serve and on the settings in which they work. According to the BLS (March 29, 2012, http://www.bls.gov/ooh/community-and-social-service/mental-health-counselors-and-marriage-and-family-therapists.htm), a master's degree is required to become a licensed counselor. In "State Licensure Information" (http://www.nbcc.org/StateLicensure/Statistics.aspx), the National Board for Certified Counselors indicates that in 2012 all 50 states and the District of Columbia had some form of counselor credentialing, licensure, certification, or registry legislation governing counselors who practice outside schools. The American Counseling Association (2012, http://www.counseling.org/AboutUs/) is the world's largest association for professional counselors and represents more than 50,000 professional counselors in various practice settings. The association has taken an active role in advocating for certification, licensure, and registry of counselors.

The BLS (March 29, 2012, http://www.bls.gov/) notes that in 2010 there were 281,400 educational, guidance, vocational, and school counselors; 129,800 rehabilitation counselors; 120,300 mental health counselors; 85,500 substance abuse and behavioral disorder counselors; and 36,000 marriage and family therapists.

Working in elementary, secondary, and postsecondary schools, educational, guidance, vocational, and school counselors work with people with disabilities and help them overcome the personal, social, and vocational effects of their disabilities. They advise people with disabilities that resulted from birth defects, illness, disease, accidents, or the stress of daily life.

Rehabilitation counselors help people with personal, social, and vocational challenges that resulted from birth defects, illness, disease, accidents, or the stress of daily life to gain independence and employment. They help design and coordinate activities for people in rehabilitation treatment facilities and perform client evaluations. Rehabilitation counselors plan and implement rehabilitation programs that may include personal and vocational counseling, training, and job placement.

Mental health counselors work in prevention programs to promote optimum mental health and provide a wide range of counseling services. They work closely with other mental health professionals, including psychiatrists, psychologists, clinical social workers, psychiatric nurses, and school counselors.

Substance abuse and behavioral disorder counselors help people overcome addictions to alcohol, drugs, gambling, and eating disorders. They counsel individuals, families, and groups in clinics, hospital-based outpatient treatment programs, community mental health centers, and inpatient chemical dependency treatment programs.

Marriage and family therapists use various techniques to intervene with individuals, families, and couples or to help them resolve emotional conflicts. They aim to modify perceptions and behavior, enhance communication and understanding among family members, and prevent family and individual crises. Individual marriage and family therapists may also offer psychotherapy to individuals, couples, and families to improve their interpersonal relationships.

Pastoral counselors offer a type of psychotherapy that combines spiritual resources with psychological understanding for healing and growth. According to the American Association of Pastoral Counselors (AAPC; 2012, http://www.aapc.org/home/mission-statement.aspx), this therapeutic modality is more than simply the comfort, support, and encouragement a religious community can offer; instead, it aims to provide "healing, hope, and wholeness to individuals, families, and communities by expanding and equipping spiritually grounded and psychologically informed care, counseling, and psychotherapy." Typically, an AAPC-certified counselor has obtained a bachelor's degree from a college or university, a three-year professional degree from a seminary, and a specialized master's or doctorate degree in the mental health field.

The AAPC asserts that demand for spiritually based counseling is on the rise, in part because interest in spirituality is on the rise in the United States. The organization also believes that despite increased interest in psychotherapy and increasing numbers of therapists, managed mental health care has reduced the availability of, and payment for, counseling services for many people. As a result, more people are turning to clergy for help with personal, marital, and family issues as well as with faith issues. For many working-poor Americans without health insurance benefits, free or low-cost counseling from pastoral counselors is the most accessible, available, affordable, and acceptable form of mental health care.

PRACTITIONERS OF COMPLEMENTARY AND ALTERNATIVE MEDICINE

The field of complementary and alternative medicine (CAM) is attracting a growing number of professionals. The National Center for Complementary and Alternative Medicine (NCCAM; July 2011, http://nccam.nih.gov/health/whatiscam/) defines alternative medicine as "a group of diverse medical and health care systems, practices, and products that are not generally considered part of conventional medicine." Even though there is some overlap between them, the NCCAM further distinguishes complementary, alternative, and integrative medicine in the following manner:

- Alternative medicine is therapy or treatment that is used instead of conventional medical treatment.

- Complementary medicine is nonstandard therapy or treatment that is used along with conventional medicine, not in place of it. Complementary medicine appears to offer health benefits, but there is less scientific evidence to support its utility than is generally available for conventional and integrative therapies.

- Integrative medicine is the combination of conventional medical treatment and CAM therapies that have been scientifically researched and have demonstrated evidence that they are both safe and effective.

In general terms, alternative therapies are often entirely untested and unproven, whereas complementary and integrative practices that are used in conjunction with mainstream medicine have substantial scientific basis of demonstrated safety and efficacy (the ability of an intervention to produce the intended diagnostic or therapeutic effect in optimal circumstances).

There is considerable enthusiasm for and use of CAM approaches and practices. Patricia M. Barnes, Barbara Bloom, and Richard L. Nahin indicate in "Complementary and Alternative Medicine Use among Adults and Children: United States, 2007" (*National Health Statistics Reports*, no. 12, December 10, 2008), the most recent publication for which comprehensive and reliable data were available as of September 2012, that in 2007, 38.3% of American adults aged 18 years and older and 11.8% of children under the age of 18 years used some form of CAM therapy within the 12 months preceding the survey. (See Figure 2.5.)

Figure 2.6 shows the 10 most frequently used CAM therapies in 2007:

- Natural products such as herbs, other botanicals, and enzymes (17.7%)

- Deep breathing (12.7%)

- Meditation (9.4%)

- Chiropractic and osteopathic care (8.6%)

FIGURE 2.5

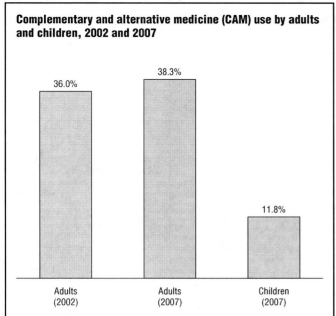

Complementary and alternative medicine (CAM) use by adults and children, 2002 and 2007

36.0%   38.3%   11.8%

Adults (2002)   Adults (2007)   Children (2007)

SOURCE: "Figure 1. CAM Use by U.S. Adults and Children," in *Downloadable Graphics on CAM Use in the United States*, National Institutes of Health, National Center for Complementary and Alternative Medicine, 2012, http://nccam.nih.gov/news/camstats/2007/graphics.htm (accessed June 13, 2012)

- Massage (8.3%)
- Yoga (6.1%)
- Diet-based therapies (3.6%)
- Progressive relaxation (2.9%)
- Guided imagery (2.2%)
- Homeopathic treatment (1.8%)

Homeopathic Medicine

Homeopathic medicine (also called homeopathy) is based on the belief that "like cures like" and uses very diluted amounts of natural substances to encourage the body's own self-healing mechanisms. Homeopathy was developed by the German physician Samuel Hahnemann (1755–1843) during the 1790s. Hahnemann found that he could produce symptoms of particular diseases by injecting small doses of various herbal substances. This discovery inspired him to administer to sick people extremely diluted formulations of substances that would produce the same symptoms they suffered from in an effort to stimulate natural recovery and regeneration.

According to Edzard Ernst of the University of Exeter, in "Bogus Arguments for Unproven Treatments" (*International Journal of Clinical Practice*, vol. 66, no. 3, March 2012), studies evaluating homeopathy find that homeopathic medicines have no effects beyond those of placebo. (A placebo is an inactive compound. The pla-

cebo effect is a health benefit, such as pain relief, that arises from the patient's expectation that the placebo will provide relief, rather than from the placebo itself.) Ernst concedes that many conventional treatments are as yet unproven but argues that "the existence of evidence gaps is no reason for introducing homeopathic placebos."

However, Peter Fisher of the Royal London Hospital for Integrated Medicine observes in "What Is Homeopathy? An Introduction" (*Frontiers in Bioscience*, no. 4, January 1, 2012) that despite widespread condemnation, homeopathy continues to be employed by thousands of conventionally trained physicians. Fisher asserts that "there is a significant body of clinical research including randomised clinical trials and meta-analyses of such trials which suggest that homeopathy has actions which are not placebo effects."

Naturopathic Medicine

As its name suggests, naturopathic medicine (also called naturopathy) uses naturally occurring substances to prevent, diagnose, and treat disease. Even though it is now considered to be an alternative medicine system, it is one of the oldest medicine systems and has its origins in Native American culture and even draws from Greek, Chinese, and East Indian ideas about health and illness.

The guiding principles of modern naturopathic medicine are "first, do no harm" and "nature has the power to heal." Naturopathy seeks to treat the whole person, because disease is seen as arising from many causes rather than from a single cause. Naturopathic physicians are taught that "prevention is as important as cure" and to view creating and maintaining health as equally important as curing disease. They are instructed to identify and treat the causes of diseases rather than to act only to relieve symptoms.

Naturopathic treatment methods include nutritional counseling; use of dietary supplements, herbs, and vitamins; hydrotherapy (water-based therapies, usually involving whirlpool or other baths); exercise; manipulation; massage; heat therapy; and electrical stimulation. Because naturopathy draws on Chinese and Indian medical techniques, naturopathic physicians often use Chinese herbs, acupuncture, and East Indian medicines to treat disease.

In "Naturopathy and the Primary Care Practice" (*Primary Care: Clinics in Office Practice*, vol. 37, no. 1, March 2010), Sara A. Fleming and Nancy C. Gutknecht of the University of Wisconsin, Madison, describe naturopathy as "a distinct type of primary care medicine that blends age-old healing traditions with scientific advances and current research. It is guided by a unique set of principles that recognize the body's innate healing capacity, emphasize disease prevention, and encourage individual responsibility to obtain optimal health." The researchers explain that "naturopathic physicians (NDs) are trained as primary care physicians in 4-year accredited,

FIGURE 2.6

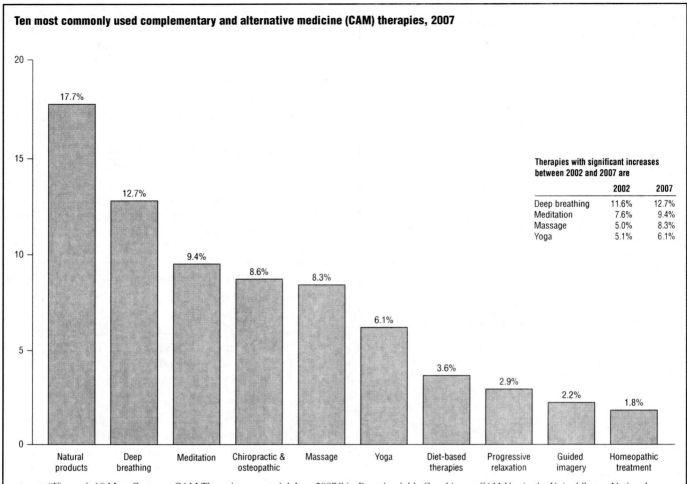

Ten most commonly used complementary and alternative medicine (CAM) therapies, 2007

Therapies with significant increases
between 2002 and 2007 are

	2002	2007
Deep breathing	11.6%	12.7%
Meditation	7.6%	9.4%
Massage	5.0%	8.3%
Yoga	5.1%	6.1%

SOURCE: "Figure 4. 10 Most Common CAM Therapies among Adults—2007," in *Downloadable Graphics on CAM Use in the United States*, National Institutes of Health, National Center for Complementary and Alternative Medicine, 2010, http://nccam.nih.gov/news/camstats/2007/graphics.htm (accessed June 13, 2012)

doctoral-level naturopathic medical schools." In 2010 there were 15 states and two U.S. territories that licensed and recognized naturopathic physicians.

Traditional Chinese Medicine

Traditional Chinese medicine (TCM) uses nutrition, acupuncture, massage, herbal medicine, and Qi Gong (exercises to improve the flow of vital energy through the body) to help people achieve balance and unity of their mind, body, and spirit. Practiced for more than 3,000 years by about a quarter of the world's population, TCM has been adopted by naturopathic physicians, chiropractors, and other CAM practitioners in the United States.

TCM views balancing *qi* (pronounced "chee"), the vital life force that flows over the surface of the body and through internal organs, as central to health, wellness, disease prevention, and treatment. This vital force or energy is thought to flow through the human body in meridians (channels). TCM practitioners believe that pain and disease develop when there is any sort of disturbance in the natural flow. TCM also seeks to balance the feminine and masculine qualities of yin and yang by using other techniques such as moxibustion, which is the stimulation of acupuncture points with heat, and cupping, in which the practitioner increases circulation by putting a heated jar on the skin of a body part. Herbal medicine is the most commonly prescribed treatment.

Acupuncture

Acupuncture is a Chinese practice that dates back more than 5,000 years. Chinese medicine describes acupuncture—the insertion of extremely thin, sterile needles to any of 360 specific points on the body—as a way to balance *qi*. When an acupuncturist determines that there is an imbalance in the flow of energy, needles are inserted at specific points along the meridians. Each point controls a different part of the body. Once the needles are in place, they are rotated gently or are briefly charged with a small electric current.

Traditional Western medicine explains the acknowledged effectiveness of acupuncture as the result of triggering the release of neurotransmitters and neuropeptides that influence brain chemistry and of pain-relieving substances called endorphins that occur naturally in the body. Besides providing lasting pain relief, acupuncture has demonstrated success in helping people with substance abuse problems, relieving nausea, heightening immunity by increasing total white blood cells and T-cell production, and assisting patients to recover from stroke and other neurological impairments. Imaging techniques confirm that acupuncture acts to alter brain chemistry and function.

Chiropractic Physicians

Chiropractic physicians treat patients whose health problems are associated mainly with the body's structural and neurological systems, especially the spine. These practitioners believe that interference with these systems can impair normal functions and lower resistance to disease. Chiropractic medicine asserts that misalignment or compression of, for example, the spinal nerves can alter many important body functions. According to the American Chiropractic Association, in "About Chiropractic" (2012, http://www.acatoday.org/level1_css.cfm?T1ID=42), the term chiropractic may be defined as "a health care profession that focuses on disorders of the musculoskeletal system and the nervous system, and the effects of these disorders on general health. Chiropractic care is used most often to treat neuromusculoskeletal complaints, including but not limited to back pain, neck pain, pain in the joints of the arms or legs, and headaches." Doctors of chiropractic medicine do not use or prescribe pharmaceutical drugs or perform surgery. Instead, they rely on adjustment and manipulation of the musculoskeletal system, particularly the spinal column.

Many chiropractors use nutritional therapy and prescribe dietary supplements; some employ a technique known as applied kinesiology to diagnose and treat disease. Applied kinesiology is based on the belief that every organ problem is associated with weakness of a specific muscle. Chiropractors who use this technique claim they can accurately identify organ system dysfunction without any laboratory or other diagnostic tests.

Besides manipulation, chiropractors also use a variety of other therapies to support healing and relax muscles before they make manual adjustments. These treatments include:

- Heat and cold therapy to relieve pain, speed healing, and reduce swelling

- Hydrotherapy to relax muscles and stimulate blood circulation

- Immobilization such as casts, wraps, traction, and splints to protect injured areas

- Electrotherapy to deliver deep tissue massage and boost circulation

- Ultrasound to relieve muscle spasms and reduce swelling

All states and the District of Columbia license chiropractors who meet the educational and examination requirements established by the state. According to the BLS (March 29, 2012, http://www.bls.gov/ooh/Health care/Chiropractors.htm), chiropractors worked at 52,600 jobs in 2010, and most were self-employed and in solo practice. In 2010 the median annual wages of salaried chiropractors were $67,200. Visits to chiropractors are most often for treatment of lower back pain, neck pain, and headaches.

INCREASE IN HEALTH CARE EMPLOYMENT

The number of people working in health care services has increased steadily since the middle of the 20th century. Figure 2.7 shows the projected increases in employment in selected health care occupations between 2006 and 2016. The largest employment increases forecasted are for RNs; personal and home care aides; home health aides; nursing aides, orderlies, and attendants; medical assistants; and licensed practical and licensed vocational nurses.

Why Is Health Care Booming?

Three major factors appear to have influenced the escalation in health care employment: advances in technology, the increasing amounts of money spent on health care, and the aging of the U.S. population. In other sectors of the economy, technology often replaces humans in the labor force. However, health care technology has increased the demand for highly trained specialists to operate the sophisticated equipment. Because of technological advances, patients are likely to undergo more tests and diagnostic procedures, take more drugs, see more specialists, and be subjected to more aggressive treatments than ever before.

The second factor involves the amount of money the nation spends on keeping its citizens in good health. The Centers for Medicare and Medicaid Services forecasts in National Health Expenditure Projections 2010–2020 (September 2011, https://www.cms.gov/) that national health expenditures will rise from an average of $9,348.80 per person in 2013 to $13,708.80 per person in 2020. For each year that the amount of money spent on health care continues to grow, employment in the field grows as well. Some health care industry observers believe that government and private financing for the health care industry, unlike most other fields, is virtually unlimited.

The third factor contributing to the rise in the number of health care workers is the aging of the nation's population. There are greater numbers of older adults in the United States than ever before, and they are living longer.

FIGURE 2.7

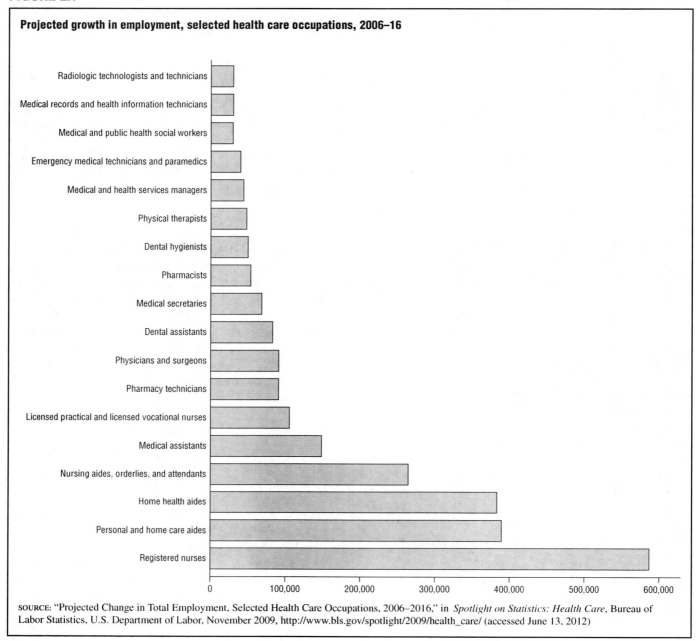

Projected growth in employment, selected health care occupations, 2006–16

SOURCE: "Projected Change in Total Employment, Selected Health Care Occupations, 2006–2016," in *Spotlight on Statistics: Health Care*, Bureau of Labor Statistics, U.S. Department of Labor, November 2009, http://www.bls.gov/spotlight/2009/health_care/ (accessed June 13, 2012)

According to the U.S. Census Bureau, in the press release "Census Bureau Reports World's Older Population: Projected to Triple by 2050" (June 23, 2009, http://www.census.gov/newsroom/releases/archives/international_population/cb09-97.html), the U.S. population aged 65 years and older will more than double by 2050, rising from 39 million in 2010 to 89 million in 2050.

The increase in the number of older people is expected to boost the demand for home health care services, assisted living, and nursing home care. Many nursing homes now offer special care for stroke patients, people with Alzheimer's disease (a progressive cognitive impairment), and people who need a respirator to breathe. To care for such patients, nursing homes need more PTs, nursing

aides, and respiratory therapists. Figure 2.7 shows the projected growth of these health care occupations.

Another factor that will likely further increase the demand for health care workers is the full implementation of the 2010 health care reform legislation, which will occur in 2014. When the millions of previously uninsured Americans obtain coverage and enter the health care system, additional health care resources (i.e., workers and facilities) will be required. The legislation may also improve the way in which physicians and other health care workers deliver care. For example, previously uninsured Americans who may have used hospital emergency departments to obtain needed medical care will be able to access preventive services in physicians' offices and clinics. This group may also seek care when the symptoms of sickness first appear, when diseases and disorders are more amenable to treatment, rather than waiting until the situation requires emergency treatment.

The James A. Baker III Institute for Public Policy of Rice University explains in "Health Reform and the Health Care Workforce" (March 2012, http://www.bakerinstitute.org/publications/HPF-pub-PolicyReport51-Web.pdf) that the PPACA and the Health Care and Education Reconciliation Act (which are commonly known as the ACA) expanded training programs for health professionals and established the National Health Care Workforce Commission to meet the growing demand for health care professionals. The ACA also creates incentives to increase primary care provider education. An estimated 30,400 physicians, 8,000 NPs, and 2,400 PAs will be needed to supply health care services. There will be a corresponding demand for services from clinical laboratory professionals, imaging technicians, pharmacists and other pharmacy personnel, and health educators. The institute avers that the ACA provisions that expand access to health insurance and promote more efficient health care delivery will be "likely to have a greater impact on the health workforce than the direct provisions of the ACA."

In the factsheet "How Does Health Reform Affect the Health Care Workforce?" (2011, http://www.rand.org/content/dam/rand/pubs/research_briefs/2011/RAND_RB9635.pdf), David M. Adamson of the RAND Corporation opines that implementation of the ACA may "accelerate the trend toward health care becoming a dominant employment sector in the economy." It may also necessitate an increase in administrative and support staff to shoulder some of the administrative burden of complying with the new requirements.

CHAPTER 3

HEALTH CARE INSTITUTIONS

A hospital is no place to be sick.

—Samuel Goldwyn

HOSPITALS

The first hospitals in the United States were established over 200 years ago. No records of hospitals in the early colonies exist, but almshouses, which sheltered the poor, also cared for those who were ill. The first almshouse opened in 1662 in the Massachusetts Bay Colony. In 1756 the Pennsylvania Hospital in Philadelphia became the first U.S. institution devoted entirely to care of the sick.

Until the late 1800s, U.S. hospitals had a bad reputation. The upper classes viewed hospitals as places for the poor who could not afford home care, and the poor saw hospitalization as a humiliating consequence of personal economic failure. People from all walks of life thought hospitals were places to go to die.

TYPES OF HOSPITALS

The American Hospital Association (AHA) notes in "Fast Facts on US Hospitals" (January 3, 2012, http://www.aha.org/aha/resource-center/Statistics-and-Studies/fast-facts.html) that in 2010 there were 5,754 hospitals in the United States that were described as short stay or long term, depending on the length of time a patient spends before being discharged. Short-stay facilities include community, teaching, and public hospitals. Sometimes short-stay hospitals are referred to as acute care facilities because the services provided within them focus on pressing problems or medical conditions, such as a heart attack, rather than on long-term chronic conditions, such as the need for rehabilitation following a head injury. Long-term hospitals are usually rehabilitation and psychiatric hospitals or facilities for the treatment of tuberculosis or other pulmonary (respiratory) diseases.

Hospitals are also distinguished by their ownership, scope of services, and whether they are teaching hospitals with academic affiliations. Hospitals may be operated as proprietary (for-profit) businesses—owned either by corporations or individuals such as the physicians on staff—or they may be voluntary—owned by not-for-profit corporations or religious organizations or operated by federal, state, or city governments. Voluntary, not-for-profit hospitals are usually governed by a board of trustees, who are selected from among community business and civic leaders and who serve without pay to oversee hospital operations.

Table 3.1 shows that the total number of U.S. hospitals declined from 7,156 in 1975 to 5,795 in 2009. Even though the number of community not-for-profit and state and local hospitals declined during this period, the number of for-profit hospitals grew, from 775 in 1975 to 998 in 2009. Occupancy rates also declined during this period.

Most community hospitals offer emergency services as well as a range of inpatient and outpatient medical and surgical services. There are more than 1,000 tertiary hospitals in the United States, which are hospitals that provide highly specialized services such as neonatal intensive care units (for care of sick newborns), trauma services, or cardiovascular surgery programs. A majority of tertiary hospitals serve as teaching hospitals.

Teaching hospitals are those community and tertiary hospitals affiliated with medical schools, nursing schools, or allied health professions training programs. Teaching hospitals are the primary sites for training new physicians, where interns and residents work under the supervision of experienced physicians. Nonteaching hospitals may also maintain affiliations with medical schools and some serve as sites for nursing and allied health professions students as well as for physicians-in-training.

TABLE 3.1

Hospitals, beds, and occupancy rates, by type of ownership and size of hospital, selected years 1975–2009

Type of ownership and size of hospital	1975	1980	1990	1995	2000	2008	2009
Hospitals				Number			
All hospitals	7,156	6,965	6,649	6,291	5,810	5,815	5,795
Federal	382	359	337	299	245	213	211
Nonfederal[a]	6,774	6,606	6,312	5,992	5,565	5,602	5,584
Community[b]	5,875	5,830	5,384	5,194	4,915	5,010	5,008
Nonprofit	3,339	3,322	3,191	3,092	3,003	2,923	2,918
For profit	775	730	749	752	749	982	998
State-local government	1,761	1,778	1,444	1,350	1,163	1,105	1,092
6–24 beds	299	259	226	278	288	389	402
25–49 beds	1,155	1,029	935	922	910	1,151	1,164
50–99 beds	1,481	1,462	1,263	1,139	1,055	995	991
100–199 beds	1,363	1,370	1,306	1,324	1,236	1,070	1,063
200–299 beds	678	715	739	718	656	596	582
300–399 beds	378	412	408	354	341	355	348
400–499 beds	230	266	222	195	182	184	192
500 beds or more	291	317	285	264	247	270	266
Beds							
All hospitals	1,465,828	1,364,516	1,213,327	1,080,601	983,628	951,045	944,277
Federal	131,946	117,328	98,255	77,079	53,067	45,992	44,772
Nonfederal[a]	1,333,882	1,247,188	1,115,072	1,003,522	930,561	905,053	899,505
Community[b]	941,844	988,387	927,360	872,736	823,560	808,069	805,593
Nonprofit	658,195	692,459	656,755	609,729	582,988	556,651	556,406
For profit	73,495	87,033	101,377	105,737	109,883	120,887	122,071
State-local government	210,154	208,895	169,228	157,270	130,689	130,531	127,116
6–24 beds	5,615	4,932	4,427	5,085	5,156	6,726	6,894
25–49 beds	41,783	37,478	35,420	34,352	33,333	37,142	37,338
50–99 beds	106,776	105,278	90,394	82,024	75,865	71,477	71,012
100–199 beds	192,438	192,892	183,867	187,381	175,778	153,488	152,655
200–299 beds	164,405	172,390	179,670	175,240	159,807	144,895	141,920
300–399 beds	127,728	139,434	138,938	121,136	117,220	122,363	120,201
400–499 beds	101,278	117,724	98,833	86,459	80,763	80,815	84,783
500 beds or more	201,821	218,259	195,811	181,059	175,638	191,163	190,790
Occupancy rate[c]				Percent			
All hospitals	76.7	77.7	69.5	65.7	66.1	68.2	67.8
Federal	80.7	80.1	72.9	72.6	68.2	67.9	69.1
Nonfederal[a]	76.3	77.4	69.2	65.1	65.9	68.2	67.8
Community[b]	75.0	75.6	66.8	62.8	63.9	66.4	65.5
Nonproit	77.5	78.2	69.3	64.5	65.5	68.4	67.4
For profit	65.9	65.2	52.8	51.8	55.9	57.8	57.7
State-local government	70.4	71.1	65.3	63.7	63.2	66.1	65.0
6–24 beds	48.0	46.8	32.3	36.9	31.7	33.8	33.6
25–49 beds	56.7	52.8	41.3	42.6	41.3	46.7	46.0
50–99 beds	64.7	64.2	53.8	54.1	54.8	56.6	55.9
100–199 beds	71.2	71.4	61.5	58.8	60.0	61.9	61.3
200–299 beds	77.1	77.4	67.1	63.1	65.0	66.4	65.5
300–399 beds	79.7	79.7	70.0	64.8	65.7	69.4	67.9
400–499 beds	81.1	81.2	73.5	68.1	69.1	74.2	70.1
500 beds or more	80.9	82.1	77.3	71.4	72.2	74.9	74.0

[a]The category of nonfederal hospitals comprises psychiatric hospitals, tuberculosis and other respiratory diseases hospitals, and long-term and short-term general and other special hospitals.

[b]Community hospitals are nonfederal short-term general and special hospitals whose facilities and services are available to the public.

[c]Estimated percentage of staffed beds that are occupied. Occupancy rate is calculated as the average daily census (from the American Hospital Association) divided by the number of hospital beds.

SOURCE: "Table 116. Hospitals, Beds, and Occupancy Rates, by Type of Ownership and Size of Hospital: United States, Selected Years 1975–2009," in *Health, United States, 2011: With Special Feature on Socioeconomic Status and Health*, U.S. Department of Health and Human Services, Centers for Disease Control and Prevention, National Center for Health Statistics, May 2012, http://www.cdc.gov/nchs/data/hus/hus11.pdf (accessed June 13, 2012). Data from American Hospital Association (AHA) Annual Survey of Hospitals.

Community Hospitals

The most common type of hospital in the United States is the community, or general, hospital. Community hospitals, where most people receive care, are typically small, with 50 to 500 beds. The AHA reports in "Fast Facts on US Hospitals" that in 2010 there were 4,985 community hospitals, with 804,943 staffed beds, in the United States. These hospitals normally provide quality care for routine medical and surgical problems. Since the 1980s many smaller hospitals have closed down because they are no longer profitable. The larger ones, usually located in cities and adjacent suburbs, are often equipped with a full complement of medical and surgical personnel and state-of-the-art equipment.

Some community hospitals are not-for-profit corporations that are supported by local funding. These include hospitals supported by religious, cooperative, or osteopathic organizations. During the 1990s increasing numbers of not-for-profit community hospitals converted their ownership status, becoming proprietary hospitals that are owned and operated on a for-profit basis by corporations. These hospitals joined investor-owned corporations because they needed additional financial resources to maintain their existence in an increasingly competitive industry. Investor-owned corporations acquire not-for-profit hospitals to build market share, expand their provider networks, and penetrate new health care markets. According to the AHA, there were 2,904 not-for-profit community hospitals and 1,013 investor-owned, for-profit community hospitals in 2010.

Teaching Hospitals

Most teaching hospitals, which provide clinical training for medical students and other health care professionals, are affiliated with a medical school and have several hundred beds. Many of the physicians on staff at the hospital also hold teaching positions at the university that is affiliated with the hospital. These physicians may serve as classroom instructors as well as teaching physicians-in-training at the bedsides of the patients. Patients in teaching hospitals understand that they may be examined by medical students and residents as well as by their primary attending physician.

One advantage of obtaining care at a university-affiliated teaching hospital is the opportunity to receive treatment from highly qualified physicians with access to the most advanced technology and equipment. A disadvantage is the inconvenience and invasion of privacy that may result from multiple examinations performed by residents and students. When compared with smaller community hospitals, some teaching hospitals have reputations for being impersonal; however, patients with complex, unusual, or difficult diagnoses usually benefit from the presence of acknowledged medical experts and more comprehensive resources that are available at these facilities.

Public Hospitals

Public hospitals are owned and operated by federal, state, or city governments. Many have a continuing tradition of caring for the poor. They are usually located in the inner cities and are often in precarious financial situations because many of their patients are unable to pay for services. These hospitals depend heavily on Medicaid payments that are supplied by federal and state agencies or on grants from local governments. Medicaid is a program run by both the federal and state governments for the provision of health care insurance to people younger than 65 years of age who cannot afford to pay for private health insurance. The federal government matches the states' contribution to provide a certain minimal level of available coverage, and the states may offer additional services at their own expense. In "Fast Facts on US Hospitals," the AHA indicates that there were 1,068 state and local government community hospitals and 213 federal government hospitals in 2010.

TREATING SOCIETY'S MOST VULNERABLE MEMBERS. Increasingly, public hospitals must bear the burden of the weaknesses in the nation's health care system. The major problems in U.S. society are readily apparent in the emergency departments and corridors of public hospitals: poverty, drug and alcohol abuse, crime-related and domestic violence, untreated or inadequately treated chronic conditions such as high blood pressure and diabetes, and infectious diseases such as acquired immunodeficiency syndrome (AIDS) and tuberculosis.

LOSING MONEY. The typical public hospital provides millions of dollars in health care and fails to recoup these costs from reimbursement by private insurance, Medicaid, and Medicare (a federal health insurance program for people aged 65 years and older and people with disabilities). Jack Zwanzige, Nasreen Khan, and Anil Bamezai note in "The Relationship between Safety Net Activities and Hospital Financial Performance" (*BMC Health Services Research*, vol. 10, no. 1, January 14, 2010) that at the close of the 20th century all U.S. hospitals were forced to take steps to reduce health care costs and faced reduced Medicare and Medicaid reimbursement. However, these changes may have disproportionately affected the nation's public hospitals, which provide "safety net" services and serve vulnerable populations such as poor and uninsured patients. (According to the Institute of Medicine [IOM], in *America's Health Care Safety Net: Intact but Endangered* [January 2000, http://www.iom.edu/], safety net services are offered by providers "that deliver a significant level of health care to uninsured, Medicaid, and other vulnerable patients." The IOM also explains that "these providers have two distinguishing characteristics: (1) either by legal mandate or explicitly adopted mission, they offer care to patients regardless of their ability to pay for those services; and (2) a substantial share of their patient mix are uninsured, Medicaid, and other vulnerable patients.") In response to these fiscal pressures, some hospitals closed and others decreased the range of services provided. Others responded by streamlining services and pursuing paying patients.

PROVIDING NEEDED SERVICES. The National Association of Public Hospitals and Health Systems (NAPH; 2012, http://www.naph.org/Main-Menu-Category/About-NAPH/About-Our-Members/Our-Members.aspx) believes the mission of public hospitals is to respond to the needs of their communities. The NAPH represents more than 100 hospitals and health care systems that provide care to patients and serve as community resources. Many of the

NAPH-member hospitals are also major academic centers, where they train medical and dental residents as well as nursing and allied health professionals.

In the press release "NAPH Annual Survey Shows Increasingly Important Role of Safety Net Hospitals" (June 7, 2012, http://www.naph.org/), the NAPH reports that in 2010 its members "provided nearly $128 billion in total inpatient and outpatient services, nearly half of which was for low-income patients." Furthermore, while its members represented a scant 2% of acute care hospitals, they provided 20% of all uncompensated care. In 2010 uncompensated care accounted for 6% of costs for U.S. hospitals, compared with 16% of costs for NAPH-member hospitals.

Following President Barack Obama's (1961–) announcement in February 2012 of his efforts to reduce the budget deficit, Bruce Siegel, the president and chief executive officer of the NAPH, issued the press release "NAPH Concerned about Health Care Cuts in President's Budget" (February 13, 2012, http://www.naph.org/Main-Menu-Category/Newsroom/2012-Press-Releases/Statement-on-Health-Care-Cut-Concerns.aspx?FT=.pdf), which opposed cuts to programs that jeopardize the nation's safety net. He explained that the "NAPH recognizes that change is necessary to create a sustainable health care system.... And we stand ready to work with the administration to develop delivery system and payment innovations that will improve care and cut costs without compromising patient access. As safety net hospitals across the nation continue to develop and implement unique, sustainable health care programs, now is not the time to cut funding for those programs."

In "How the Affordable Care Act Supports a High-Performance Safety Net" (January 16, 2012, http://www.commonwealthfund.org/Blog/2012/Jan/Affordable-Care-Act-Safety-Net.aspx), Pamela Riley, Julia Berenson, and Cara Dermody explain that the provisions of the Patient Protection and Affordable Care Act and the Health Care and Education Reconciliation Act (which are commonly known as the ACA) present challenges and opportunities for safety net hospitals. The challenges include reduced supplemental funding for some safety net providers and reductions in Medicare and Medicaid payments, which may compromise the providers' ability to offer needed services. However, the impact of reduced funding may be offset by the fact that the ACA will reduce the number of uninsured, which may mean that safety net providers will not have to provide as much uncompensated care and may receive greater revenues from newly insured patients.

Under the ACA safety net providers will have opportunities to coordinate care and serve as medical homes—sources of patient-centered, comprehensive, and coordinated care. The ACA approved the creation of the Center for Medicare and Medicaid Innovation, which will test and disseminate innovative payment and delivery system models, such as medical homes. The law also offers states the option to receive federal matching funds to implement or expand health home programs for Medicaid beneficiaries with chronic conditions, which are akin to medical homes. Furthermore, the law funds initiatives to pilot and assess novel delivery system and payment models, especially those that incentivize providers to coordinate and integrate care for vulnerable populations. For example, the Medicare Shared Savings Program creates incentives for providers to work together in accountable care organizations to improve health care quality and efficiency.

Hospital Emergency Departments: More Than They Can Handle

For many Americans, the hospital emergency department (ED) has replaced the physician's office as the place to seek health care services. With no insurance and little money, many people go to the only place that will take them without question. Insurance companies and health care planners estimate that more than half of all ED visits are for nonemergency treatment.

Among children under the age of 18 years of all races, those whose families lived below 100% of the poverty level (30.6%) or between 100% and 199% of the poverty level (25.7%) were more likely to visit EDs in 2010 than those whose families lived at 400% or more above the poverty level (15.9%). (See Table 3.2.) In 2010, 30% of children on Medicaid visited EDs at least once, as opposed to 17.1% of children who were privately insured and 19.4% of uninsured children. In the 18 years and older age group, 30.6% of people living below 100% of the poverty level and 25.6% of those living between 100% and 199% of the poverty level made at least one visit to the ED in 2010. (See Table 3.3.) Of adults aged 18 to 64 years, 17.4% of people who were privately insured visited the ED at least once in 2010, as opposed to 40.2% of those who had Medicaid and 21.3% of those who were uninsured.

MAJORITY OF ED PATIENTS HAVE HEALTH INSURANCE. Because people without health insurance or a usual source of care often resort to using hospital EDs, industry observers sometimes assume that the crowding and long waits in the ED are at least in part caused by uninsured patients seeking care for routine problems such as colds, allergies, or back pain. In "Frequent Users of Emergency Departments: The Myths, the Data, and the Policy Implications" (*Annals of Emergency Medicine*, vol. 56, no. 1, July 2010), Eduardo LaCalle and Elaine Rabin of the Mount Sinai School of Medicine refute this hypothesis and characterize frequent users of emergency medical care (adults who make four or more ED visits in one year) as people with insurance who also make frequent use of other health care services such as clinics and

TABLE 3.2

Emergency department visits within the past 12 months among children under 18, by selected characteristics, 1997, 2009, and 2010

Characteristic	Under 18 years			Under 6 years			6–17 years		
	1997	2009	2010	1997	2009	2010	1997	2009	2010
	Percent of children with one or more emergency department visits								
All children[a]	19.9	20.8	22.1	24.3	25.9	27.8	17.7	18.2	19.1
Sex									
Male	21.5	22.2	23.3	25.2	25.6	29.3	19.6	20.3	20.1
Female	18.3	19.4	20.9	23.3	26.2	26.3	15.7	15.9	18.2
Race[b]									
White only	19.4	19.8	21.2	22.6	24.6	26.6	17.8	17.3	18.4
Black or African American only	24.0	26.9	27.6	33.1	34.2	34.0	19.4	23.2	24.2
American Indian or Alaska Native only	24.1	23.1	20.9	24.3	*	35.4	24.0	20.7	*
Asian only	12.6	11.4	15.0	20.8	14.0	18.4	8.6	10.0	13.3
Native Hawaiian or other Pacific Islander only	—	*	*	—	*	*	—	*	*
2 or more races	—	25.2	27.2	—	28.6	34.9	—	22.9	21.6
Hispanic origin and race[b]									
Hispanic or Latino	21.1	20.2	23.6	25.7	27.5	30.2	18.1	15.7	19.4
Not Hispanic or Latino	19.7	21.0	21.7	24.0	25.3	27.0	17.6	18.8	19.0
White only	19.2	19.8	20.4	22.2	23.7	25.1	17.7	18.0	18.2
Black or African American only	23.6	26.5	27.2	32.7	33.1	34.4	19.2	23.2	23.3
Percent of poverty level[c]									
Below 100%	25.1	26.6	30.6	29.5	33.9	35.4	22.2	21.9	27.6
100%–199%	22.0	23.3	25.7	28.0	28.9	31.6	19.0	20.4	22.3
200%–399%	18.0	18.9	18.4	21.4	23.3	22.7	16.4	16.8	16.4
400% or more	16.3	16.0	15.9	19.1	17.9	21.7	15.1	15.1	13.3
Hispanic origin and race and percent of poverty level[b, c]									
Hispanic or Latino:									
Percent of poverty level:									
Below 100%	21.9	24.6	27.0	25.0	29.9	32.0	19.6	20.9	23.4
100%–199%	20.8	18.7	23.3	28.8	27.3	31.6	15.6	13.6	18.0
200%–399%	21.4	16.9	19.5	24.6	26.1	25.2	19.6	12.2	16.1
400% or more	17.7	16.5	21.4	20.2	22.7	28.6	16.4	12.2	18.0
Not Hispanic or Latino:									
White only:									
Percent of poverty level:									
Below 100%	25.5	27.8	33.7	27.2	36.1	37.4	24.4	22.6	31.6
100%–199%	22.3	24.7	26.3	25.8	29.0	29.2	20.7	22.5	24.7
200%–399%	17.8	18.3	17.6	20.9	21.8	21.2	16.3	16.6	15.9
400% or more	16.5	16.2	15.5	19.0	17.4	21.0	15.4	15.7	13.2
Black or African American only:									
Percent of poverty level:									
Below 100%	29.3	28.4	32.4	39.5	39.4	41.6	23.0	21.1	26.6
100%–199%	22.5	26.8	27.5	31.7	27.6	34.5	18.5	26.4	23.7
200%–399%	18.5	27.9	22.3	23.9	32.1	24.6	16.3	26.1	21.4
400% or more	16.1	16.9	18.9	18.8	19.6	24.1	15.2	15.7	16.1
Health insurance status at the time of interview[d]									
Insured	19.8	21.1	22.3	24.4	25.7	28.1	17.5	18.7	19.2
Private	17.5	16.6	17.1	20.9	18.7	21.8	15.9	15.6	14.9
Medicaid	28.2	27.8	30.0	33.0	32.7	35.5	24.1	24.4	26.4
Uninsured	20.2	16.8	19.4	23.0	27.4	24.0	18.9	13.0	17.6
Health insurance status prior to interview[d]									
Insured continuously all 12 months	19.6	20.8	22.2	24.1	25.4	28.1	17.3	18.3	19.1
Uninsured for any period up to 12 months	24.0	25.8	23.7	27.1	32.4	28.0	21.9	22.5	21.3
Uninsured more than 12 months	18.4	14.2	17.6	19.3	24.1	21.3	18.1	11.4	16.7

*Estimates are considered unreliable.
—Data not available.
[a]Includes all other races not shown separately and unknown health insurance status.
[b]The race groups, white, black, American Indian or Alaska Native, Asian, Native Hawaiian or Other Pacific Islander, and 2 or more races, include persons of Hispanic and non-Hispanic origin. Persons of Hispanic origin may be of any race. Starting with 1999 data, race-specific estimates are tabulated according to the 1997 Revisions to the Standards for the Classification of Federal Data on Race and Ethnicity and are not strictly comparable with estimates for earlier years. The five single-race categories plus multiple-race categories shown in the table conform to the 1997 Standards. Starting with 1999 data, race-specific estimates are for persons who reported only one racial group; the category 2 or more races includes persons who reported more than one racial group. Prior to 1999, data were tabulated according to the 1977 Standards with four racial groups, and the Asian only category included Native Hawaiian or Other Pacific Islander. Estimate for single-race categories prior to 1999 included persons who reported one race or, if they reported more than one race, identified one race as best representing their race. Starting with 2003 data, race responses of the race and unspecified multiple race were treated as missing, and then race was imputed if these were the only race responses. Almost all persons with a race response of other race were of Hispanic origin.
[c]Percent of poverty level is based on family income and family size and composition using U.S. Census Bureau poverty thresholds. Missing family income data were imputed for 1997 and beyond.

TABLE 3.2

Emergency department visits within the past 12 months among children under 18, by selected characteristics, 1997, 2009, and 2010

[CONTINUED]

dHealth insurance categories are mutually exclusive. Persons who reported both Medicaid and private coverage are classified as having private coverage. Starting with 1997 data, state-sponsored health plan coverage is included as Medicaid coverage. Starting with 1999 data, coverage by the Children's Health Insurance Program (CHIP) is included with Medicaid coverage. In addition to private and Medicaid, the insured category also includes military, other government, and Medicare coverage. Persons not covered by private insurance, Medicaid, CHIP, state-sponsored or other government-sponsored health plans (starting in 1997), Medicare, or military plans are considered to have no health insurance coverage. Persons with only Indian Health Service coverage are considered to have no health insurance coverage.

SOURCE: Adapted from "Table 93. Emergency Department Visits within the Past 12 Months among Children under 18 Years of Age, by Selected Characteristics: United States, 1997–2010," in *Health, United States, 2011: With Special Feature on Socioeconomic Status and Health*, U.S. Department of Health and Human Services, Centers for Disease Control and Prevention, National Center for Health Statistics, May 2012, http://www.cdc.gov/nchs/data/hus/hus11.pdf (accessed June 13, 2012)

physicians' offices. The researchers conclude that "frequent ED users are a heterogeneous group along many dimensions and defy popular assumptions...and many frequent users present with true medical needs, which may explain why existing attempts to address the phenomena have had mixed success at best."

Renee M. Gindi, Robin A. Cohen, and Whitney K. Kirzinger confirm in "Emergency Room Use among Adults Aged 18–64: Early Release of Estimates from the National Health Interview Survey, January–June 2011" (May 2012, http://www.cdc.gov/nchs/data/nhis/earlyrelease/emergency_room_use_january-june_2011.pdf) that many ED visits could be prevented if people had better access to other providers such as urgent care centers or physicians with extended office hours. A CDC survey finds that 79.7% of adults visiting the ED who were not admitted to the hospital said they sought care in the ED because other care was inaccessible. Almost half claimed they had "no other place to go" (46.3%) or the ED "is [their] closest provider" (45.8). Nearly one-fifth (17.7%) said the ED was their usual source of care.

HOSPITALS TRY TO EASE THE PAIN OF WAITING. In an effort to distinguish themselves from competitors and increase patient satisfaction with care, some hospitals are promising ED patients that they will not have to wait for more than 30 minutes to be seen. In "Emergency Department: Hospitals Aim to Help Patients Pick an ED by Posting Wait Times on the Web" (*Hospitals and Health Networks*, vol. 84, no. 2, February 2010), Denene Brox reports that some hospitals post "up-to-the-minute ED wait times on the Internet." By using these websites, health care consumers with urgent, but not life-threatening, medical problems can choose the area hospital with the shortest wait time. Participating hospitals hope that informing prospective patients about wait times will result in higher levels of patient satisfaction.

HOSPITALS CATER TO SPECIAL POPULATIONS. Because more older adults than children make ED visits, some hospitals are creating special areas in the ED or even dedicating EDs to meet their needs. For example,

Anemona Hartocollis reports in "For the Elderly, Emergency Rooms of their Own" (*New York Times*, April 9, 2012) that the Mount Sinai Hospital in New York City is among a growing number of hospitals with an ED dedicated to serving older adults. Also known as a "geri-ed," it looks more like a clinic than an ED and has features such as nonskid floors, wall rails, reclining chairs, and thicker mattresses to improve the comfort of patients aged 65 years and older. Volunteers interact with patients in a calm environment that is designed to allay anxiety and enhance patient satisfaction. Patients use iPads to initiate two-way conversations with nurses and can order lunch, pain medication, or music using the touchscreen.

HOSPITALIZATION

In *Health, United States, 2011: With Special Feature on Socioeconomic Status and Health* (May 2012, http://www.cdc.gov/nchs/data/hus/hus11.pdf), the National Center for Health Statistics (NCHS) reports that the discharge rate increased among people aged 65 years and older between 1990 and 2005, decreased between 2005 and 2007, and then rose again in 2008–09. The discharge rates for all other age groups steadily declined during this period until 2007. In 2008–09 the discharge rates increased slightly for people aged 45 to 64 years but declined or remained relatively stable for other age groups.

According to the NCHS, in 2008–09 the hospital discharge rate was 1,149.8 per 10,000 population. The rate for females was 1,307.6 per 10,000 population, and for males it was 1,000.9 per 10,000 population. Male patients had longer average lengths of stay (ALOS) than female patients—5.4 days compared with 4.4 days. ALOS and discharge rates varied by geography—ALOS ranged from 4.4 days in the Midwest to 5.5 days in the Northeast. Furthermore, the discharge rate per 10,000 population ranged from 959.7 in the West to 1,322.5 in the Northeast.

Organ Transplants

Organ transplants are a viable means of saving lives, and according to the United Network for Organ

TABLE 3.3

Emergency department visits within the past 12 months among adults, by selected characteristics, selected years 1997–2010

Characteristic	One or more emergency department visits				Two or more emergency department visits			
	1997	2000	2009	2010	1997	2000	2009	2010
	Percent of adults with emergency department visits							
18 years and over, age-adjusted[a, b]	19.6	20.2	21.4	21.4	6.7	6.9	8.1	7.8
18 years and over, crude[a]	19.6	20.1	21.2	21.3	6.7	6.8	8.0	7.7
Age								
18–44 years	20.7	20.5	22.0	22.0	6.8	7.0	8.8	8.4
18–24 years	26.3	25.7	24.6	25.4	9.1	8.8	9.1	9.6
25–44 years	19.0	18.8	21.1	20.7	6.2	6.4	8.7	8.0
45–64 years	16.2	17.6	18.4	19.2	5.6	5.6	6.8	6.7
45–54 years	15.7	17.9	18.0	18.6	5.5	5.8	7.0	6.6
55–64 years	16.9	17.0	18.9	19.8	5.7	5.3	6.5	6.8
65 years and over	22.0	23.7	24.9	23.7	8.1	8.6	8.4	7.7
65–74 years	20.3	21.6	21.6	20.7	7.1	7.4	6.7	6.4
75 years and over	24.3	26.2	28.8	27.4	9.3	10.0	10.4	9.4
Sex[b]								
Male	19.1	18.7	19.9	18.5	5.9	5.7	7.1	6.0
Female	20.2	21.6	22.9	24.3	7.5	7.9	9.1	9.6
Race[b, c]								
White only	19.0	19.4	20.4	20.7	6.2	6.4	7.6	7.2
Black or African American only	25.9	26.5	31.1	28.6	11.1	10.8	13.2	12.6
American Indian or Alaska Native only	24.8	30.3	23.5	22.6	13.1	12.6	10.2	11.8
Asian only	11.6	13.6	13.2	13.3	2.9	3.8	3.2	3.3
Native Hawaiian or other Pacific Islander only	—	*	*	*	—	*	*	*
2 or more races	—	32.5	23.6	29.7	—	11.3	10.7	11.1
American Indian or Alaska Native; white	—	33.9	28.0	31.1	—	9.4	13.9	15.2
Hispanic origin and race[b, c]								
Hispanic or Latino	19.2	18.3	19.5	19.8	7.4	7.0	7.2	6.9
Mexican	17.8	17.4	16.9	18.1	6.4	7.1	6.1	6.1
Not Hispanic or Latino	19.7	20.6	21.9	21.9	6.7	6.9	8.4	8.1
White only	19.1	19.8	20.8	21.1	6.2	6.4	7.9	7.4
Black or African American only	25.9	26.5	31.3	29.0	11.0	10.8	13.3	12.7
Percent of poverty level[b, d]								
Below 100%	28.1	29.0	31.5	30.6	12.8	13.3	15.7	14.9
100%–199%	23.8	23.9	26.6	25.6	9.3	9.6	11.0	10.5
200%–399%	18.3	19.8	20.8	20.4	5.9	6.3	7.8	6.8
400% or more	15.9	16.8	16.3	17.0	3.9	4.5	4.7	4.7
Hispanic origin and race and percent of poverty level[b, c, d]								
Hispanic or Latino:								
Below 100%	22.1	22.4	23.9	23.6	9.8	9.7	10.8	11.5
100%–199%	19.2	18.1	20.0	19.9	8.1	6.7	7.6	6.3
200%–399%	18.5	17.3	19.0	18.1	6.0	7.4	6.2	5.2
400% or more	14.6	16.4	13.5	18.8	3.8	4.3	4.0	5.5
Not Hispanic or Latino:								
White only:								
Below 100%	29.5	30.1	32.4	33.3	13.0	13.9	15.3	15.5
100%–199%	24.3	25.5	28.3	26.8	9.1	10.4	12.2	11.2
200%–399%	18.1	20.1	20.6	20.3	5.8	6.3	8.3	6.5
400% or more	15.8	16.3	16.1	16.9	3.8	4.1	4.8	4.9
Black or African American only:								
Below 100%	34.6	35.4	41.8	36.9	17.5	17.4	24.1	20.2
100%–199%	29.2	28.5	34.1	33.5	12.8	12.2	14.5	15.9
200%–399%	20.8	23.2	28.7	25.7	8.1	8.0	9.4	10.2
400% or more	18.2	22.6	22.7	18.8	5.9	8.8	7.3	4.0
Health insurance status at the time of interview[e, f]								
18–64 years:								
Insured	18.8	19.5	20.5	20.8	6.1	6.4	7.8	7.5
Private	16.9	17.6	16.7	17.4	4.7	5.1	5.1	5.2
Medicaid	37.6	42.2	41.5	40.2	19.7	21.0	22.9	21.1
Uninsured	20.0	19.3	21.2	21.3	7.5	6.9	9.0	8.9
Health insurance status prior to interview[e, f]								
18–64 years:								
Insured continuously all 12 months	18.3	19.0	19.8	20.2	5.8	6.1	7.4	7.1
Uninsured for any period up to 12 months	25.5	28.2	27.3	26.0	9.4	10.3	11.7	12.5
Uninsured more than 12 months	18.9	17.3	20.2	20.6	7.1	6.4	8.8	8.1

TABLE 3.3

Emergency department visits within the past 12 months among adults, by selected characteristics, selected years 1997–2010 [CONTINUED]

Characteristic	One or more emergency department visits				Two or more emergency department visits			
	1997	2000	2009	2010	1997	2000	2009	2010
Percent of poverty level and health insurance status prior to interview[d, e, f]	Percent of adults with emergency department visits							
18–64 years:								
Below 100%:								
Insured continuously all 12 months	30.2	31.6	35.0	35.2	14.7	15.4	20.3	18.3
Uninsured for any period up to 12 months	34.1	43.7	36.8	34.2	16.1	18.1	18.1	16.5
Uninsured more than 12 months	20.8	20.5	24.1	23.4	8.1	9.1	9.9	11.7
100%–199%:								
Insured continuously all 12 months	24.5	25.5	27.6	26.1	8.9	10.2	11.3	10.8
Uninsured for any period up to 12 months	28.7	27.7	31.7	29.7	12.3	11.7	14.9	15.6
Uninsured more than 12 months	19.0	17.4	20.7	21.2	8.3	6.4	7.9	7.8
200%–399%:								
Insured continuously all 12 months	17.5	19.5	20.3	19.6	5.3	6.3	7.1	6.0
Uninsured for any period up to 12 months	21.6	24.6	21.2	25.4	6.6	7.3	9.4	12.2
Uninsured more than 12 months	16.8	15.6	18.1	17.6	5.9	4.5	9.6	5.7
400% or more:								
Insured continuously all 12 months	14.9	15.5	14.4	15.9	3.7	3.7	3.9	4.5
Uninsured for any period up to 12 months	18.0	20.1	22.2	12.5	3.1	6.4	*	*
Uninsured more than 12 months	19.1	15.8	15.0	19.4	*	5.2	5.6	*
Disability measure[b, g]								
Any basic actions difficulty or complex activity limitation	30.8	32.0	35.9	34.9	13.5	14.6	17.9	16.8
Any basic actions difficulty	30.5	32.4	36.0	35.0	13.5	14.9	18.2	17.2
Any complex activity limitation	39.7	41.5	44.8	43.8	19.9	21.2	25.0	24.5
No disability	14.5	15.3	15.3	16.1	3.7	3.9	4.4	4.4
Geographic region[b]								
Northeast	19.5	20.0	21.0	22.6	6.9	6.2	8.2	8.4
Midwest	19.3	20.1	22.2	22.3	6.2	6.9	8.6	8.2
South	20.9	21.2	22.6	22.1	7.3	7.6	9.1	8.0
West	17.7	18.6	19.1	18.9	6.0	6.3	6.2	6.7
Location of residence[b]								
Within MSA[h]	19.1	19.6	20.9	20.8	6.4	6.6	7.8	7.5
Outside MSA[h]	21.5	22.5	24.0	25.5	7.8	7.8	9.6	9.8

Notes: Data for additional years are available.
*Estimates are considered unreliable.
—Data not available.
[a]Includes all other races not shown separately, unknown health insurance status, and unknown disability status.
[b]Estimates are for persons 18 years of age and over and are age-adjusted to the year 2000 standard population using five age groups: 18–44 years, 45–54 years, 55–64 years, 65–74 years, and 75 years and over.
[c]The race groups, white, black, American Indian or Alaska Native, Asian, Native Hawaiian or Other Pacific Islander, and 2 or more races, include persons of Hispanic and non-Hispanic origin. Persons of Hispanic origin may be of any race. Starting with 1999 data, race-specific estimates are tabulated according to the 1997 Revisions to the Standards for the Classification of Federal Data on Race and Ethnicity and are not strictly comparable with estimates for earlier years. The five single-race categories plus multiple-race categories shown in the table conform to the 1997 Standards. Starting with 1999 data, race-specific estimates are for persons who reported only one racial group; the category 2 or more races includes persons who reported more than one racial group. Prior to 1999, data were tabulated according to the 1977 Standards with four racial groups, and the Asian only category included Native Hawaiian or Other Pacific Islander. Estimates for single-race categories prior to 1999 included persons who reported one race or, if they reported more than one race, identified one race as best representing their race. Starting with 2003 data, race responses of other race and unspecified multiple race were treated as missing, and then race was imputed if these were the only race responses. Almost all persons with a race response of other race were of Hispanic origin.
[d]Percent of poverty level is based on family income and family size and composition using U.S. Census Bureau poverty thresholds. Missing family income data were imputed for 1997 and beyond.
[e]Estimates for persons 18–64 years of age are age-adjusted to the year 2000 standard population using three age groups: 18–44 years, 45–54 years, and 55–64 years.
[f]Health insurance categories are mutually exclusive. Persons who reported both Medicaid and private coverage are classified as having private coverage. Starting with 1997 data, state-sponsored health plan coverage is included as Medicaid coverage. Starting with 1999 data, coverage by the Children's Health Insurance Program (CHIP) is included with Medicaid coverage. In addition to private and Medicaid, the insured category also includes military plans, other government-sponsored health plans, and Medicare, not shown separately. Persons not covered by private insurance, Medicaid, CHIP, state-sponsored or other government-sponsored health plans (starting in 1997), Medicare, or military plans are considered to have no health insurance coverage. Persons with only Indian Health Service coverage are considered to have no health insurance coverage.
[g]Any basic actions difficulty or complex activity limitation is defined as having one or more of the following limitations or difficulties: movement difficulty, emotional difficulty, sensory (seeing or hearing) difficulty, cognitive difficulty, self-care (activities of daily living or instrumental activities of daily living) limitation, social limitation, or work limitation. Starting with 2007 data, the hearing question, a component of the basic actions difficulty measure, was revised. Consequently, data prior to 2007 are not comparable with data for 2007 and beyond.
[h]MSA is metropolitan statistical area. Starting with 2006 data, MSA status is determined using 2000 census data and the 2000 standards for defining MSAs.

SOURCE: Adapted from "Table 94. Emergency Department Visits within the Past 12 Months among Adults 18 Years of Age and over, by Selected Characteristics: United States, Selected Years 1997–2010," in *Health, United States, 2011: With Special Feature on Socioeconomic Status and Health*, U.S. Department of Health and Human Services, Centers for Disease Control and Prevention, National Center for Health Statistics, May 2012, http://www.cdc.gov/nchs/data/hus/hus11.pdf (accessed June 13, 2012)

Sharing's (UNOS) Organ Procurement and Transplantation Network (OPTN; August 24, 2012, http://optn.transplant.hrsa.gov/), 28,538 transplants were performed in 2011. The UNOS compiles data on organ transplants, distributes organ donor cards, and maintains a registry of patients waiting for organ transplants. It reports that as of August 24, 2012, 118,579 Americans were waiting for a transplant. Because demand for organs continues to outpace supply, many patients die waiting for an organ transplant.

In February 2004 the UNOS/OPTN revised and strengthened its policies to guard against potential medical errors in transplant candidate and donor matching. The policy revisions were developed in response to a systematic review of a medical error in February 2003, when a teenager named Jésica Sántillan (1985–2003) died after receiving a heart-lung transplant from a blood-type incompatible donor at Duke University Medical Center. News of this tragic error immediately prompted transplant centers throughout the United States to perform internal audits of their protocols and procedures to ensure appropriate donor-recipient matching.

The key policy revisions included stipulations that:

- The blood type of each transplant candidate and donor must be independently verified by two staff members at the institution involved at the time blood type is entered into the national database.

- Each transplant program and organ procurement organization (OPO) must establish a protocol to ensure blood-type data for transplant candidates, and donors are accurately entered into the national database and communicated to transplant teams. The UNOS will verify the existence and effective use of these protocols during routine audits of OPOs and transplant programs.

- Organs must only be offered to candidates specifically identified on the computer-generated list of medically suitable transplant candidates for a given organ offer. If the organ offer is not accepted for any candidate on a given match run, an OPO may give transplant programs the opportunity to update transplant candidate data and rerun a match to see if any additional candidates are identified.

The UNOS resolved to continuously review national policies and procedures for organ placement and to recommend policy and procedure enhancements to maximize the efficiency of organ placement and the safety of transplant candidates and recipients. As of September 2012, there were no further reported occurrences of unintentional blood-type incompatible transplants.

The risks associated with organ transplant were, however, publicized once again in 2005 and 2006, when two transplant recipients from the same organ donor contracted West Nile virus, a potentially serious illness that is transmitted by mosquitoes. Even though 28,117 transplants were performed in the United States in 2005, according to the OPTN (August 24, 2012, http://optn .transplant.hrsa.gov/), and these two recipients were the only ones reported to have become ill from West Nile virus, they suffered the worst possible outcome. Both developed encephalitis (a brain infection), fell into coma, and died. These cases catalyzed transplant physicians and public health officials to intensify organ safety protocols and procedures.

Following a review of more than 200 reports of unexpected disease transmission through organ transplantation, Debbie L. Seem et al. published "PHS Guideline for Reducing Transmission of Human Immunodeficiency Virus (HIV), Hepatitis B Virus (HBV), and Hepatitis C Virus (HCV) through Solid Organ Transplantation" (September 21, 2011, http://www.regulations.gov/ #!docketDetail;dct=FR%252BPR%252BN%252BO% 252BSR;rpp=10;po=0;D=CDC-2011-0011) to reduce the risk and occurrence of unintended disease in organ recipients. The guidelines recommend enhancing donor screening practices and improving organ testing procedures to enable patients and physicians to make more informed risk-benefit decisions about organs that are available for transplant.

SURGICAL CENTERS AND URGENT CARE CENTERS

Ambulatory surgery centers (also called surgicenters) are equipped to perform routine surgical procedures that do not require an overnight hospital stay. A surgical center requires less sophisticated and expensive equipment than a hospital operating room. Minor surgery, such as biopsies, abortions, hernia repair, and many cosmetic surgery procedures, are performed at outpatient surgical centers. Most procedures are done under local anesthesia, and patients go home the same day.

Most ambulatory surgery centers are freestanding, but some are located on hospital campuses or are next to physicians' offices or clinics. Facilities are licensed by their state and must be equipped with at least one operating room, an area for preparing patients for procedures, a patient recovery area, and x-ray and clinical laboratory services. Also, surgical centers must have a registered nurse on the premises when patients are in the facility.

Urgent care centers (also called urgicenters) are usually operated by private, for-profit organizations and provide up to 24-hour care on a walk-in basis. These centers fill several special needs in a community. They provide convenient, timely, and easily accessible care in an emergency when the nearest hospital is miles away. The centers are normally open during the hours when most physicians' offices are closed, and they are economical to operate because they do not provide hospital beds. They usually treat problems such as cuts that require sutures, sprains and bruises from accidents, and various infections. Many provide inexpensive immunizations, and some offer routine health care for people who do not have a regular source of medical care. Urgent care may be more expensive than a visit to the family physician, but an urgent care center visit is usually less expensive than treatment from a traditional hospital ED.

Clinics in Stores and Malls

Christine K. Cassel of the American Board of Internal Medicine in Philadelphia, Pennsylvania, observes in "Retail Clinics and Drugstore Medicine" (*Journal of the American Medical Association*, vol. 307, no. 20, May 23, 2012) that the number of retail-based clinics has grown at a rate of about 20% per year to nearly 1,400 in 2012. Studies suggest that the care the clinics provide is comparable and costs less than care in other settings such as hospital EDs and produces high levels of patient satisfaction.

Retail-based clinics offer more than simply convenient locations. Many welcome walk-in patients and offer urgent care as well as extended hours, flat fees for physician visits, low-cost immunizations, and comfortable surroundings. They also emphasize unscheduled care much more than do most primary care practices. Furthermore, some clinics telephone 100% of their patients within 48 hours of being seen for care, a measure that serves to improve both quality of care and patient satisfaction.

Cassel notes that retail-based clinics are taking steps to better integrate into the health care system by sending electronic messages to the patient's physician following each visit and by forging relationships with other health care providers. She explains that critics of the retail-based clinics worry about potential conflicts of interest arising from clinics operating in commercial buildings in close proximity to pharmacies selling prescription and over-the-counter drugs, but observes that "these conflicts are inherent in many aspects of health care delivery" and "can and should be managed by transparency, oversight, and payment incentives that reward value rather than volume."

LONG-TERM-CARE FACILITIES

Families are still the major caretakers of older, dependent, and disabled members of American society. However, the number of people aged 65 years and older living in long-term-care facilities such as nursing homes is rising because the population in this age group is increasing rapidly. Even though many older people now live longer, healthier lives, the increase in overall length of life has expanded the need for long-term-care facilities.

Growth of the home health care industry during the early 1990s only slightly slowed the increase in the numbers of Americans entering nursing homes. Assisted-living and continuing-care retirement communities offer other alternatives to nursing home care. When it is possible, many older adults prefer to remain in the community and receive health care in their home.

Types of Nursing Homes

Nursing homes fall into three broad categories: residential care facilities, intermediate care facilities, and skilled nursing facilities. Each provides a different range and intensity of services:

- A residential care facility (RCF) normally provides meals and housekeeping for its residents, plus some basic medical monitoring, such as administering medications. This type of home is for people who are fairly independent and do not need constant medical attention but need help with tasks such as laundry and cleaning. Many RCFs also provide social activities and recreational programs for their residents.

- An intermediate care facility (ICF) offers room and board and nursing care as necessary for people who can no longer live independently. As in the RCF, exercise and social programs are provided, and some ICFs also offer physical therapy and rehabilitation programs.

- A skilled nursing facility (SNF) provides around-the-clock nursing care, plus on-call physician coverage. The SNF is for patients who need intensive nursing care and services such as occupational therapy, physical therapy, respiratory therapy, and rehabilitation.

Nursing Home Beds, Residents, and Occupancy Rates

The National Nursing Home Survey (NNHS) was a continuing series of national sample surveys of nursing homes, their residents, and their staff. The surveys were conducted in 1973–74, 1977, 1985, 1995, 1997, 1999, and 2004. Even though each survey focused on different aspects of care, they all provided some common basic information about nursing homes, their residents, and their staff from two perspectives: the provider of services and the recipient. Data about the facilities included characteristics such as size, ownership, Medicare/Medicaid certification, occupancy rate, number of days of care provided, and expenses. The surveys gathered demographic data, health status, and services received by nursing home residents. The last NNHS was conducted in 2004 and its results were published in *2004 National Nursing Home Survey* (December 2006, http://www.cdc.gov/nchs/data/nnhsd/nursinghomefacilities2006.pdf). The nursing homes included in this survey had at least three beds and were either certified (by Medicare or Medicaid) or had a state license to operate as a nursing home.

The National Center for Health Statistics (NCHS) reports in *Health, United States, 2011* that in 2010 the nation's 15,690 certified nursing homes housed more than 1.7 million beds and had occupancy rates of 82%. (See Table 3.4.) Besides certified nursing homes, there were 6,424 ICFs operating in 2010; of these, 438 provided long-term care.

The NNHS found that most residents of nursing homes are the "oldest old" (people aged 85 years and older). Out of the total 1.3 million nursing home residents aged 65 years and older in 2004, the so-called oldest old accounted for 674,500 (52%) of all nursing home residents.

TABLE 3.4

Nursing home beds, residents, and occupancy rates, selected years 1995–2010

State	Nursing homes				Beds			
	1995	2000	2009	2010	1995	2000	2009	2010
United States	**16,389**	**16,886**	**15,700**	**15,690**	**1,751,302**	**1,795,388**	**1,705,808**	**1,703,398**
Alabama	221	225	231	227	23,353	25,248	26,854	26,656
Alaska	15	15	15	15	814	821	716	682
Arizona	152	150	135	139	16,162	17,458	16,073	16,460
Arkansas	256	255	230	232	29,952	25,715	24,413	24,548
California	1,382	1,369	1,252	1,239	140,203	131,762	121,699	121,167
Colorado	219	225	210	213	19,912	20,240	19,867	20,259
Connecticut	267	259	240	239	32,827	32,433	29,306	29,255
Delaware	42	43	46	47	4,739	4,906	4,953	4,990
District of Columbia	19	20	19	19	3,206	3,078	2,765	2,775
Florida	627	732	676	678	72,656	83,365	81,887	82,226
Georgia	352	363	360	360	38,097	39,817	39,993	39,960
Hawaii	34	45	47	48	2,513	4,006	4,241	4,303
Idaho	76	84	79	79	5,747	6,181	6,176	6,153
Illinois	827	869	794	787	103,230	110,766	102,123	101,061
Indiana	556	564	504	506	59,538	56,762	57,450	57,721
Iowa	419	467	447	443	39,959	37,034	33,301	32,842
Kansas	429	392	341	340	30,016	27,067	25,732	25,598
Kentucky	288	307	287	285	23,221	25,341	25,996	26,063
Louisiana	337	337	282	281	37,769	39,430	35,602	36,098
Maine	132	126	109	109	9,243	8,248	7,113	7,127
Maryland	218	255	231	231	28,394	31,495	29,100	29,004
Massachusetts	550	526	429	427	54,532	56,030	49,126	49,175
Michigan	432	439	428	428	49,473	50,696	47,271	47,054
Minnesota	432	433	385	385	43,865	42,149	32,956	32,339
Mississippi	183	190	202	203	16,059	17,068	18,458	18,589
Missouri	546	551	513	514	52,679	54,829	55,361	55,393
Montana	100	104	90	88	7,210	7,667	7,053	6,991
Nebraska	231	236	225	222	18,169	17,877	16,214	16,065
Nevada	42	51	49	50	3,998	5,547	5,719	5,856
New Hampshire	74	83	80	79	7,412	7,837	7,742	7,692
New Jersey	300	361	360	360	43,967	52,195	51,159	51,101
New Mexico	83	80	70	70	6,969	7,289	6,760	6,769
New York	624	665	640	635	107,750	120,514	121,769	117,984
North Carolina	391	410	423	424	38,322	41,376	44,106	44,392
North Dakota	87	88	84	85	7,125	6,954	6,339	6,438
Ohio	943	1,009	961	960	106,884	105,038	93,359	93,043
Oklahoma	405	392	316	314	33,918	33,903	29,269	28,932
Oregon	161	150	137	137	13,885	13,500	12,313	12,218
Pennsylvania	726	770	711	710	92,625	95,063	88,861	88,829
Rhode Island	94	99	86	86	9,612	10,271	8,818	8,802
South Carolina	166	178	177	184	16,682	18,102	19,085	19,474
South Dakota	114	114	109	110	8,296	7,844	6,900	7,932
Tennessee	322	349	318	318	37,074	38,593	37,185	37,279
Texas	1,266	1,215	1,165	1,173	123,056	125,052	128,984	130,665
Utah	91	93	96	99	7,101	7,651	8,027	8,255
Vermont	23	44	40	40	1,862	3,743	3,293	3,276
Virginia	271	278	281	286	30,070	30,595	31,972	32,152
Washington	285	277	233	229	28,464	25,905	22,050	21,837
West Virginia	129	139	128	127	10,903	11,413	10,843	10,840
Wisconsin	413	420	391	392	48,754	46,395	36,482	36,113
Wyoming	37	40	38	38	3,035	3,119	2,974	2,965

In December 2008 the Centers for Medicare and Medicaid Services (CMS) began the Five-Star Quality Rating System (https://www.cms.gov/CertificationandComplianc/13_FSQRS.asp) for the nation's certified nursing homes. The CMS also provides a nursing home checklist (http://www.medicare.gov/Nursing/Checklist.pdf) to help consumers assess and compare nursing homes. Furthermore, the CMS offers the website "Nursing Home Compare" (http://www.medicare.gov/NHCompare/Include/DataSection/Questions/ProximitySearch.asp), which contains detailed information about every Medicare- and Medicaid-certified nursing home in the country.

Diversification of Nursing Homes

To remain competitive with home health care and the increasing array of alternative living arrangements for the elderly, many nursing homes offer alternative services and programs. These services include adult day care and visiting nurse services for people who still live at home. Other programs include respite plans that allow caregivers who need to travel for business or vacation to leave an elderly relative in the nursing home temporarily.

One of the most popular nontraditional services is subacute care, which is comprehensive inpatient treatment

TABLE 3.4

Nursing home beds, residents, and occupancy rates, selected years 1995–2010 [CONTINUED]

State	Residents				Occupancy rate*			
	1995	2000	2009	2010	1995	2000	2009	2010
United States	**1,479,550**	**1,480,076**	**1,401,718**	**1,396,473**	**84.5**	**82.4**	**82.2**	**82.0**
Alabama	21,691	23,089	23,186	22,968	92.9	91.4	86.3	86.2
Alaska	634	595	633	641	77.9	72.5	88.4	94.0
Arizona	12,382	13,253	11,908	11,878	76.6	75.9	74.1	72.2
Arkansas	20,823	19,317	17,801	17,864	69.5	75.1	72.9	72.8
California	109,805	106,460	102,747	102,591	78.3	80.8	84.4	84.7
Colorado	17,055	17,045	16,288	16,302	85.7	84.2	82.0	80.5
Connecticut	29,948	29,657	26,253	25,972	91.2	91.4	89.6	88.8
Delaware	3,819	3,900	4,256	4,145	80.6	79.5	85.9	83.1
District of Columbia	2,576	2,858	2,531	2,595	80.3	92.9	91.5	93.5
Florida	61,845	69,050	71,657	71,907	85.1	82.8	87.5	87.5
Georgia	35,933	36,559	34,899	34,704	94.3	91.8	87.3	86.8
Hawaii	2,413	3,558	3,841	3,880	96.0	88.8	90.6	90.2
Idaho	4,697	4,640	4,419	4,388	81.7	75.1	71.6	71.3
Illinois	83,696	83,604	75,673	75,224	81.1	75.5	74.1	74.4
Indiana	44,328	42,328	39,190	39,167	74.5	74.6	68.2	67.9
Iowa	27,506	29,204	25,814	25,463	68.8	78.9	77.5	77.5
Kansas	25,140	22,230	19,029	18,985	83.8	82.1	74.0	74.2
Kentucky	20,696	22,730	23,318	23,252	89.1	89.7	89.7	89.2
Louisiana	32,493	30,735	25,077	25,198	86.0	77.9	70.4	69.8
Maine	8,587	7,298	6,485	6,417	92.9	88.5	91.2	90.0
Maryland	24,716	25,629	25,025	24,816	87.0	81.4	86.0	85.6
Massachusetts	49,765	49,805	43,227	42,880	91.3	88.9	88.0	87.2
Michigan	43,271	42,615	40,306	39,894	87.5	84.1	85.3	84.8
Minnesota	41,163	38,813	30,073	29,434	93.8	92.1	91.3	91.0
Mississippi	15,247	15,815	16,294	16,489	94.9	92.7	88.3	88.7
Missouri	39,891	38,586	37,588	37,839	75.7	70.4	67.9	68.3
Montana	6,415	5,973	5,077	4,943	89.0	77.9	72.0	70.7
Nebraska	16,166	14,989	12,627	12,630	89.0	83.8	77.9	78.6
Nevada	3,645	3,657	4,699	4,735	91.2	65.9	82.2	80.9
New Hampshire	6,877	7,158	6,941	6,932	92.8	91.3	89.7	90.1
New Jersey	40,397	45,837	45,788	45,917	91.9	87.8	89.5	89.9
New Mexico	6,051	6,503	5,569	5,555	86.8	89.2	82.4	82.1
New York	103,409	112,957	109,867	109,044	96.0	93.7	90.2	92.4
North Carolina	35,511	36,658	37,587	37,199	92.7	88.6	85.2	83.8
North Dakota	6,868	6,343	5,777	5,629	96.4	91.2	91.1	87.4
Ohio	79,026	81,946	80,185	79,234	73.9	78.0	85.9	85.2
Oklahoma	26,377	23,833	19,209	19,227	77.8	70.3	65.6	66.5
Oregon	11,673	9,990	7,708	7,549	84.1	74.0	62.6	61.8
Pennsylvania	84,843	83,880	80,562	81,014	91.6	88.2	90.7	91.2
Rhode Island	8,823	9,041	8,040	8,043	91.8	88.0	91.2	91.4
South Carolina	14,568	15,739	17,148	17,133	87.3	86.9	89.9	88.0
South Dakota	7,926	7,059	6,476	6,497	95.5	90.0	93.9	81.9
Tennessee	33,929	34,714	31,876	31,927	91.5	89.9	85.7	85.6
Texas	89,354	85,275	90,534	91,099	72.6	68.2	70.2	69.7
Utah	5,832	5,703	5,358	5,361	82.1	74.5	66.8	64.9
Vermont	1,792	3,349	2,980	2,931	96.2	89.5	90.5	89.5
Virginia	28,119	27,091	28,392	28,314	93.5	88.5	88.8	88.1
Washington	24,954	21,158	18,188	18,065	87.7	81.7	82.5	82.7
West Virginia	10,216	10,334	9,613	9,557	93.7	90.5	88.7	88.2
Wisconsin	43,998	38,911	31,619	30,618	90.2	83.9	86.7	84.8
Wyoming	2,661	2,605	2,380	2,427	87.7	83.5	80.0	81.9

—Data not available.

*Percentage of beds occupied (number of nursing home residents per 100 nursing home beds).

Notes: Annual numbers of nursing homes, beds, and residents are based on the Online Survey Certification and Reporting Database reporting cycle. Data for additional years are available.

SOURCE: "Table 120. Nursing Homes, Beds, Residents, and Occupancy Rates, by State: United States, Selected Years 1995–2010," in *Health, United States, 2011: With Special Feature on Socioeconomic Status and Health*, U.S. Department of Health and Human Services, Centers for Disease Control and Prevention, National Center for Health Statistics, May 2012, http://www.cdc.gov/nchs/data/hus/hus11.pdf (accessed June 13, 2012). Nongovernment data from the Cowles Research Group.

for people recovering from acute illnesses such as pneumonia, injuries such as a broken hip, and chronic diseases such as arthritis that do not require intensive, hospital-level treatment. This level of care also enables nursing homes to expand their markets by offering services to younger patients.

Innovation Improves Quality of Nursing Home Care

Even though industry observers and the media frequently raise concerns about the care provided in nursing homes and publicize instances of elder abuse and other quality of care issues, several organizations have actively sought to develop models of health service delivery that improve the clinical care and quality of life for nursing home residents. In *Evaluation of the Wellspring Model for Improving Nursing Home Quality* (August 2002, http://www.cmwf.org/usr_doc/stone_wellspringevaluation.pdf), a benchmark report that examines one such model in eastern Wisconsin, Robyn Stone et al. evaluate the Wellspring model of nursing home quality improvement.

Wellspring is a group of not-for-profit nursing homes that are governed by a group called the Wellspring Alliance. Founded in 1994, the alliance aims to improve the clinical care delivered to its nursing home residents and the work environment for its employees. Based on the Wellspring philosophy that education and collaboration are paramount to success, the program began by equipping nursing home personnel with the skills needed to perform their jobs and by organizing employees in teams working toward shared goals. The Wellspring model of service delivery uses a multidisciplinary clinical team approach (nurse practitioners, social service professionals, food service personnel, nursing assistants, and facility and housekeeping personnel) to solve problems and develop approaches to better meet residents' needs. Each of these teams represents an important innovation because it allows health professionals and other workers to interact as peers and share resources, information, and decision making in a cooperative, supportive environment.

Stone et al. observe that there was more cooperation, responsibility, and accountability within the teams and the institutions than what was noted at other comparable facilities. Besides finding a strong organizational culture that seemed committed to quality patient care, the researchers document measurable improvements in specific areas including:

- Wellspring facilities had lower rates of staff turnover than comparable Wisconsin facilities during the same period, probably because Wellspring workers felt valued by management and experienced greater job satisfaction than other nursing home personnel

- The Wellspring model did not require additional resources to institute, and Wellspring facilities operated at lower costs than comparable facilities

- Wellspring facilities' performance, as measured by a federal survey, improved

- Wellspring personnel appeared more attentive to residents' needs and problems and sought to anticipate and promptly resolve problems

- An organizational commitment to training and shared decision making, along with improved quality of interactions and relationships among staff and between staff and residents, significantly contributed to enhanced quality of life for residents

In *A Process Evaluation of the Implementation of the Lutheran Wellspring Alliance of the Carolinas* (August 2008, http://www.leadingage.org/), a report that examines the evolution and implementation of the Wellspring model of nursing home quality improvement, Natasha Bryant, Janice Heineman, and Robyn Stone evaluate how adopting the Wellspring model changed the lives of residents, staff, and families in nine Lutheran Carolina nursing homes. The researchers assert, "The nursing home workers interviewed believed that the Wellspring program improved the quality of life and care for residents. The Wellspring program provided workers with best practices and tools that enabled them to better care for residents. The staff, therefore, has a better understanding of the overall care process for the resident and can provide better care." Bryant, Heineman, and Stone also observe that a higher percentage of family members rated the facilities as "excellent" or "good" after the Wellspring model was implemented.

Mary Jane Koren of the Commonwealth Fund enumerates in "Person-Centered Care for Nursing Home Residents: The Culture-Change Movement" (*Health Affairs*, vol. 29, no. 2, February 2010) the principles of the culture-change movement championed by organizations such as Wellspring. These include:

- Resident direction—supporting residents to make their own choices and decisions about personal issues such as food choices, clothing, and activities

- Homelike environment—using strategies such as replacing larger institutional units with smaller groups of residents and eliminating public address systems

- Relationship cultivation—improving continuity of care by having the same staff provide care to a resident

- Staff empowerment—by providing necessary training and granting them authority, staff are better able to respond to residents' needs

- Collaborative decision making—direct caregivers, working in teams, should have the authority to make decisions about residents' care

- Quality improvement—culture change should be understood as continuous performance improvement

Koren observes that about one-third of nursing homes have adopted some culture-change practices and an additional one-third are planning to make some changes. She encourages policy changes to support the wider adoption of comprehensive culture change.

MENTAL HEALTH FACILITIES

In earlier centuries mental illness was often considered to be a sign of possession by the devil or, at best, a moral weakness. A change in these attitudes began during the late 18th century, when mental illness was perceived to be a treatable condition. It was then that the concept of asylums was developed, not only to lock the mentally ill away but also to provide them with "relief" from the conditions they found troubling.

In the 21st century mental health care is provided in a variety of treatment settings by different types of organizations. The following mental health organizations offer diagnostic and therapeutic mental health services:

- A psychiatric hospital (public or private) provides 24-hour inpatient care to people with mental illnesses in a hospital setting. It may also offer 24-hour residential care and less than 24-hour care, but these are not requirements. Psychiatric hospitals are operated under state, county, private for-profit, and private not-for-profit auspices.

- General hospitals with separate psychiatric services, units, or designated beds are under governmental or nongovernmental auspices and maintain assigned staff for 24-hour inpatient care, 24-hour residential care, and less than 24-hour care (outpatient care or partial hospitalization) to provide mental health diagnosis, evaluation, and treatment.

- Veterans Administration (VA) hospitals are operated by the U.S. Department of Veterans Affairs and include VA general hospital psychiatric services and VA psychiatric outpatient clinics that exclusively serve people entitled to VA benefits.

- Outpatient mental health clinics that provide only ambulatory mental health services. Generally, a psychiatrist has overall medical responsibility for clients and establishes the philosophy and orientation of the mental health program.

- Community mental health centers were funded under the Federal Community Mental Health Centers Act of 1963 and subsequent amendments to the act. During the early 1980s, when the federal government reverted to funding mental health services through block grants to the states rather than by funding them directly, the federal government stopped tracking these mental health organizations individually, and statistical reports include them in the category "all other mental health organizations." This category also includes freestanding psychiatric outpatient clinics, freestanding partial care organizations, and multiservice mental health organizations such as residential treatment centers. These so-called community mental health centers have sliding scale fees and accept Medicaid, Medicare, private health insurance, and private fee-for-service (paid for each visit, procedure, or treatment that is delivered) payment. Mental health care is also available from not-for-profit mental health or counseling services offered by health and social service agencies, such as Catholic Social Services, family and children's service agencies,

Jewish Family Services, and Lutheran Social Services, that are staffed by qualified mental health professionals to provide counseling services.

- Residential treatment centers for emotionally disturbed children serve children and youth primarily under the age of 18 years, provide 24-hour residential services, and offer a clinical program that is directed by a psychiatrist, psychologist, social worker, or psychiatric nurse who holds a master's or doctorate degree.

Where Are the Mentally Ill?

The chronically mentally ill reside in mental hospitals, in intermediate care facilities, or in community settings, such as with families, in boarding homes and shelters, in single-room-occupancy hotels (usually inexpensive hotels or boardinghouses), in prison, or even on the streets as part of the homeless population. The institutionalized mentally ill are those people with psychiatric diagnoses who have lived in mental hospitals for more than one year or those with diagnosed mental illness who are living in nursing homes.

Declining mental health expenditures have resulted in fewer available services for specific populations of the mentally ill, particularly those who could benefit from inpatient or residential care. Even for people without conditions requiring institutional care there are barriers to access. The U.S. surgeon general's landmark report *Mental Health: A Report of the Surgeon General, 1999* (1999, http://profiles.nlm.nih.gov/ps/retrieve/Resource Metadata/NNBBHS) describes the U.S. mental health service system as largely uncoordinated and fragmented, in part because it involves so many different sectors—health and social welfare agencies, public and private hospitals, housing, criminal justice, and education—and because it is funded through many different sources. Finally, inequalities in insurance coverage for mental health, coupled with the stigma associated with mental illness and treatment, have also limited access to services.

The NCHS reveals in *Health, United States, 2011* that the number of mental health organizations for 24-hour inpatient treatment steadily declined from 3,942 in 1990 to 3,130 in 2008. (See Table 3.5.) Except for Department of Veterans Affairs medical centers and residential treatment centers for children, all other service sites and types of organizations diminished in capacity. The number of beds per 100,000 civilian population fell from 128.5 in 1990 to just 78.6 in 2008. There was a similar decline in the number of ICFs specializing in psychiatric care—the number of beds declined from 689 in 1995 to 508 in 2010. This decline was not necessarily a result of better treatment for the mentally ill but a consequence of reduced funding for inpatient facilities. Many of the patients who were once housed in mental institutions (including some who had been lifelong residents in these facilities) were forced to fend for themselves on the streets or in prison.

TABLE 3.5

Mental health organizations and beds for 24-hour hospital and residential treatment, by type of organization, selected years 1986–2008

Type of organization	1986	1990	1994	2000	2002	2004	2008[a]
	Number of mental health organizations						
All organizations	3,512	3,942	3,853	3,211	3,044	2,891	3,130
State psychiatric hospitals	285	278	270	229	227	237	241
Private psychiatric hospitals	314	464	432	271	255	264	256
Nonfederal general hospitals with psychiatric services	1,351	1,577	1,539	1,325	1,231	1,230	1,292
Department of Veterans Affairs medical centers[b]	139	131	136	134	132	—	130
Residential treatment centers for children with emotional disturbance	437	501	472	476	510	458	538
All other organizations[c]	986	991	1,004	776	689	702	673
	Number of beds						
All organizations	267,613	325,529	293,139	214,186	211,040	212,231	239,014
State psychiatric hospitals	119,033	102,307	84,063	61,833	57,314	57,034	37,450
Private psychiatric hospitals	30,201	45,952	42,742	26,402	24,996	28,422	25,406
Nonfederal general hospitals with psychiatric services	45,808	53,576	53,455	40,410	40,520	41,403	54,390
Department of Veterans Affairs medical centers[b]	26,874	24,779	21,346	8,989	9,581	—	11,991
Residential treatment centers for children with emotional disturbance	24,547	35,170	32,691	33,508	39,407	33,835	50,063
All other organizations[c]	21,150	63,745	58,842	43,044	39,222	51,536	59,715
	Beds per 100,000 civilian population[d]						
All organizations	111.7	128.5	110.9	74.8	72.2	71.2	78.6
State psychiatric hospitals	49.7	40.4	31.8	21.6	19.6	19.1	12.3
Private psychiatric hospitals	12.6	18.1	16.2	9.2	8.6	9.5	8.4
Nonfederal general hospitals with psychiatric services	19.1	21.2	20.2	14.1	13.9	13.9	17.9
Department of Veterans Affairs medical centers[b]	11.2	9.8	8.1	3.1	3.3	—	3.9
Residential treatment centers for children with emotional disturbance	10.3	13.9	12.4	11.7	13.5	11.4	16.5
All other organizations[c]	8.8	25.2	22.2	15.0	13.4	17.3	19.6

Notes: Data for additional years are available.
—Data not available.
[a]Data for 2008 are not strictly comparable with data for earlier years due to the survey redesign, including a new name, National Survey of Mental Health Treatment Facilities.
[b]Department of Veterans Affairs medical centers (VA general hospital psychiatric services and VA psychiatric outpatient clinics) were not included in the 2004 survey.
[c]Includes residential treatment facilities for adults, freestanding psychiatric outpatient clinics, partial care organizations, and multiservice mental health organizations.
[d]Civilian population estimates for 2000 and beyond are based on the 2000 census as of July 1; population estimates for 1992–1998 are 1990 postcensal estimates.

SOURCE: "Table 117. Mental Health Organizations and Beds for 24-Hour Hospital and Residential Treatment, by Type of Organization: United States, Selected Years 1986–2008," in *Health, United States, 2011: With Special Feature on Socioeconomic Status and Health*, U.S. Department of Health and Human Services, Centers for Disease Control and Prevention, National Center for Health Statistics, May 2012, http://www.cdc.gov/nchs/data/hus/hus11.pdf (accessed June 13, 2012)

Besides mental health units or beds in acute care medical/surgical hospitals and physicians' offices, mental health care and treatment is offered in the offices of other mental health clinicians such as psychologists, clinical social workers, and marriage and family therapists, as well as in other settings. Private psychiatric hospitals provide outpatient mental health evaluation and therapy in day programs as well as inpatient care. Like acute care hospitals, these facilities are accredited by the Joint Commission on Accreditation of Healthcare Organizations and may offer outpatient services by way of referral to a local network of qualified mental health providers.

National Goals for Mental Health Service Delivery

Healthy People 2020 (December 2010, http://healthy people.gov/2020/topicsobjectives2020/pdfs/HP2020objec tives.pdf) is a set of health objectives for the United States to achieve during the first two decades of the 21st century. Twelve of the 600 health objectives

enumerated in *Healthy People 2020* relate to mental health and mental disorders. Even though nearly all the objectives intend to reduce the incidence and prevalence of mental illness in the United States and improve access to care and treatment, several address new emerging health problems in specific populations such as veterans who have experienced physical and mental trauma and people affected by natural disasters, and mental health disorders of older adults such as mood disorders and dementia (impaired memory, reasoning, planning, and behavior resulting from the gradual death of brain cells).

Emphasizing prevention and access to appropriate, quality mental health treatment is intended to:

• Reduce the suicide rate

• Reduce suicide attempts by adolescents

• Increase the proportion of homeless adults with mental health problems who receive mental health services

- Reduce the proportion of adolescents who engage in disordered eating behaviors in an attempt to control their weight

- Reduce the proportion of persons who experience major depressive episode [a serious depression with symptoms such as despondency, feelings of worthlessness, and even suicidal thoughts]

- Increase the proportion of primary care facilities that provide mental health treatment onsite or by paid referral

- Increase the proportion of children with mental health problems who receive treatment

- Increase the proportion of juvenile residential facilities that screen admissions for mental health problems

- Increase the proportion of persons with serious mental illness who are employed

- Increase the proportion of adults with mental disorders who receive treatment

- Increase the proportion of persons with co-occurring substance abuse and mental disorders who receive treatment for both disorders

- Increase the proportion of homeless adults with mental health problems who receive mental health services

- Increase depression screening by primary care providers

HOME HEALTH CARE

The concept of home health care began as postacute care after hospitalization, an alternative to longer, costlier lengths of stay in regular hospitals. Home health care services have grown tremendously since the 1980s, when prospective payment (payments made before, rather than after, care is received) for Medicare patients sharply reduced hospital lengths of stay. During the mid-1980s Medicare began reimbursing hospitals using a rate scale based on diagnosis-related groups—hospitals received a fixed amount for providing services to Medicare patients based on their diagnoses. This form of payment gave hospitals powerful financial incentives to use fewer resources because they could keep the difference between the prospective payment and the amount they actually spent to provide care. Hospitals experienced losses when patients had longer lengths of stay and used more services than were covered by the standardized diagnosis-related group prospective payment.

According to the article "Home Health Care" (*Family Economics and Nutrition Review*, Spring 1996), home health care grew faster during the early 1990s than any other segment of health services. Its growth may be attributable to the observation that in many cases caring for patients at home is preferable to and more cost effective than care provided in a hospital, nursing home, or some other residential facility. Oftentimes, older adults are more comfortable and much happier living in their own home or with family members. Disabled people may also be able to function better at home with limited assistance than in a residential setting with full-time monitoring.

Home health care agencies provide a wide variety of services. Services range from helping with activities of daily living, such as bathing, doing light housekeeping, and making meals, to skilled nursing care, such as the nursing care needed by AIDS or cancer patients. The number of Medicare-certified home health agencies has varied in response to reimbursement, growing from 2,924 in 1980 to 8,437 in 1996, then declining to 6,928 in 2003. (See Table 3.6.) In 2009 the number of Medicare-certified home health agencies rose to 10,184, the highest it has ever been.

In 1972 Medicare extended home health care coverage to people under 65 years of age only if they were disabled or suffered from end-stage renal disease. Before 2000 Medicare coverage for home health care was limited to patients immediately following discharge from the hospital. By 2000 Medicare covered beneficiaries' home health care services with no requirement for previous hospitalization. There were also no limits to the number of professional visits or to the length of coverage. As long as the patient's condition warranted it, the following services were provided:

- Part-time or intermittent skilled nursing and home health aide services

- Speech-language pathology services

- Physical and occupational therapy

- Medical social services

- Medical supplies

- Durable medical equipment (with a 20% co-payment)

Over time, the population receiving home health care services has changed. Since 2000 much of home health care is associated with rehabilitation from critical illnesses, and fewer users are long-term patients with chronic conditions. This changing pattern of utilization reflects a shift from longer-term care for chronic conditions to short-term, postacute care. Compared with postacute care users, the long-term patients are older, more functionally disabled, more likely to be incontinent, and more expensive to serve.

Medicare Limits Home Health Care Services

The Balanced Budget Act of 1997 cut approximately $16.2 billion from the federal government's home health care expenditures over a period of five years. The act sought to return home health care to its original concept of short-term care plus skilled nursing and therapy

TABLE 3.6

Medicare-certified providers and suppliers, selected years 1975–2009

Providers or suppliers	1975	1980	1985	1990	1996	2000	2003	2005	2007	2009
					Number of providers or suppliers					
Skilled nursing facilities	—	5,052	6,451	8,937	—	14,841	14,838	15,006	15,054	15,071
Home health agencies	2,242	2,924	5,679	5,730	8,437	7,857	6,928	8,090	9,024	10,184
Clinical Laboratory Improvement Amendments facilities	—	—	—	—	159,907	171,018	176,947	196,296	206,065	218,139
End-stage renal disease facilities	—	999	1,393	1,937	2,876	3,787	4,309	4,755	5,095	5,476
Outpatient physical therapy	117	419	854	1,195	2,302	2,867	2,961	2,962	2,915	2,640
Portable X-ray	132	216	308	443	555	666	641	553	550	546
Rural health clinics	—	391	428	551	2,775	3,453	3,306	3,661	3,781	3,752
Comprehensive outpatient rehabilitation facilities	—	—	72	186	307	522	587	634	539	406
Ambulatory surgical centers	—	—	336	1,197	2,112	2,894	3,597	4,445	4,964	5,260
Hospices	—	—	164	825	1,927	2,326	2,323	2,872	3,255	3,405

—Data not available.
Notes: Data for 1975–1990 are as of July 1. Data for 1996–1999 and 2004–2009 are as of December 31. Data for 2001, 2002, and 2003 are as of December 2000, December 2001, and December 2002, respectively. Data for additional years are available.

SOURCE: "Table 122. Medicare-Certified Providers and Suppliers: United States, Selected Years 1975–2009," in *Health, United States, 2011: With Special Feature on Socioeconomic Status and Health*, U.S. Department of Health and Human Services, Centers for Disease Control and Prevention, National Center for Health Statistics, May 2012, http://www.cdc.gov/nchs/data/hus/hus11.pdf (accessed June 13, 2012)

services. As a result of this shift away from personal care and "custodial care" services and toward short-term, skilled nursing services, some Medicare beneficiaries who received home health care lost coverage for certain personal care services, such as assistance with bathing, dressing, and eating.

The Balanced Budget Act sharply curtailed the growth in home health care spending, which affected health care providers. Nonetheless, the aging population and the financial imperative to prevent or minimize institutionalization (hospitalization or placement in a long-term-care facility) combined to generate increasing expenditures for home health care services. Medicare expenditures for home health care rose from $4 billion in 2000 to $7 billion in 2010, which represented 2.8% of Medicare expenditures. (See Table 3.7.) In contrast, payments to SNFs accounted for 10.8% ($26.9 billion) of expenditures in 2010, and inpatient hospital expenditures were 54.9% ($136.1 billion) of the total.

HOSPICE CARE

In medieval times hospices were refuges for the sick, the needy, and travelers. The modern hospice movement developed in response to the need to provide humane care to terminally ill patients, while at the same time offering support to their families. British physician Cicely Saunders (1918–2005) pioneered the hospice concept in Britain during the late 1960s and helped introduce it in the United States during the 1970s. The care provided by hospice workers is called palliative care, and it aims to relieve patients' pain and the accompanying symptoms of terminal illness without seeking to cure the illness.

Hospice is a philosophy, an approach to care for the dying, and it is not necessarily a physical facility. Hospice may refer to a place—a freestanding facility or a designated floor in a hospital or nursing home—or to a program such as hospice home care, where a team of health professionals helps the dying patient and family at home. Hospice teams may involve physicians, nurses, social workers, pastoral counselors, and trained volunteers. The goal of hospice care is to provide support and care for people at the end of life, enabling them to remain as comfortable as possible.

Hospice workers consider the patient and family as the "unit of care" and focus their efforts on attending to emotional, psychological, and spiritual needs as well as to physical comfort and well-being. The programs provide respite care, which offers relief at any time for families who may be overwhelmed and exhausted by the demands of caregiving and may be neglecting their own needs for rest and relaxation. Finally, hospice programs work to prepare relatives and friends for the loss of their loved ones. Hospice offers bereavement support groups and counseling to help deal with grief and may even help with funeral arrangements.

The hospice concept is different from most other health care services because it focuses on care rather than on cure. Hospice workers try to minimize the two greatest fears associated with dying: fear of isolation and fear of pain. Potent, effective medications are offered to patients in pain, with the goal of controlling pain without impairing alertness so that patients may be as comfortable as possible.

Hospice care also emphasizes living life to its fullest. Patients are encouraged to stay active for as long as

TABLE 3.7

Medicare enrollees and expenditures by type of service, selected years 1970–2010

Medicare program and type of service	1970	1980	1990	1995	2000	2003	2004	2005	2008	2009[a]	2010[a]
Enrollees					Number in millions						
Total Medicare[b]	**20.4**	**28.4**	**34.3**	**37.6**	**39.7**	**41.2**	**41.9**	**42.6**	**45.5**	**46.6**	**47.5**
Hospital insurance	20.1	28.0	33.7	37.2	39.3	40.7	41.5	42.2	45.1	46.2	47.1
Supplementary medical insurance (SMI)[c]	19.5	27.3	32.6	35.6	37.3	38.6	—	—	—	—	—
Part B	19.5	27.3	32.6	35.6	37.3	38.6	39.1	39.8	42.0	42.9	43.8
Part D[d]	—	—	—	—	—	—	1.2	1.8	32.4	33.5	34.5
Expenditures					Amount in billions						
Total Medicare	**$7.5**	**$36.8**	**$111.0**	**$184.2**	**$221.8**	**$280.8**	**$308.9**	**$336.4**	**$468.1**	**$509.0**	**$522.8**
Total hospital insurance (HI)	5.3	25.6	67.0	117.6	131.1	154.6	170.6	182.9	235.6	242.5	247.9
HI payments to managed care organizations[e]	—	0.0	2.7	6.7	21.4	19.5	20.8	24.9	50.6	59.4	60.7
HI payments for fee-for-service utilization	5.1	25.0	63.4	109.5	105.1	134.5	146.5	156.6	172.8	179.5	183.3
Inpatient hospital	4.8	24.1	56.9	82.3	87.1	109.1	117.0	123.3	130.2	134.0	136.1
Skilled nursing facility	0.2	0.4	2.5	9.1	11.1	14.8	17.2	19.3	24.6	26.3	26.9
Home health agency	0.1	0.5	3.7	16.2	4.0	4.9	5.4	6.0	6.7	7.0	7.0
Hospice	—	—	0.3	1.9	2.9	5.7	6.8	8.0	11.3	12.2	13.2
Other[f]	—	—	—	—	—	—	—	—	—	—	0.1
Home health agency transfer[g]	—	—	—	—	1.7	−2.2	—	—	—	—	—
Medicare Advantage premiums[h]	—	—	—	—	—	—	—	—	0.1	0.1	0.2
Accounting error (Calendar year 2005–2008)[i]	—	—	—	—	—	—	—	−1.9	8.5	—	—
Administrative expenses[j]	0.2	0.5	0.9	1.4	2.9	2.8	3.3	3.3	3.6	3.5	3.8
Total supplementary medical insurance (SMI)[c]	2.2	11.2	44.0	66.6	90.7	126.1	138.3	153.5	232.6	266.5	274.9
Total Part B	2.2	11.2	44.0	66.6	90.7	126.1	137.9	152.4	183.3	205.7	212.9
Part B payments to managed care organizations[e]	0.0	0.2	2.8	6.6	18.4	17.3	18.7	22.0	48.1	53.4	55.2
Part B payments for fee-for-service utilization[k]	1.9	10.4	39.6	58.4	72.2	104.3	116.2	125.0	140.5	149.0	154.3
Physician/supplies[l]	1.8	8.2	29.6	—	—	—	—	—	—	—	—
Outpatient hospital[m]	0.1	1.9	8.5	—	—	—	—	—	—	—	—
Independent laboratory[n]	0.0	0.1	1.5	—	—	—	—	—	—	—	—
Physician fee schedule	—	—	—	31.7	37.0	48.3	54.1	57.7	60.6	62.4	64.5
Durable medical equipment	—	—	—	3.7	4.7	7.5	7.7	8.0	8.6	8.0	8.3
Laboratory[o]	—	—	—	4.3	4.0	5.5	6.1	6.3	7.2	8.1	8.4
Other[p]	—	—	—	9.9	13.6	22.6	25.0	26.7	29.6	31.9	32.6
Hospital[q]	—	—	—	8.7	8.4	15.3	17.4	19.3	24.2	27.0	28.4
Home health agency	0.0	0.2	0.1	0.2	4.5	5.1	5.9	7.1	10.3	11.6	12.1
Home health agency transfer[g]	—	—	—	—	−1.7	2.2	—	—	—	—	—
Medicare Advantage premiums[h]	—	—	—	—	—	—	—	—	0.1	0.1	0.2
Accounting error (Calendar year 2005–2008)[i]	—	—	—	—	—	—	—	1.9	−8.5	—	—
Administrative expenses[j]	0.2	0.6	1.5	1.6	1.8	2.4	2.8	2.8	3.1	3.2	3.2
Part D start-up costs[r]	—	—	—	—	—	—	0.2	0.7	0.0	—	—
Total Part D[d]	—	—	—	—	—	—	0.4	1.1	49.3	60.8	62.0
					Percent distribution of expenditures						
Total hospital insurance (HI)	100.0	100.0	100.0	100.0	100.0	100.0	100.0	100.0	100.0	100.0	100.0
HI payments to managed care organizations[e]	—	0.0	4.0	5.7	16.3	12.6	12.2	13.6	21.5	24.5	24.5
HI payments for fee-for-service utilization	97.0	97.9	94.6	93.1	80.2	87.0	85.9	85.6	73.4	74.0	73.9
Inpatient hospital	91.4	94.3	85.0	70.0	66.4	70.6	68.6	67.4	55.3	55.3	54.9
Skilled nursing facility	4.7	1.5	3.7	7.8	8.5	9.6	10.1	10.6	10.5	10.9	10.8
Home health agency	1.0	2.1	5.5	13.8	3.1	3.1	3.2	3.3	2.8	2.9	2.8
Hospice	—	—	0.5	1.6	2.2	3.7	4.0	4.4	4.8	5.0	5.3
Other	—	—	—	—	—	—	—	—	—	—	0.1
Home health agency transfer[g]	—	—	—	—	1.3	−1.4	—	—	—	—	—
Medicare Advantage premiums[h]	—	—	—	—	—	—	—	—	0.0	0.1	0.1
Accounting error (Calendar year 2005–2008)[i]	—	—	—	—	—	—	—	−1.0	3.6	—	—
Administrative expenses[j]	3.0	2.1	1.4	1.2	2.2	1.8	2.0	1.8	1.5	1.4	1.5

possible, to do things they enjoy, and to learn something new each day. Quality of life, rather than length of life, is the focus. In addition, whenever it is possible, family and friends are urged to be the primary caregivers in the home. Care at home helps both patients and family members enrich their lives and face death together.

Ira Byock, the former president of the American Academy of Hospice and Palliative Medicine, explains the concept of hospice care in *Dying Well: The Prospect for Growth at the End of Life* (1997): "Hospice care differs noticeably from the modern medical approach to dying. Typically, as a hospice patient nears death, the medical details become almost automatic and attention focuses on the personal nature of this final transition—what the patient and family are going through emotionally and spiritually. In the more established system, even as people die, medical procedures remain the first priority. With hospice, they move to the background as the personal comes to the fore."

—Category not applicable or data not available.
0.0 = Quantity more than zero but less than 0.05.
aPreliminary estimates.
bAverage number enrolled in the hospital insurance (HI) and/or supplementary medical insurance (SMI) programs for the period.
cStarting with 2004 data, the SMI trust fund consists of two separate accounts: Part B (which pays for a portion of the costs of physicians' services, outpatient hospital services, and other related medical and health services for voluntarily enrolled individuals) and Part D (Medicare Prescription Drug Account, which pays private plans to provide prescription drug coverage.
dThe Medicare Modernization Act, enacted on December 8, 2003, established within SMI two Part D accounts related to prescription drug benefits: the Medicare Prescription Drug Account and the Transitional Assistance Account. The Medicare Prescription Drug Account is used in conjunction with the broad, voluntary prescription drug benefits that began in 2006. The Transitional Assistance Account was used to provide transitional assistance benefits, beginning in 2004 and extending through 2005, for certain low-income beneficiaries prior to the start of the new prescription drug benefit. The amounts shown for Total Part D expenditures—and thus for total SMI expenditures and total Medicare expenditures—for 2006 and later years include estimated amounts for premiums paid directly from Part D beneficiaries to Part D prescription drug plans.
eMedicare-approved managed care organizations.
fReflects Community Based Care Transition Program ($25 million in 2010) and Electronic Health Records Incentive Program ($113 million in 2010).
gFor 1998 to 2003 data, reflects annual home health HI to SMI transfer amounts.
hWhen a beneficiary chooses a Medicare Advantage plan whose monthly premium exceeds the benchmark amount, the additional premiums (that is, amounts beyond those paid by Medicare to the plan) are the responsibility of the beneficiary. Beneficiaries subject to such premiums may choose to either reimburse the plans directly or have the additional premiums deducted from their Social Security checks. The amounts shown here are only those additional premiums deducted from Social Security checks. These amounts are transferred to the HI trust and SMI trust funds and then transferred from the trust funds to the plans.
iRepresents misallocation of benefit payments between the HI trust fund and the Part B account of the SMI trust fund from May 2005 to September 2007, and the transfer made in June 2008 to correct the misallocation.
jIncludes expenditures for research, experiments and demonstration projects, peer review activity (performed by Peer Review Organizations from 1983 to 2001 and by Quality Review Organizations from 2002 to present), and to combat and prevent fraud and abuse.
kType-of-service reporting categories for fee-for-service reimbursement differ before and after 1991.
lIncludes payment for physicians, practitioners, durable medical equipment, and all suppliers other than independent laboratory through 1990. Starting with 1991 data, physician services subject to the physician fee schedule are shown. Payments for laboratory services paid under the laboratory fee schedule and performed in a physician office are included under Laboratory beginning in 1991. Payments for durable medical equipment are shown separately beginning in 1991. The remaining services from the Physician/supplies category are included in Other.
mIncludes payments for hospital outpatient department services, skilled nursing facility outpatient services, Part B services received as an inpatient in a hospital or skilled nursing facility setting, and other types of outpatient facilities. Starting with 1991 data, payments for hospital outpatient department services, except for laboratory services, are listed under Hospital. Hospital outpatient laboratory services are included in the Laboratory line.
nStarting with 1991 data, those independent laboratory services that were paid under the laboratory fee schedule (most of the independent laboratory category) are included in the Laboratory line; the remaining services are included in the Physician fee schedule and Other lines.
oPayments for laboratory services paid under the laboratory fee schedule performed in a physician office, independent laboratory, or in a hospital outpatient department.
pIncludes payments for physician-administered drugs; freestanding ambulatory surgical center facility services; ambulance services; supplies; freestanding end-stage renal disease (ESRD) dialysis facility services; rural health clinics; outpatient rehabilitation facilities; psychiatric hospitals; and federally qualified health centers.
qIncludes the hospital facility costs for Medicare Part B services that are predominantly in the outpatient department, with the exception of hospital outpatient laboratory services, which are included on the Laboratory line. Physician reimbursement is included on the Physician fee schedule line.
rPart D start-up costs were funded through the SMI Part B account in 2004–2008.
Notes: All data shown are estimates and are subject to revision. Percents may not sum to totals because of rounding. Estimates are for Medicare-covered services furnished to Medicare enrollees residing in the United States, Puerto Rico, Virgin Islands, Guam, other outlying areas, foreign countries, and unknown residence.

SOURCE: Adapted from "Table 143. Medicare Enrollees and Expenditures and Percent Distribution, by Medicare Program and Type of Service: United States and Other Areas, Selected Years 1970–2010," in *Health, United States, 2011: With Special Feature on Socioeconomic Status and Health*, U.S. Department of Health and Human Services, Centers for Disease Control and Prevention, National Center for Health Statistics, May 2012, http://www.cdc.gov/nchs/data/hus/hus11.pdf (accessed June 13, 2012)

According to the National Hospice and Palliative Care Organization (NHPCO), in *NHPCO Facts and Figures: Hospice Care in America* (January 2012, http://www.nhpco.org/files/public/Statistics_Research/2011_Facts_Figures.pdf), the use of hospice care is increasing in the United States. The NHPCO estimates that in 2010, 1.6 million patients received hospice care and over 1 million patients died in hospice programs. In 2010 Medicare and Medicaid expenditures for hospice care totaled $13.2 billion and accounted for 5.3% of Medicare expenditures. (See Table 3.7.)

MANAGED CARE ORGANIZATIONS

Managed health care is the sector of the health insurance industry in which health care providers are not independent businesses run by, for example, private medical practitioners but are instead administrative firms that manage the allocation of health care benefits. In contrast to conventional indemnity insurers that do not govern the provision of medical care services and simply pay for them, managed care firms have a significant voice in how services are administered to enable them to exert better control over health care costs. (Indemnity insurance is traditional fee-for-service coverage in which providers are paid according to the service performed.)

Managed care, which has a primary purpose of controlling service utilization and costs, represents a rapidly growing segment of the health care industry. The beneficiaries of employer-funded health plans (people who receive health benefits from their employers), as well as Medicare and Medicaid recipients, often find themselves in this type of health care program. The term *managed care organization* covers several types of health care delivery systems, such as health maintenance organizations (HMOs), preferred provider organizations (PPOs), and utilization review groups that oversee diagnoses, recommend treatments, and manage costs for their beneficiaries.

Health Maintenance Organizations

HMOs began to grow during the 1970s as alternatives to traditional health insurance, which was becoming increasingly expensive. The HMO Act of 1973 was a federal law requiring employers with more than 24 employees to offer an alternative to conventional indemnity insurance in the form of a federally qualified HMO. The intent of the act was to stimulate HMO development, and the federal government has been promoting HMOs since the administration of President Richard M. Nixon (1913–1994), maintaining that groups of physicians following certain rules of practice can slow rising medical costs and improve health care quality.

HMOs are health insurance programs organized to provide complete coverage for subscribers' (also known as enrollees or members) health needs for negotiated, prepaid prices. The subscribers (and/or their employers) pay a fixed amount each month; in turn, the HMO group provides, at no extra charge or at a minimal charge, preventive care, such as routine checkups, screening, and immunizations, and care for any illness or accident. The monthly fee also covers inpatient hospitalization and referral services. HMO members benefit from reduced out-of-pocket costs (they do not pay deductibles), they do not have to file claims or fill out insurance forms, and they generally pay only nominal co-payments for each office visit. Members are usually locked into the plan for a specified period—usually one year. If the necessary service is available within the HMO, patients must normally use an HMO doctor. There are several types of HMOs:

- Staff model—the "purest" form of managed care. All primary care physicians are employees of the HMO and practice in a centralized location such as an outpatient clinic that may also house a laboratory, pharmacy, and facilities for other diagnostic testing. The staff model offers the HMO the greatest opportunity to manage both cost and quality of health care services.

- Group model—in which the HMO contracts with a group of primary care and multispecialty health providers. The group is paid a fixed amount per patient to provide specific services. The administration of the medical group determines how the HMO payments will be distributed among the physicians and other health care providers. Group model HMOs are usually located in hospitals or in clinic settings and have on-site pharmacies. Participating physicians usually do not have any fee-for-service patients.

- Network model—in which the HMO contracts with two or more groups of health providers that agree to provide health care at negotiated prices to all members enrolled in the HMO.

- Independent practice association (IPA) model—in which the HMO contracts with individual physicians or medical groups that then provide medical care to HMO members at their own offices. The individual physicians agree to follow the practices and procedures of the HMO when caring for the HMO members; however, they generally also maintain their own private practices and see fee-for-service patients as well as HMO members. IPA physicians are paid by capitation (literally, per head) for the HMO patients and by conventional methods for their fee-for-service patients. Physician members of the IPA guarantee that the care for each HMO member for which they are responsible will be delivered within a fixed budget. They guarantee this by allowing the HMO to withhold an amount of their payments (usually about 20% per year). If at year's end the physician's cost for providing care falls within the preset amount, then the physician receives all the monies withheld. If the physician's costs of care exceed the agreed-on amount, the HMO may retain any portion of the monies it has withheld. This arrangement places physicians and other providers such as hospitals, laboratories, and imaging centers at risk for keeping down treatment costs, and this at-risk formula is the key to HMO cost-containment efforts.

Some HMOs offer an open-ended or point-of-service (POS) option that allows members to choose their own physicians and hospitals, either within or outside the HMO. However, a member who chooses an outside provider will generally have to pay a larger portion of the expenses. Physicians not contracting with the HMO but who see HMO patients are paid according to the services performed. POS members are given an incentive to seek care from contracted network physicians and other health care providers through comprehensive coverage offerings.

The Kaiser Family Foundation indicates in "Number of HMOs" (http://www.statehealthfacts.org/comparetable.jsp?ind=347&cat=7&sub=85&yr=208&typ=1&sort=a) that as of July 2011, 70.2 million HMO members were served by 564 HMOs operating in the United States. In *Health, United States, 2007: With Chartbook on Trends in the Health of Americans* (2007, http://www.cdc.gov/nchs/data/hus/hus07.pdf), the NCHS notes that HMO enrollment grew during the 1990s and reached about 30% of the U.S. population in 2000. However, the Kaiser Family Foundation states that by July 2011 HMO enrollment had declined to just 22.5% of the U.S population.

HMO enrollment varies by geographic region, with the highest levels of enrollment in the New England states, Wisconsin, Michigan, and the far West. According to the Kaiser Family Foundation, 43.5% of the populations in the District of Columbia, 53% in Hawaii, 42.9% in California, and 34.5% in Massachusetts were enrolled in HMOs as of July 2011. In contrast, 0.1% of the populations in Alaska and 1.1% in Wyoming were covered by HMOs.

HMOs Have Fans and Critics

HMOs have been the subject of considerable debate among physicians, payers, policy makers, and health care consumers. Many physicians feel HMOs interfere in the physician-patient relationship and effectively prevent them from practicing medicine the way they have traditionally practiced. These physicians claim they know their patients' conditions and are, therefore, in the best position to recommend treatment. The physicians resent being advised and overruled by insurance administrators. (Physicians can recommend the treatment they believe is best, but if the insurance company will not cover the costs, patients may be unwilling to undergo the recommended treatment.)

The HMO industry counters that its evidence-based determinations (judgments about the appropriateness of care that reflect scientific research) are based on the experiences of many thousands of physicians and, therefore, it knows which treatment is most likely to be successful. The industry maintains that, in the past, physician-chosen treatments were not scrutinized or even assessed for effectiveness, and as a result most physicians did not really know whether the treatment they prescribed was optimal for the specific medical condition.

Furthermore, the HMO industry cites the slower increase in health care expenses as another indicator of its management success. Industry spokespeople note that any major change in how the industry is run would lead to increasing costs. They claim that HMOs and other managed care programs are bringing a more rational approach to the health care industry while maintaining health care quality and controlling costs.

Still, many physicians resent that, with a few exceptions, HMOs are not financially liable for their decisions. When a physician chooses to forgo a certain procedure and negative consequences result, the physician may be held legally accountable. When an HMO informs a physician that it will not cover a recommended procedure and the HMO's decision is found to be wrong, it cannot be held directly liable. Many physicians assert that because HMOs make such choices, they are practicing medicine and should, therefore, be held accountable. The HMOs counter that these are administrative decisions and deny that they are practicing medicine.

The legal climate, however, began to change for HMOs during the mid-1990s. Both the Third Circuit Federal Court of Appeals in *Dukes v. U.S. Healthcare* (57 F.3d 350 [1995]) and the 10th Circuit Federal Court of Appeals in *PacifiCare of Oklahoma, Inc. v. Burrage* (59 F.3rd 151 [1995]) agreed that HMOs were liable for malpractice and negligence claims against the HMO and HMO physicians. In *Frappier Estate v. Wishnov* (678 So.2d 884 [1996]), the Florida District Court of Appeals, Fourth District, agreed with the earlier findings. It appeared that these court decisions would be backed by a new federal law when both houses of Congress passed legislation (the Patients' Bill of Rights) that would give patients more recourse to contest the decisions of HMOs, even though the U.S. House of Representatives and the U.S. Senate disagreed about the specific rights and actions patients could take to enforce their rights. However, by August 2002 the prospects for a patients' rights law passing by the end of that year dimmed as the House and Senate failed to resolve their differences about the legislation. The central issue that stalled the negotiations about the bill was the question of how much recourse patients should have in court when they believe their HMO has not provided adequate care.

In June 2004 the U.S. Supreme Court struck down a law in California and in several other states that allowed patients to sue their health plans for denying them health care services. Even though patients can still sue in federal court for reimbursement of denied benefits, they are no longer able to sue for damages in federal or state courts.

California Is the First State to Limit HMO Wait Times

In response to complaints from California HMO members about delays in obtaining appointments with HMO physicians, state regulators established guidelines in January 2010 to reduce wait times. Duke Helfand reports in "California Limits HMO Wait Times" (*Los Angeles Times*, January 19, 2010) that HMOs were given until January 2011 to implement the new guidelines, which require that people seeking care from a primary care physician be seen within 10 business days of requesting an appointment and within 15 days of requesting an appointment with a physician specialist. As of September 2012, no other state had chosen to follow California's lead.

PPOs

In response to HMOs and other efforts by insurance groups to cut costs, physicians began forming or joining PPOs during the 1990s. PPOs are managed care organizations that offer integrated delivery systems (networks of providers) available through a wide array of health plans and are readily accountable to purchasers for access, cost, quality, and services of their networks. They use provider selection standards, utilization management, and quality assessment programs to complement negotiated fee reductions (discounted rates from participating physicians, hospitals, and other health care providers) as effective strategies for long-term cost control. Under a PPO benefit plan, covered people retain the freedom of choice of providers but are offered financial incentives such as lower out-of-pocket costs to use the preferred provider network. PPO members may use other physicians and hospitals, but they usually have to pay a higher proportion of the costs. PPOs are marketed directly to employers and to third-party administrators who then market PPOs to their employer clients.

Exclusive provider organizations (EPOs) are a more restrictive variation of PPOs in which members must seek care from providers on the EPO panel. If a member visits an outside provider who is not on the EPO panel, then the EPO will offer either limited or no coverage for the office or hospital visit.

According to the Kaiser Family Foundation, in "Employer Health Benefits: 2011 Summary of Findings" (September 2011, http://ehbs.kff.org/pdf/8226.pdf), 55% of U.S. workers were enrolled in PPO plans in 2011. By contrast, only 17% of U.S. workers were enrolled in HMO plans and 10% in POS plans.

Health Care Reform Will Affect Managed Care Plans

Brian Boyle, David Deaton, and Michael Maddigan of O'Melveny & Myers LLP note in "United States: The Health Care Reform Legislation and Its Impact on the Health Care and Life Sciences Industries" (March 30, 2010, http://www.mondaq.com/unitedstates/article.asp?articleid=97086) that the ACA will have a significant impact on the benefits provided by managed care plans and other insurers. In the short term, the legislation requires insurers to change certain underwriting practices and benefit structures. The act requires the plans to cover children with preexisting conditions, forbids them from canceling coverage when enrollees require costly treatment, prohibits caps on lifetime benefits, and permits children to remain on their parents' insurance until they turn 27 years old.

Boyle, Deaton, and Maddigan explain that other changes will occur in 2014. When the requirement that most Americans will have to obtain health coverage or face penalties takes effect, managed care plans and other insurers will doubtless experience increased enrollment. Because the act limits the extent to which premiums can vary in response to enrollee characteristics, such as age, tobacco use, and whether coverage is for an individual or family, the plans may experience reduced revenue from premiums. Presumably, this reduced revenue would be offset by larger numbers of enrollees.

According to Boyle, Deaton, and Maddigan, plans that offer coverage to Medicaid and Medicare beneficiaries will also experience changes in enrollment. Because the act extends Medicaid eligibility to more low-income people, Medicaid managed care plans will experience increased enrollment. By contrast, the act reduces reimbursement to Medicare managed care plans, and these will lose enrollees should they decrease benefits in response to the diminished reimbursement.

In the article "Experts Talk Health-Care Reform Bill Impact" (*BusinessWeek*, March 22, 2010), Phillip Seligman of Standard & Poor's Equity Research opines that the health care reform legislation will ultimately have a favorable effect on managed care organizations. Seligman believes that even though managed care plans "will face fees, which are delayed until 2014, and will have restrictions such as the ban on rescissions, no lifetime caps, and inability to bar coverage based on health status, which can pressure margins," these potential losses will "be offset by enrollment gains, providing economies of scale, leverage over general and administrative costs, and greater negotiating clout with providers. We also see potential opportunities for consolidation."

In "ACA's Effect on Employer-Sponsored Insurance" (*Managed Care*, July 2011), Miryam Frieder of Avalere Health, a consulting firm that is dedicated to improving the health care system, opines that the impact of full implementation of the ACA on employer-sponsored insurance (ESI)—primarily PPOs and HMOs—will be minimal. In sharp contrast, the same article reports that the results of a 2011 McKinsey & Co. market research study suggest that "30% of employers will 'definitely or probably stop offering ESI in the years after 2014.'"

CHAPTER 4

RESEARCHING, MEASURING, AND MONITORING THE QUALITY OF HEALTH CARE

There are hundreds of agencies, institutions, and organizations dedicated to researching, quantifying (measuring), monitoring, and improving health in the United States. Some are federally funded public entities such as the many institutes and agencies governed by the U.S. Department of Health and Human Services (HHS). Others are professional societies and organizations that develop standards of care, represent the views and interests of health care providers, and ensure the quality of health care facilities such as the American Medical Association and the Joint Commission on Accreditation of Healthcare Organizations. Still other voluntary health organizations, such as the American Heart Association, the American Cancer Society, and the March of Dimes, promote research and education about prevention and treatment of specific diseases.

U.S. DEPARTMENT OF HEALTH AND HUMAN SERVICES

The HHS is the nation's lead agency for ensuring the health of Americans by planning, operating, and funding delivery of essential human services, especially for society's most vulnerable populations. According to the HHS, in "HHS: What We Do" (2012, http://www.hhs.gov/about/whatwedo.html/), it consists of over 300 programs that are operated by 11 divisions—eight agencies in the U.S. Public Health Service and three human services agencies. It is the largest grant-making agency in the federal government, funding several thousand grants each year as well as the HHS Medicare program, the nation's largest health insurer, which processes over 1 billion claims per year. For fiscal year (FY) 2013, the HHS had a budget of $940.9 billion, which was an increase of $69 billion from FY 2012. (See Table 4.1.)

HHS Milestones

The HHS notes in "Historical Highlights" (2012, http://www.hhs.gov/about/hhshist.html) that it began with the 1798 opening of the first Marine Hospital in Boston, Massachusetts, to care for sick and injured merchant seamen. Under President Abraham Lincoln (1809–1865) the agency that would become the U.S. Food and Drug Administration was established in 1862. The National Institutes of Health (NIH) dates back to 1887 and eventually became part of the Public Health Service. The 1935 enactment of the Social Security Act spurred the development of the Federal Security Agency in 1939 to direct programs in health, human services, insurance, and education. In 1946 the Communicable Disease Center, which would become the Centers for Disease Control and Prevention (CDC), was established, and 19 years later, in 1965, Medicare (a federal health insurance program for people aged 65 years and older and people with disabilities) and Medicaid (a state and federal health insurance program for low-income people) were enacted to improve access to health care for older, disabled, and low-income Americans. That same year the Head Start program was developed to provide education, health, and social services to preschool-aged children.

In 1970 the National Health Service Corps was established to help meet the health care needs of underserved areas and populations. The following year the National Cancer Act became law, which established cancer research as a national research priority. In 1984 the human immunodeficiency virus (HIV), the virus that causes acquired immunodeficiency syndrome (AIDS), was identified by the Public Health Service and French research scientists. The National Organ Transplant Act became law in 1984, and in 1990 the Human Genome Project was initiated.

In 1994 NIH-funded research isolated the genes responsible for inherited breast cancer, colon cancer, and the most frequently occurring type of kidney cancer. In 1998 efforts were launched to eliminate racial and ethnic disparities (differences) in health, and in 2000

TABLE 4.1

U.S. Department of Health and Human Services budget, fiscal years 2011–13

[Dollars in millions]

	2011	2012	2013	2013 +/− 2012
Budget authority	882,993	866,017	932,234	+66,217
Total outlays	**891,323**	**871,924**	**940,927**	**+69,003**
Full-Time Equivalents (FTE)	73,704	74,948	76,341	+1,393

SOURCE: "FY 2013 President's Budget for HHS," in *U.S. Department of Health and Human Services Budget in Brief, Fiscal Year 2013*, U.S. Department of Health and Human Services, 2012, http://www.hhs.gov/budget/budget-brief-fy2013.pdf (accessed June 19, 2012)

the human genome sequencing was published. In 2001 the Health Care Financing Administration was replaced by the Centers for Medicaid and Medicare Services, and the HHS responded to the first reported cases of bioterrorism (the 2001 anthrax attacks) and developed new strategies to detect and prevent threats of bioterrorism. In 2003 the Medicare Prescription Drug Improvement and Modernization Act expanded Medicare and included prescription drug benefits. In 2010 the landmark health care reform legislation—the Patient Protection and Affordable Care Act and the Health Care and Education Reconciliation Act (which are now commonly known as the ACA)—was enacted.

According to the HHS, in *U.S. Department of Health and Human Services Budget in Brief, Fiscal Year 2013: Advancing the Health, Safety, and Well-Being of Our Nation* (February 2012, http://www.hhs.gov/budget/budget-brief-fy2013.pdf), significant initiatives funded in the FY 2013 budget include implementing the ACA, which entails expanding access to health insurance coverage, developing new models of service delivery to improve quality of care and reduce costs, and advancing the use of health information technology. The budget includes $66 million to accelerate the adoption of health information technology and promote the use of electronic health records to not only improve the health of individuals but also to improve the health care system as a whole.

HHS Agencies and Institutes Provide Comprehensive Health and Social Services

Besides the CDC and the NIH, the HHS explains in *U.S. Department of Health and Human Services Budget in Brief, Fiscal Year 2013* that the following agencies research, plan, direct, oversee, administer, and provide health care services:

- The Administration on Aging (AoA) provides services aimed at helping older Americans retain their independence. The AoA develops policies that support older adults and directs programs that provide transportation, in-home services, and other health and

social services. For FY 2013 the AoA planned for a budget of nearly $2 billion and 135 employees.

- The Administration for Children and Families (ACF) provides services for families and children in need, administers Head Start, and works with state foster care and adoption programs. The ACF was allotted a budget of $50.3 billion and 1,362 employees for FY 2013.

- The Agency for Healthcare Research and Quality (AHRQ) researches access to health care, quality of care, and efforts to control health care costs. It also looks at the safety of health care services and the ways to prevent medical errors. Figure 4.1 shows how the AHRQ researches health system problems by performing a continuous process of needs assessment, gaining knowledge, interpreting and communicating information, and evaluating the effects of this process on the health problem. Figure 4.2 shows the process that transforms new information about health care issues into actions to improve access, costs, outcomes (how patients fare as a result of the care they receive), and quality. For FY 2013 the AHRQ planned for a budget of $409 million and 333 employees. The AHRQ budgeted $63 million for patient safety research and activities and $93 million for research about how to improve health care quality, effectiveness, and efficiency.

- The Agency for Toxic Substances and Disease Registry seeks to prevent exposure to hazardous waste. The agency's FY 2013 budget of $76 million represented no change from FY 2012.

- The Centers for Medicare and Medicaid Services (CMS) administers programs that provide health insurance for about 52 million Americans who are either aged 65 years and older or in financial need. It also operates the Children's Health Insurance Program, which covers about 10 million uninsured children, and regulates all laboratory testing, except testing performed for research purposes, in the United States. For FY 2013 the CMS planned for a budget of $829.4 billion. Figure 4.3 shows the allocation of the CMS budget—62.8% was devoted to Medicare, 34.1% to Medicaid, and 1.2% each to the Children's Health Insurance Plan and administration.

- The U.S. Food and Drug Administration (FDA) acts to ensure the safety and efficacy (the ability of an intervention to produce the intended diagnostic or therapeutic effect in optimal circumstances) of dietary supplements, pharmaceutical drugs, and medical devices and monitors food safety and purity. The FDA planned for a budget of nearly $4.5 billion in FY 2013 and 14,828 employees. The FDA budget included an increase of $658 million over the FY 2012 budget of $3.8 billion to ensure the safety and security of the food supply and to provide other biodefense activities.

FIGURE 4.1

Cycle of health care research

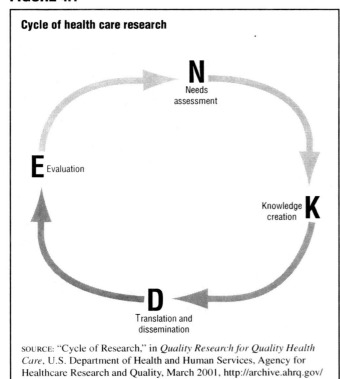

SOURCE: "Cycle of Research," in *Quality Research for Quality Health Care*, U.S. Department of Health and Human Services, Agency for Healthcare Research and Quality, March 2001, http://archive.ahrq.gov/about/qr4qhc/chart4.htm (accessed June 19, 2012)

FIGURE 4.2

Health care research pipeline

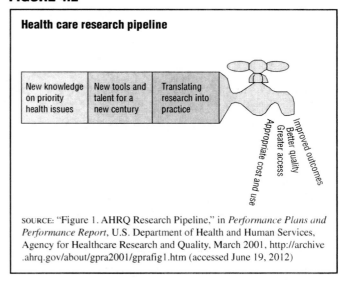

SOURCE: "Figure 1. AHRQ Research Pipeline," in *Performance Plans and Performance Report*, U.S. Department of Health and Human Services, Agency for Healthcare Research and Quality, March 2001, http://archive.ahrq.gov/about/gpra2001/gprafig1.htm (accessed June 19, 2012)

FIGURE 4.3

Budgeted net outlays, Centers for Medicare and Medicaid Services (CMS), fiscal year 2013

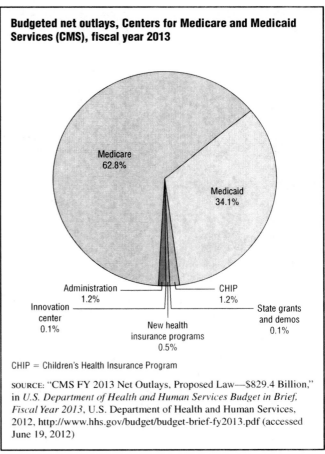

CHIP = Children's Health Insurance Program

SOURCE: "CMS FY 2013 Net Outlays, Proposed Law—$829.4 Billion," in *U.S. Department of Health and Human Services Budget in Brief, Fiscal Year 2013*, U.S. Department of Health and Human Services, 2012, http://www.hhs.gov/budget/budget-brief-fy2013.pdf (accessed June 19, 2012)

- The Health Resources and Services Administration (HRSA) provides services for medically underserved populations such as migrant workers, the homeless, and public housing residents. The HRSA oversees the nation's organ transplant program, directs efforts to improve maternal and child health, and delivers services to people with AIDS through the Ryan White CARE Act. In FY 2013 it planned to have 1,818 employees and a budget of $6 billion.

- The Indian Health Service (IHS) serves nearly 560 tribes through a network of 45 hospitals, 287 health stations, and 320 health centers. In FY 2013 the IHS planned to employ 15,773 workers and have a budget of $5.5 billion.

- The General Departmental Management provides the HHS's leadership and oversees the 12 staff divisions and offices of the HHS. It also advises the president about health, welfare, human service, and income security issues. In FY 2013 it was allotted 1,446 employees and a budget of $567 million.

- The Substance Abuse and Mental Health Services Administration (SAMHSA) seeks to improve access to, and availability of, substance abuse prevention and treatment programs as well as other mental health services. SAMHSA was budgeted $3.4 billion in FY 2013 and had 574 employees.

The HHS agencies work with state, local, and tribal governments as well as with public and private organiza-tions to coordinate and deliver a wide range of services including:

- Conducting preventive health services such as surveillance to detect outbreaks of disease and immunization programs through efforts directed by the CDC and the NIH

- Ensuring food, drug, and cosmetic safety through efforts of the FDA

- Improving maternal and child health and preschool education in programs such as Head Start, which served more than 1.1 million children in 2010, according to the National Head Start Association, in "Basic Head Start Facts" (2012, http://www.nhsa.org/)

- Preventing child abuse, domestic violence, and substance abuse, as well as funding substance abuse treatment through programs directed by the ACF

- Ensuring the delivery of health care services to about 2 million Native Americans and Alaskan Natives through the IHS, a network of hospitals, health centers, and other programs and facilities (2012, http://www.ihs.gov/PublicAffairs/IHSBrochure/QuickLook.asp)

- Administering Medicare and Medicaid via the CMS

- Providing financial assistance and support services for low-income and older Americans, such as home-delivered meals (Meals on Wheels) coordinated by the AoA

SUBSTANTIAL BUDGET HELPS THE HHS TO ACHIEVE ITS OBJECTIVES. Table 4.2 displays how the FY 2013 HHS budget was allocated and provides comparisons between 2011, 2012, and 2013 outlays. The FY 2013 budget is a net increase of $69 billion over the FY 2012 budget and aims to provide funds to help improve access to and quality of health care, prevent disease, and support scientific research. In *U.S. Department of Health and Human Services Budget in Brief, Fiscal Year 2013*, the HHS explains that it provides funds "to expand the capacity and improve the training and distribution of primary care, dental, and pediatric health providers [and] will support the placement of more than 7,100 primary care providers in underserved areas." Furthermore, the HHS reiterates that it "is also working to ensure that the most vulnerable in our Nation have full access to seamless, high-quality health care."

U.S. PUBLIC HEALTH SERVICE COMMISSIONED CORPS. The U.S. Public Health Service Commissioned Corps (November 22, 2011, http://www.usphs.gov/aboutus/history.aspx) was originally the uniformed service component of the early Marine Hospital Service, which adopted a military model for a group of career health professionals who traveled from one marine hospital to another as their services were needed. It also assisted the Marine Hospital Service to prevent infectious diseases from entering the country by examining newly arrived immigrants and directing state quarantine (the period and place where people suspected of having contagious diseases are detained and isolated) functions. A law enacted in 1889 established this group as the Commissioned Corps, and in 1912 the Marine Hospital Service was renamed the Public Health Service (PHS) to reflect its broader scope of activities.

Throughout the 20th century the corps grew to include a wide range of health professionals. Besides physicians, the corps employed nurses, dentists, research scientists, planners, pharmacists, sanitarians, engineers, and other public health professionals. These PHS-commissioned officers played important roles in disease prevention and detection, acted to ensure food and drug safety, conducted research, provided medical care to underserved groups such as Native Americans and Alaskan Natives, and assisted in disaster relief programs. As one of the seven uniformed services in the United States (the other six are the U.S. Navy, the U.S. Army, the U.S. Marine Corps, the U.S. Air Force, the U.S. Coast Guard, and the National Oceanic and Atmospheric Administration Commissioned Corps), the PHS Commissioned Corps continues to perform all these functions and identifies environmental threats to health and safety, promotes healthy lifestyles for Americans, and is involved with international agencies to help address global health problems.

The Office of the Surgeon General notes in "Mission of the U.S. Public Health Service Commissioned Corps" (http://www.surgeongeneral.gov/about/corps/index.html) that as of 2012 the PHS Commissioned Corps numbered approximately 6,500 health professionals. These people report to the U.S. surgeon general, who holds the rank of vice admiral in the PHS. Corps officers work in PHS agencies and in other agencies including the U.S. Bureau of Prisons, the U.S. Coast Guard, the U.S. Environmental Protection Agency, and the Commission on Mental Health of the District of Columbia. The surgeon general is a physician who is appointed by the U.S. president to serve in a medical leadership position for a four-year term of office. The surgeon general reports to the assistant secretary of health, and the Office of the Surgeon General (2012, http://www.surgeongeneral.gov/aboutoffice.html) is part of the Office of Public Health and Science. Eighteen surgeons general have served since the 1870s. In January 2010 Vice Admiral Regina M. Benjamin (1956–; http://www.surgeongeneral.gov/about/biographies/biosg.html) began her term as the surgeon general.

CENTERS FOR DISEASE CONTROL AND PREVENTION

The CDC is the primary HHS agency responsible for ensuring the health and safety of the nation's citizens in the United States and abroad. The CDC's responsibilities include researching and monitoring health, detecting and investigating health problems, researching and instituting prevention programs, developing health policies, ensuring environmental health and safety, and offering education and training.

TABLE 4.2

Health and Human Services budget, by operating division, 2011–13

	Mandatory and discretionary dollars in millions			
	Fiscal year 2011	Fiscal year 2012	Fiscal year 2013	Fiscal years 2013 +/− 2012
Food and Drug Administration				
Budget authority	2,404	2,508	2,519	+11
Outlays	1,985	2,574	2,499	−75
Health Resources and Services Administration				
Budget authority	9,867	8,377	8,576	+199
Outlays	8,780	9,113	8,651	−462
Indian Health Service				
Budget authority	4,228	4,464	4,581	+117
Outlays	4,176	4,972	4,722	−250
Centers for Disease Control and Prevention				
Budget authority	6,473	6,857	6,218	−629
Outlays	6,740	6,760	6,400	−360
National Institutes of Health				
Budget authority	30,620	30,852	30,852	—
Outlays	34,353	31,567	30,464	−1,103
Substance Abuse and Mental Health Services Administration				
Budget authority	3,467	3,435	3,257	−178
Outlays	3,413	3,434	3,405	−29
Agency for Healthcare Research and Quality				
Program level	392	405	409	+4
Outlays	115	294	145	−149
Centers for Medicare & Medicaid Services[a]				
Budget authority	773,825	757,220	823,166	+65,946
Outlays	773,504	757,068	829,307	+72,239
Administration for Children and Families[b]				
Budget authority	50,908	50,139	50,308	+169
Outlays	54,208	50,722	50,902	+180
Administration on Aging				
Budget authority	1,507	1,492	1,949	+457
Outlays	1,555	1,491	1,752	+261
Office of the National Coordinator				
Budget authority	42	16	26	+10
Outlays	463	971	419	−552
Medicare Hearings and Appeals				
Budget authority	72	87	84	−3
Outlays	71	72	84	+12
Office for Civil Rights				
Budget authority	43	41	39	−2
Outlays	41	42	40	−2
Departmental Management				
Budget authority	694	529	541	+2
Outlays	371	657	440	−217
Prevention and Wellness				
Recovery act budget authority	—	—	—	—
Outlays	22	18	—	−18
Health Insurance Reform Implementation Fund[c]				
Budget authority	—	—	—	—
Outlays	208	411	344	−67
Public Health and Social Services Emergency Fund				
Budget authority	−584	568	642	+74
Outlays	1,702	1,898	1,881	−17
Office of Inspector General				
Budget authority	50	50	59	+9
Outlays	94	75	60	−15
Program Support Center (Retirement pay, medical benefits, misc. trust funds)				
Budget authority	556	606	626	+20
Outlays	701	1,009	621	−388
Offsetting Collections				
Budget authority	−1,179	−1,224	−1,209	+15
Outlays	−1,179	−1,224	−1,209	+15
Total, Health and Human Services				
Budget authority	**882,993**	**866,017**	**932,234**	**+66,217**
Outlays	**891,323**	**871,924**	**940,927**	**+69,003**
Full-Time Equivalents	73,704	74,948	76,341	+1,393

In "CDC Fact Sheet" (February 25, 2010, http://www.cdc.gov/about/resources/facts.htm), the CDC indicates that it employs over 15,000 people in 168 disciplines and in 50 countries. Besides research scientists, physicians, nurses, and other health practitioners, the CDC employs epidemiologists, who study disease in

TABLE 4.2

	Dollars in millions			
	Fiscal year 2011	Fiscal year 2012	Fiscal year 2013	Fiscal years 2013 +/− 2012
Discretionary programs (budget authority):[d]				
Food and Drug Administration	2,457	2,506	2,517	†12
Program level	3,690	3,832	4,486	+654
Health Resources and Services Administration[e]	6,272	6,215	6,077	−138
Program level	9,665	8,203	8,431	+288
Indian Health Service	4,069	4,307	4,422	+116
Program level	5,140	5,386	5,502	+116
Centers for Disease Control and Prevention	5,726	5,732	5,068	−664
Program level	10,995	11,196	11,236	+39
National Institutes of Health[f]	30,767	30,702	30,702	—
Program level	30,926	30,860	30,860	—
Substance Abuse and Mental Health Services Administration	3,380	3,347	3,152	−196
Program level	3,599	3,565	3,423	−142
Agency for Healthcare Research and Quality	—	—	—	—
Program level	392	405	409	+4
Centers for Medicare & Medicaid Services[f,g]	3,587	3,820	4,821	+1,001
Program level	5,027	4,687	6,040	+1,353
Administration for Children and Families	17,235	16,489	16,181	−309
Program level	17,241	16,495	16,186	−309
Administration on Aging[f]	1,998	1,971	1,978	+7
Program level	2,015	2,005	2,012	+7
Office of the Secretary:				
General Departmental Management	480	474	306	−168
Program level	598	587	567	−21
Office of Medicare Hearing and Appeals	70	72	84	+12
Office of the National Coordinator	42	16	26	+10
Program level	61	61	66	+5
Office of Inspector General	50	50	59	+8
Program level	290	356	370	+14
Office for Civil Rights	41	41	39	−2
Public Health and Social Services Emergency Fund	675	568	642	+74
Program level	1,090	983	1,057	+74
Discretionary HCFAC[h]	310	581	610	+29
Accrual for Commissioned Corps Medical Benefits	38	36	26	−10
Prevention fund activities across HHS	—	20	100	+80
Discretionary total[i]	**77,198**	**76,928**	**76,711**	**−218**
One-time rescissions[j]	−6,984	−6,768	−6,706	+62
Discretionary total adjusted for rescissions	**70,214**	**70,160**	**70,005**	**−156**
Mandatory programs (outlays):				
Medicare	480,202	479,553	523,749	+44,196
Medicaid	274,964	255,263	282,819	+27,556
Temporary Assistance for Needy Families[k]	19,072	17,855	17,699	−156
Foster Care and Permanency	6,860	6,795	7,170	+375
Children's Health Insurance Program[l]	8,633	9,903	10,227	+324
Child Support Enforcement	4,182	3,869	3,873	+4
Child Care	3,100	2,868	3,286	+418
Social Services Block Grant	1,787	1,908	1,792	−116
Other mandatory programs	7,185	10,987	10,929	−58
Offsetting collections	−1,179	−1,224	−1,209	+15
Subtotal, mandatory outlays	804,806	787,777	860,335	+72,558
Total, HHS outlays	**891,323**	**871,924**	**940,927**	**+69,003**

populations as opposed to individuals. Epidemiologists measure disease occurrences, such as incidence and prevalence of disease, and work with clinical researchers to answer questions about causation (how particular diseases arise and the factors that contribute to their development), whether new treatments are effective, and how to prevent specific diseases.

The CDC states in "CDC Organization" (February 17, 2012, http://www.cdc.gov/about/organization/cio.htm) that it is home to 15 national centers and various institutes and offices. Among the best known are the National

Center for Health Statistics, which collects vital statistics, and the National Institute for Occupational Safety and Health, which seeks to prevent workplace injuries and accidents through research and prevention. Thomas R. Frieden (1960–) was named the director of the CDC in June 2009. Figure 4.4 shows the organization and leadership of the CDC in 2012.

CDC Actions to Protect the Health of the Nation

The CDC is part of the first response to natural disasters, outbreaks of disease, other public health

TABLE 4.2

Health and Human Services budget, by operating division, 2011–13 [CONTINUED]

[a]Budget Authority includes Non-CMS budget authority for Hospital Insurance and Supplementary Medical Insurance for the Social Security Administration and Medicare Payment Advisory Commission.
[b]Includes rescission of $25 million in prior year Refugee funds.
[c]Includes outlays for all agencies receiving resources from the fund.
[d]Program level includes non-discretionary funding for activities traditionally funded with discretionary funding.
[e]The fiscal year 2013 budget transfers the Health Education Assistance Loan (HEAL) program to the Department of Education. Funding is requested in HHS for fiscal year 2013 and will be used to administer HEAL until the point of transfer. The funding level for HRSA without HEAL in fiscal year 2013 is $6.074 billion.
[f]Figures for fiscal year 2011 and fiscal year 2012 include program transfers for comparability to the fiscal year 2013 budget.
[g]Fiscal year 2011 figure includes $176 million transfer from GDM. In fiscal year 2011 and fiscal year 2012, High-Risk Pool grants are displayed as discretionary funding for comparability with fiscal year 2013.
[h]The president's budget assumes an increase in the 2012 base funding to $311 million (which is fully offset) and the provision of an additional $270 million in funding allowed by the cap adjustment, consistent with the Budget Control Act of 2011.
[i]Includes amounts that count toward the discretionary caps, other than one-time rescissions.
[j]Fiscal year 2011 rescissions include $2.2B from CO-Ops, $3.5B from the Children's Health Insurance Program Reauthorization Act of 2009 (CHIPRA) performance bonuses, $1.3B in flu balances and $25M from ACF. Fiscal year 2012 rescissions include $400M from CO-OPs and $6.37B from CHIPRA performance bonuses. The fiscal year 2013 federal budget includes by $6.706B in proposed rescissions to CHIPRA performance bonuses. The fiscal year 2013 budget also includes general provision language that would redirect $13M in unused abstinence education funding from ACF.
[k]Includes outlays for the TANF Contingency Fund and the Recovery Act's TANF Emergency Contingency Fund.
[l]Includes outlays for the Child Enrollment Contingency Fund.

SOURCE: "HHS Budget by Operating Division," in *U.S. Department of Health and Human Services Budget in Brief, Fiscal Year 2013*, U.S. Department of Health and Human Services, 2012, http://www.hhs.gov/budget/budget-brief-fy2013.pdf (accessed June 19, 2012)

emergencies, and urgent public health problems. For example, the agency produces *Public Health Grand Rounds* (http://www.publichealthgrandrounds.unc.edu/), a monthly webcast that is intended to stimulate discussion of significant public health issues. Each session describes a specific health challenge and considers leading-edge scientific evidence and the possible impact of different interventions. In 2012 the series focused on a variety of topics, including preventing injuries, alcohol abuse, heart attacks, multidrug-resistant gonorrhea, intimate partner violence, HIV prevention, and global tobacco control.

The CDC also monitors and plans responses to the emerging threat of seasonal influenza and other influenza viruses. In 2009 the CDC tracked and reported the H1N1 flu outbreak. Figure 4.5 compares influenza cases in selected seasons including the 2009–10 pandemic flu and reveals that the 2011–12 season was mild compared with the other years.

Among the many recent CDC initiatives to combat the obesity epidemic is the documentary film series *The Weight of the Nation*, which was developed in partnership with the Institute of Medicine and the NIH. The series debuted on HBO and was shown at the CDC's Weight of the Nation Conference (http://www.cdc.gov/won/overview/index.htm) in Washington, D.C., in May 2012. The conference focused on changes in policies, systems, and environments that have the potential to improve health or have demonstrated success for improving three population level measures: nutrition, physical activity, and the prevalence of obesity.

The CDC LEAN Works identifies and promotes worksite interventions to combat obesity as well as interventions that target school-age children and women. The CDC also educates and communicates vital health information via its publications *Morbidity and Mortality Weekly Report* and *Emerging Infectious Disease Journal*, which alert the medical community to the presence of health risks, outbreaks, and preventive measures. Besides providing vital statistics (births, deaths, and related health data), the CDC monitors Americans' health using surveys to measure the frequency of behaviors that increase health risk (such as smoking, substance abuse, and physical inactivity) and compiles data about the use of health care resources (such as inpatient hospitalization rates and visits to hospital emergency departments).

The CDC partners with national, state, local, public, and private agencies and organizations to deliver services. Examples of these collaborative efforts include the global battle against HIV/AIDS via the Leadership and Investment in Fighting an Epidemic initiative and the CDC Coordinating Center for Health Information and Service, which was created to improve public health through increased efficiencies and to foster stronger collaboration between the CDC and international health foundations, health care practitioners, community and philanthropic organizations, schools and universities, nonprofit and voluntary organizations, and state and local public health departments.

NATIONAL INSTITUTES OF HEALTH

The NIH (April 23, 2012, http://www.nih.gov/about/history.htm) began as a one-room laboratory in 1887 and eventually became the world's premier medical research center. The NIH conducts research in its own facilities and supports research in universities, medical schools,

FIGURE 4.4

Centers for Disease Control and Prevention organization and leadership, 2012

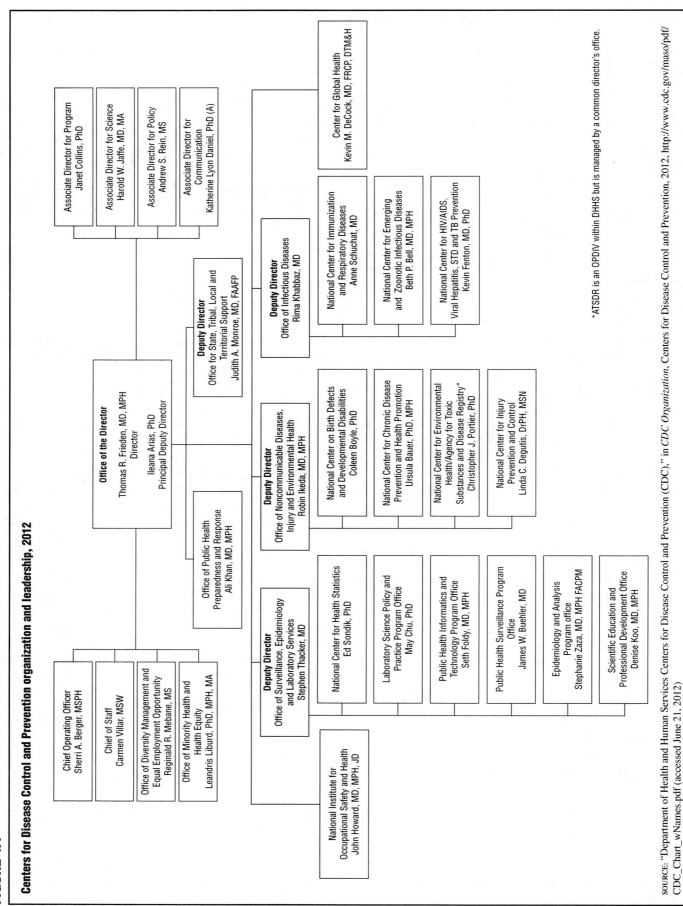

SOURCE: "Department of Health and Human Services Centers for Disease Control and Prevention (CDC)," in *CDC Organization*, Centers for Disease Control and Prevention, 2012, http://www.cdc.gov/maso/pdf/CDC_Chart_wNames.pdf (accessed June 21, 2012)

FIGURE 4.5

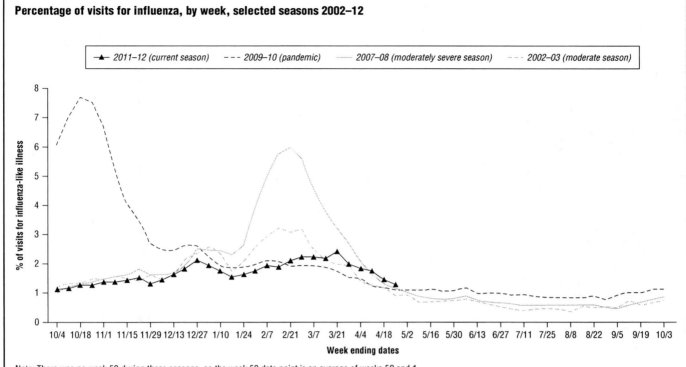

Percentage of visits for influenza, by week, selected seasons 2002–12

Note: There was no week 53 during these seasons, so the week 53 data point is an average of weeks 52 and 1.

SOURCE: "Percentage of Visits for Influenza-like Illness (ILI) Reported by the U.S. Outpatient Influenza-like Illness Surveillance Network (ILINet), Weekly National Summary, Selected Seasons," in *2011–2012 Flu Season Draws to a Close*, Centers for Disease Control and Prevention, National Center for Immunization and Respiratory Diseases (NCIRD), June 14, 2012, http://www.cdc.gov/flu/spotlights/2011-2012-flu-season-wrapup.htm (accessed June 21, 2012)

and hospitals throughout and outside the United States. The NIH trains research scientists and other investigators and serves to communicate medical and health information to professional and consumer audiences.

The NIH (October 14, 2011, http://www.nih.gov/about/organization.htm) consists of 27 centers and institutes and is housed in more than 75 buildings on a 300-acre (121-ha) campus in Bethesda, Maryland. Among the better-known centers and institutes are the National Cancer Institute, the National Human Genome Research Institute, the National Institute of Mental Health, and the National Center for Complementary and Alternative Medicine.

In "Facts at a Glance" (September 9, 2011, http://clinicalcenter.nih.gov/about/welcome/fact.shtml), the NIH explains that patients arrive at the NIH Warren Grant Magnuson Clinical Center in Bethesda to participate in clinical research trials. About 6,000 patients per year are treated as inpatients, and an additional 95,000 receive outpatient treatment. The National Library of Medicine (NLM)—which produces the *Index Medicus*, a monthly listing of articles from the world's top medical journals, and maintains MEDLINE, a comprehensive medical bibliographic database—is in the NIH Lister Hill Center. According to the NIH, in "The NIH Almanac:

Chronology of Events" (March 27, 2012, http://www.nih.gov/about/almanac/historical/chronology_of_events.htm), in 2010 the NLM released ReUnite, an iPhone application to improve postdisaster family reunification. ReUnite was downloaded by more than 1,000 people during the first week of its release.

The NIH also notes that the health care reform law signed by President Barack Obama (1961–) in 2010 redesignated the National Center on Minority Health and Health Disparities to an institute. The new institute plans, coordinates, reviews, and evaluates all minority health and health disparities research activities that are conducted by the NIH. In September 2010 the National Cancer Institute (NCI) began construction of a new, expanded campus that will accommodate about 2,100 NCI staff. The new campus was slated to open in 2013.

The NIH budget for FY 2013 was $30.7 billion. Table 4.3 shows NIH funding allocation by institute. In "About the National Institutes of Health" (2010, http://science.education.nih.gov/supplements/nih1/Genetic/about/about-nih.htm), the NIH states that it works to achieve its ambitious research objectives "to acquire new knowledge to help prevent, detect, diagnose, and treat disease and disability, from the rarest genetic disorder to the common

TABLE 4.3

National Institutes of Health total funding, fiscal years 2011–13

[Dollars in millions]

	2011	2012	2013	2013 +/− 2012
Institutes				
National Cancer Institute	5,050	5,066	5,069	+3
National Heart, Lung and Blood Institute	3,065	3,075	3,076	+1
National Institute of Dental and Craniofacial Research	409	410	408	−2
Natl Inst. of Diabetes & Digestive & Kidney Diseases	1,939	1,945	1,942	−3
National Institute of Neurological Disorders and Stroke	1,619	1,624	1,625	—
National Institute of Allergy and Infectious Diseases	4,768	4,485	4,495	+10
National Institute of General Medical Sciences	2,368	2,427	2,379	−48
Eunice K. Shriver Natl Inst. of Child Health & Human Dev	1,316	1,320	1,321	+1
National Eye Institute	700	702	693	−9
National Institute of Environmental Health Sciences:				
Labor/HHS Appropriation	683	685	684	−1
Interior Appropriation	79	79	79	—
National Institute on Aging	1,099	1,102	1,103	+1
Natl Inst. of Arthritis & Musculoskeletal & Skin Diseases	533	535	536	—
Natl Inst. on Deafness and Communication Disorders	414	416	417	+2
National Institute of Mental Health	1,475	1,479	1,479	+1
National Institute on Drug Abuse	1,049	1,052	1,054	+2
National Institute on Alcohol Abuse and Alcoholism	458	459	457	−2
National Institute of Nursing Research	144	145	144	—
National Human Genome Research Institute	511	512	511	−1
Natl Institute of Biomedical Imaging and Bioengineering	345	338	337	−1
Natl Institute on Minority Health and Health Disparities	276	276	279	+3
Natl Center for Complementary and Alternative Medicine	127	128	128	—
National Center for Advancing Translational Sciences	554	575	639	+64
Fogarty International Center	69	70	70	—
National Library of Medicine	371	373	381	+8
Office of the Director	1,454	1,457	1,429	−28
Buildings and Facilities	50	125	125	—
Total, program level	**30,926**	**30,860**	**30,860**	**—**
Less funds allocated from other sources				
Public health services evaluation funds (NLM)	−8	−8	−8	—
Type 1 diabetes research (NIDDK)*	−150	−150	−150	—
Total, discretionary budget authority	**30,767**	**30,702**	**30,702**	**—**
Labor/HHS Appropriation	**30,688**	**30,623**	**30,623**	**—**
Interior Appropriation	**79**	**79**	**79**	
FTE	18,573	18,573	18,387	−186

*These mandatory funds were pre-appropriated in P.L. 110–275, the Medicare Improvements for Patients and Providers Act of 2008, and P.L. 111–309, the Medicare and Medicaid Extenders Act of 2010.
HHS = Department of Health and Human Services
FTE = Full-time Equivalent
NLM = National Library of Medicine
NIDDK = National Institute of Diabetes and Digestive and Kidney Diseases

SOURCE: "National Institutes of Health," in *U.S. Department of Health and Human Services Budget in Brief, Fiscal Year 2013*, U.S. Department of Health and Human Services, 2012, http://www.hhs.gov/budget/budget-brief-fy2013.pdf (accessed June 19, 2012)

cold" by investing in promising biomedical research. The NIH makes grants and contracts to support research and training in every state in the country, at more than 2,000 institutions. The NIH allocated more than half (53.3%) of its FY 2013 budget to research project grants, 11.1% to intramural research, 10% to research and development contracts, and 9.6% to research centers. (See Figure 4.6.)

Establishing Research Priorities

By law, all 27 institutes of the NIH must be funded, and each institute must allocate its funding to specific areas and aspects of research within its domain. About half of each institute's budget is dedicated to supporting the best research proposals presented, in terms of their potential to contribute to advances that will combat the diseases the institute is charged with researching. Some of the other criteria that are used to determine research priorities include:

- Public health need—the NIH responds to health problems and diseases based on their incidence (the rate of development of a disease in a group during a given period) and severity and on the costs associated with them. Examples of other measures used to weigh and assess need are the mortality rate (the number of deaths caused by disease), the morbidity rate (the degree of disability caused by disease), the economic and social consequences of the disease, and whether rapid action is required to control the spread of the disease.

FIGURE 4.6

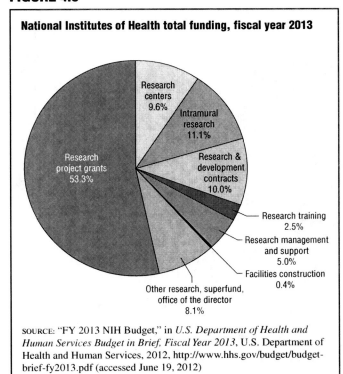

National Institutes of Health total funding, fiscal year 2013

SOURCE: "FY 2013 NIH Budget," in *U.S. Department of Health and Human Services Budget in Brief, Fiscal Year 2013*, U.S. Department of Health and Human Services, 2012, http://www.hhs.gov/budget/budget-brief-fy2013.pdf (accessed June 19, 2012)

- Rigorous peer review—proposals are scrutinized by accomplished researchers to determine their potential return on the investment of resources.

- Flexibility and expansiveness—the NIH experience demonstrates that important findings for commonly occurring diseases may come from research on rarer ones. The NIH attempts to fund the broadest possible array of research opportunities to stimulate creative solutions to pressing problems.

- Commitment to human resources and technology—the NIH invests in people and equipment in the pursuit of scientific advancement.

Because not even the most gifted scientists can accurately predict the next critical discovery or stride in biomedical research, the NIH must analyze each research opportunity in terms of competition for the same resources, public interest, scientific merit, and the potential to build on current knowledge. Figure 4.7 shows all the stakeholders whose interests and opinions are considered when NIH resource allocation and grant funding decisions are made.

NIH Achievements

The HHS notes in *U.S. Department of Health and Human Services Budget in Brief, Fiscal Year 2013* that in FY 2013 the NIH had 18,387 employees. The NIH recruits and attracts the most capable research scientists in the world. In fact, the NIH indicates in "The NIH Almanac: Nobel Laureates" (August 6, 2012, http://www.nih.gov/about/almanac/nobel/index.htm) that as of August 2012, 136 scientists who conducted NIH research or were supported by NIH grants had received Nobel Prizes. Several Nobel Prize winners made their prize-winning discoveries in NIH laboratories.

Equally important, NIH research has contributed to great improvements in the health of the nation. The following are some of the NIH's (March 27, 2012, http://www.nih.gov/about/almanac/historical/chronology_of_events.htm) recent achievements (from 2009 to 2010):

- NIH released its final "Guidelines for Human Stem Cell Research" on July 6, after officials spent several weeks reviewing more than 49,000 public comments on the draft guidelines.

- NIH launched the first clinical trials of 2009 H1N1 vaccine candidates on July 22.

- [National Institute of Child Health and Human Development] began a research program to enhance newborn screening, which can identify serious, often fatal, disorders at birth so that treatment can begin.

- By evaluating the entire genome of a 40-year-old man, scientists pinpointed gene variants linked to cardiovascular disease and several other conditions in the man's family, as well as diseases not known to be in his family. Some variants predicted the man's likely responses to common medications, including certain heart medications. This NIH-funded study provides a glimpse into how whole-genome sequencing might one day be used in the clinic.

- An independent panel convened by the NIH Office of Medical Applications of Research determined there is currently no conclusive evidence that taking any substance or engaging in any activity can prevent or delay Alzheimer's disease or cognitive decline.

- A computer model of heart disease in U.S. adults suggested that reducing salt intake by 3 grams per day could cut the number of new cases of coronary heart disease each year by as many as 120,000, stroke by 66,000 and heart attack by nearly 100,000. It could also prevent up to 92,000 deaths and save up to $24 billion in health care costs a year, the NIH-funded researchers estimated.

- NIH launched a multi-year study to look at potential health effects from the oil spill in the Gulf region. The Gulf Worker Study is a response to the largest oil spill in U.S. history.

- Nearly 40% of the energy consumed by 2- to 18-year-olds comes in the form of "empty" calories, according to a study by NIH scientists. Half of those empty calories come from the solid fats and added sugars in just 6 sources: soda, fruit drinks, dairy desserts, grain

FIGURE 4.7

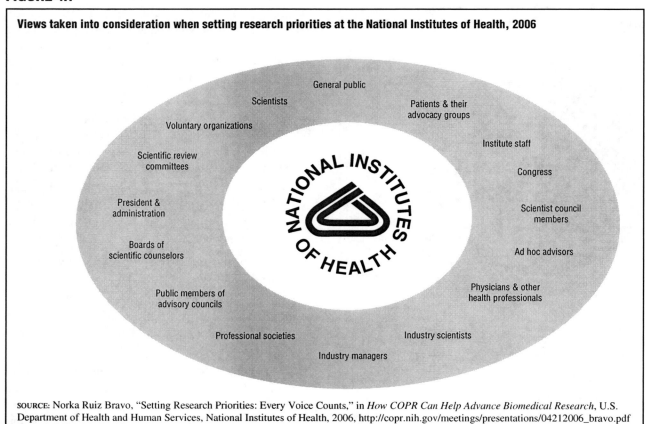

Views taken into consideration when setting research priorities at the National Institutes of Health, 2006

SOURCE: Norka Ruiz Bravo, "Setting Research Priorities: Every Voice Counts," in *How COPR Can Help Advance Biomedical Research*, U.S. Department of Health and Human Services, National Institutes of Health, 2006, http://copr.nih.gov/meetings/presentations/04212006_bravo.pdf (accessed June 19, 2012)

desserts, pizza and whole milk. Experts recommend that kids limit their intake of empty calories to 20% or less of their total calories.

- NIH-supported scientists developed a technique to regenerate damaged leg joints in rabbits. The researchers created porous scaffolds in the shape of leg bone tips and added a gel to aid cartilage development. By 3 to 4 weeks after surgery, the rabbits could move around almost as well as normal rabbits. Within 4 months, both bone and cartilage had regenerated. The accomplishment could point the way toward joint renewal in humans.

In "Francis Collins: 3 Scientific Breakthroughs Changing Medicine" (February 15, 2012, http://www.medscape.com/viewarticle/758435), an interview by John C. Reed for the program *Medscape One-on-One*, Francis S. Collins (1950–), the director of the NIH, explains that personalized medicine—understanding how family history and genetics influence an individual's risk of developing specific diseases—can help people take specific actions to reduce their risk of developing certain diseases. Collins also discusses the potential of genomic medicine to help physicians customize prevention programs for their patients. He observes that preventive medicine not only reduces the risk for and occurrence of disease but also serves to reduce health care

costs. There are several NIH websites where people can assess their risk and learn about actions to reduce risk:

- Smoking—http://www.cancer.gov/cancertopics/smoking offers smokers information about the risks that are associated with tobacco use and how to quit

- Breast cancer—http://www.cancer.gov/bcrisktool helps women assess their risk of developing breast cancer and http://www.cancer.gov/cancertopics/factsheet/Risk/BRCA provides information about cancer risk and genetic testing

- Colorectal cancer—http://www.cancer.gov/colorectalcancerrisk helps individuals assess their risks of developing colorectal cancer

- Cancer risk—http://www.cancer.gov/cancertopics/prevention-genetics-causes offers people at increased risk of developing cancer updated information about prevention and early detection

ACCREDITATION

Accreditation of health care providers (facilities and organizations) offers consumers, payers, and other stakeholders the assurance that accredited facilities and organizations have been certified as meeting or exceeding predetermined standards. Accreditation refers to both the process during which the quality of care delivered is measured and the resulting official endorsement that quality standards have been met. Besides promoting accreditation to health care consumers and other purchasers of care such as employer groups, accreditation assists health care facilities and organizations to recruit and retain qualified staff, increase organizational efficiencies to reduce costs, identify ways to improve service delivery, and reduce liability insurance premiums.

Joint Commission on Accreditation of Healthcare Organizations

The Joint Commission on Accreditation of Healthcare Organizations (JCAHO; September 12, 2012, http://www.jointcommission.org/about_us/about_the_joint_commission_main.aspx) surveys and accredits more than 19,000 health care organizations and programs throughout the United States. The JCAHO is a not-for-profit organization and is headquartered in Oakbrook Terrace, Illinois, with a satellite office in Washington, D.C. The JCAHO notes in "Facts about the Joint Commission" (January 2012, http://www.jointcommission.org/assets/1/18/The%20Joint%20Commission%203%207%20111.PDF) that it has more than 1,000 surveyors—physicians, nurses, pharmacists, hospital and health care organization administrators, and other health professionals—who are qualified and trained to evaluate specific aspects of health care quality.

Working closely with medical and other professional societies, purchasers of health care services, and management experts as well as with other accrediting organizations, the JCAHO develops the standards that health care organizations are expected to meet. Besides developing benchmarks and standards of organizational quality, the JCAHO is credited with promoting improvement in infection control, safety, and patients' rights.

THE JCAHO GROWS TO BECOME THE PREEMINENT ACCREDITING BODY. In *The Joint Commission History* (February 2012, http://www.jointcommission.org/assets/1/6/Joint_Commission_History_2012.pdf), the JCAHO explains that early efforts to standardize and evaluate care delivered in hospitals began in 1913 by the American College of Surgeons. Thirty-eight years later, in 1951, the Joint Commission on Accreditation of Hospitals (JCAH) was established. In 1966 the JCAH began offering accreditation to long-term care facilities, and in 1972 the Social Security Act was amended to require the U.S. secretary of health and human services to validate JCAH findings and include them in the HHS annual report to Congress. In subsequent years the JCAH's mandate was expanded to include a variety of other health care facilities, and in 1987 it was renamed the Joint Commission on Accreditation of Healthcare Organizations.

In 1992 the JCAHO instituted a requirement that accredited hospitals prohibit smoking in the hospital, and in 1993 it began performing random, surprise surveys (unannounced site visits) on 5% of accredited organizations. The JCAHO also moved to emphasize performance improvement standards by revising its policies on medical errors.

In 1999 the JCAHO required hospitals to begin collecting and reporting data about the care they provide for five specific diagnoses: acute myocardial infarction (heart attack), congestive heart failure, pneumonia, pregnancy and related medical conditions, and surgical procedures and complications. The JCAHO calls these diagnoses "core measure data" and uses these data to compare facilities and assess the quality of service delivered. In 2002 the JCAHO moved to make its recommendations more easily understood by consumers so they can make informed choices about health care providers.

In 2006 the JCAHO shifted to an unannounced survey program—meaning that organizations receive no advanced notice of their survey date. Before this policy change, the leaders of the nation's more than 4,500 Medicare-participating hospitals had ample notice and time to prepare for JCAHO visits and inspections. The policy change was intended to shift hospitals' orientation from preparing for the next JCAHO survey to preparing for the next patient. The policy also required hospitals to conduct an annual periodic performance review using their own internal evaluators to assess their own level of standards compliance and to communicate the results of their audit to the JCAHO.

This policy change, presumably implemented to improve hospital vigilance about safety, care, and quality, coincided with another, seemingly contradictory JCAHO policy change, which allowed hospitals to accumulate a higher number of deficiencies (patient care lapses and other violations) before sanctions are imposed on them. The JCAHO defends this practice by explaining that it would rather identify more problems and have hospitals resolve them than deny hospitals accreditation.

In "Statement from the Joint Commission Regarding Enactment of Health Care Reform Bill" (*Joint Commission Perspectives*, vol. 30, no. 5, May 2010), a statement about the Patient Protection and Affordable Care Act of 2010, the JCAHO asserts that "the United States has the most technologically sophisticated care in the world, and a cadre of dedicated and skilled health professionals beyond rival. At the same time, there are persistent issues in health care delivery that keep the health care system from attaining the highest achievable levels of quality and safety for every patient in every setting." The JCAHO explains that it is working with health care facilities, providers, the CMS, safety advocates, Congress, and other stakeholders to effectively address urgent health and safety issues.

The JCAHO's 2011 annual report on quality and safety, *Improving America's Hospitals: The Joint Commission's Annual Report on Quality and Safety* (November 2011, http://www.jointcommission.org/assets/1/6/TJC_Annual_Report_2011_9_13_11_.pdf), named and ranked hospitals distinguished as top performers in the use of evidence-based care processes (approaches and methods based on the results of research), which are closely linked to positive patient outcomes (how patients fare as a result of treatment). Stephen P. Schmaltz et al. demonstrate in "Hospital Performance Trends on National Quality Measures and the Association with Joint Commission Accreditation" (*Journal of Hospital Medicine*, vol. 6, no. 8, October 2011) that hospitals accredited by the JCAHO outperform non-accredited hospitals on nationally standardized quality measures.

National Committee for Quality Assurance

The National Committee for Quality Assurance (NCQA) is another well-respected accrediting organization that focuses its attention on the managed care industry. The NCQA began surveying and accrediting managed care organizations (MCOs) in 1991. The NCQA notes in the press release "PPOs Rising: Report Finds PPOs Catching up to HMOs on Quality" (2011, http://www.ncqa.org/tabid/1427/Default.aspx) that by 2011 most health maintenance organizations (HMOs) in the United States had been reviewed by the NCQA and that more than 118 million Americans (two-fifths of the U.S. population) enrolled in health plans were covered by NCQA-accredited plans. In addition, the NCQA's 15th annual *The State of Health Care Quality 2011* (2011, http://www.ncqa.org/LinkClick.aspx?fileticket=J8kEuhuPqxk%3d&tabid=836) compares for the first time HMOs and preferred provider organizations (PPOs) across all measures. This is a significant milestone because prior to this report some PPOs measured, but only a few disclosed their results. The NCQA commends PPOs' willingness to engage in self-evaluation, particularly in view of the fact that one-third of Americans are enrolled in PPOs.

When an MCO undergoes an NCQA survey, it is assessed by more than 60 different standards, each focusing on a specific aspect of health plan operations. The standards address access and service, the qualifications of providers, the organization's commitment to prevention programs and health maintenance, the quality of care delivered to members when they are ill or injured, and the organization's approach to helping members manage chronic diseases such as diabetes, heart disease, and asthma. To ensure fair comparisons between managed health care plans and to track their progress and improvement over time, the NCQA considers many standards, including:

- Management of asthma and effective use of medication

- Controlling hypertension (high blood pressure)

- Effective and appropriate use of antidepressant medications

- The frequency and consistency with which smokers are counseled to quit

- Rates of breast cancer screening

- The frequency and consistency with which beta blockers (drug treatment) are used following heart attack

- Rates of immunization among children and teens

The NCQA combines the Healthcare Effectiveness Data and Information Set (HEDIS) with national and regional benchmarks of quality in a national database called the Quality Compass. This national database enables employers and health care consumers to compare health plans to one another and make choices about coverage based on quality and value rather than simply on price and participating providers (physicians, hospitals, and other providers that offer services to the managed care plan members).

The NCQA issues health plan report cards that rate HMOs and MCOs, and health care consumers and other stakeholders can access them at the NCQA website. After the NCQA review, the plans may be granted the NCQA's full accreditation for three years, indicating a level of excellence that exceeds NCQA standards. Those that need some improvement are granted one-year accreditation with recommendations about areas that need improvement, and those MCOs that meet some but not all NCQA standards may be denied accreditation or granted provisional accreditation.

In *State of Health Care Quality 2011*, the NCQA acknowledges that "we find encouraging signs of rising quality. Across diverse measures of care, performance is improving, and insurers can be proud of what they have accomplished. We also note that some insurers are not reporting and that for some measures, we have not seen the gains in performance we would like." The NCQA explains, "Of the 32 HEDIS Effectiveness of Care measures, 23 show clear trends of improvement. While year-to-year gains are often quite small, they are steady over time." An example of a successful measure is that the percentage of HMO members who received colorectal cancer screening rose by 2% between 2009 and 2010. Less successful is avoidance of antibiotic treatment in adults with acute bronchitis (cough lasting longer than five days that is caused by a virus in 90% of cases). Antibiotics continue to be prescribed for 60% of cases of bronchitis, and of this percentage, 80% of antibiotic prescriptions were deemed unnecessary by the CDC because antibiotics are not effective against viral infections and their misuse may contribute to antibiotic resistance (making the drugs less effective).

Accreditation Association for Ambulatory Health Care

Another accrediting organization, the Accreditation Association for Ambulatory Health Care (AAAHC), was formed in 1979 and focuses exclusively on ambulatory (outpatient) facilities and programs. Outpatient clinics, group practices, student health services, occupational medicine clinics, and ambulatory surgery centers are among the organizations that are evaluated by the AAAHC. The AAAHC accreditation process involves a self-assessment by the organization seeking accreditation and a survey that is conducted by AAAHC surveyors who are all practicing professionals. The AAAHC grants accreditation for periods ranging from six months to three years.

In 2002 the AAAHC and the JCAHO signed a collaborative accreditation agreement that permits ambulatory health care organizations to use their AAAHC accreditation to satisfy the JCAHO's requirements. That same year the CMS granted the AAAHC authority to review health plans that provide coverage for Medicare beneficiaries. HMOs, PPOs, and ambulatory surgery centers are now considered to be Medicare-certified on their receipt of accreditation from the AAAHC.

In 2009 the AAAHC established standards for reviewing so-called medical homes—primary care practices that aim to serve as centralized overseers of all the health care needs of individuals. The term *medical home* is a relatively new descriptor of the long-standing practice of having a primary care practitioner (for adults usually an internist or family practitioner and for children a pediatrician) provide and coordinate needed care. By 2012 the AAAHC (http://www.aaahc.org/en/about/) was accrediting over 5,000 organizations.

National Quality Forum

In 2006 two other national quality organizations, the National Quality Forum and the National Committee on Quality Health Care, merged to become a new organization, also named the National Quality Forum (NQF; http://www.qualityforum.org/). The NQF is a private, not-for-profit membership organization created to develop and implement a national strategy for health care quality measurement and reporting. Its mission is to improve U.S. health care through the endorsement of consensus-based national standards for measurement and public reporting of health care performance data that provide meaningful information about whether care is safe, timely, beneficial, patient centered, equitable, and efficient.

In the press release "NQF Approves Expansion of Settings for Nursing Home Measures" (May 7, 2012, http://www.qualityforum.org/), the NQF states that it aims to improve the quality of U.S. health care by "building consensus on national priorities and goals for performance improvement and working in partnership to achieve them; endorsing national consensus standards for measuring and publicly reporting on performance; [and] promoting the attainment of national goals through education and outreach programs."

PROFESSIONAL SOCIETIES

There are professional and membership organizations and societies for all health professionals, such as physicians, nurses, psychologists, and hospital administrators, as well as for institutional health care providers, such as hospitals, managed care plans, and medical groups. These professional organizations represent the interests and concerns of their members, advocate on their behalf, and frequently compile data and publish information about working conditions, licensing, accreditation, compensation, and scientific advancements of interest to members.

American Medical Association

The American Medical Association (AMA) is a powerful voice for U.S. physicians' interests. The AMA concerns itself with a wide range of health-related issues including medical ethics, medical education, physician and patient advocacy, and development of national health policy. The AMA publishes the highly regarded *Journal of the American Medical Association* and the *AMNews*, as well as journals in 10 specialty areas called *Archives Journals*.

Founded in 1847, the AMA has worked to upgrade medical education by expanding medical school curricula and establishing standards for licensing and accreditation of practitioners and postgraduate training programs. Recent activities of the AMA include campaigning to avert a Medicare pay cut for physicians, combating childhood obesity, and supporting the 2010 health care reform legislation. In the speech "Focus and Impact: The AMA's Long-Range Strategic Plan" (http://www.ama-assn.org/ama/pub/news/speeches/2012-06-16-madara-annual-address.page), which was given during the AMA's annual meeting in Chicago on June 16, 2012, James L. Madera, the executive vice president and chief executive officer of the AMA, explains that the organization is focusing on "improving health outcomes, accelerating change in medical education, and shaping delivery and payment models that demonstrate high quality care and value while enhancing physician satisfaction and practice sustainability."

American Nurses Association

The American Nurses Association (ANA; 2012, http://www.nursingworld.org/FunctionalMenuCategories/About ANA) is a professional organization that represents more than 3.1 million registered nurses and promotes high standards of nursing practice and education as well as the roles and responsibilities of nurses in the workplace and the community. On behalf of its members, the ANA works to protect patients' rights, lobbies to advocate for nurses' interests, champions workplace safety, and provides career and continuing education opportunities. The ANA publishes the *American Journal of Nursing* and actively seeks to improve the public image of nurses among health professionals and the community at large.

American Hospital Association

The American Hospital Association (AHA; 2012, http://www.aha.org/aha/about/index.html) represents nearly 5,000 hospitals, health care systems, networks, and other health care providers and 40,000 individual members. Originally established as a membership organization for hospital superintendents in 1898, the AHA eventually expanded its mission to address all facets of hospital care and quality. Besides national advocacy activities and participation in the development of health policy, the AHA oversees research and pilot programs to improve health service delivery. It also gathers and disseminates hospital and other related health care data, publishes information of interest for its members, and sponsors educational opportunities for health care managers and administrators.

VOLUNTARY HEALTH ORGANIZATIONS
American Heart Association

The American Heart Association's mission is to decrease disability and death from cardiovascular disease and stroke. The association's national headquarters is in Dallas, Texas, and eight regional affiliate offices serve the balance of the United States. The American Heart Association explains in "History of the American Heart Association" (March 7, 2011, http://www.heart.org/HEART ORG/General/History-of-the-American-Heart-Association _UCM_308120_Article.jsp) that it was started by a group of physicians and social workers in New York City in 1915. The early efforts of this group, called the Association for the Prevention and Relief of Heart Disease, were to educate physicians and the general public about heart disease. The first fund-raising efforts were launched in 1948 during a radio broadcast, and since then the association has raised millions of dollars to fund research, education, and treatment programs.

Besides research, fund-raising, and generating public awareness about reducing the risk of developing heart disease, the American Heart Association has published many best-selling cookbooks that feature heart-healthy recipes and meal planning ideas. The association is also considered to be one of the world's most trusted authorities about heart health among physicians and scientists. It publishes five print journals and one online professional journal, including *Circulation, Stroke, Hypertension*, and *Atherosclerosis, Thrombosis, and Vascular Biology*.

The American Heart Association supports many initiatives to prevent heart disease and educate the community-at-large. For example, in the press release "American Heart Association's New Heart-Check Meal Certification Offers Consumer Confidence on Healthy Choices" (June 4, 2012 http://newsroom.heart.org/pr/aha/american-heart-association-s-new-234696.aspx), the association announces the expansion of its heart check program, the Heart-Check Meal Certification, that aims to help consumers choose heart-healthy meals when they dine out. For the last 17 years the same heart-check mark has assisted consumers to identify heart-healthy products in grocery stores.

The American Heart Association also educates consumers about the importance of seeking medical care immediately when symptoms arise. For example, in the press release "Heart Attack Patients Taken to PCI Hospitals First Treated Faster" (May 10, 2012, http://newsroom.heart.org/pr/aha/heart-attack-patients-taken-to-233120.aspx), the association indicates that patients taken directly to hospitals that treat heart attacks using percutaneous coronary intervention (PCI is a nonsurgical procedure that is used to restore blood flow to the coronary arteries that supply the heart) received lifesaving treatments earlier—on average 31 minutes sooner than patients first taken to a hospital without PCI capability.

American Cancer Society

The American Cancer Society (ACS; 2012, http://www.cancer.org/AboutUs/WhoWeAre/index) is headquartered in Atlanta, Georgia, and has more than 900 local offices across the country. The ACS's (November 11, 2008, http://www.cancer.org/AboutUs/WhoWeAre/acsmissionstatements) mission is "eliminating cancer as a major health problem by preventing cancer, saving lives, and diminishing suffering from cancer, through research, education, advocacy, and service."

The ACS is the biggest source of private, not-for-profit funding for cancer research—second only to the federal government. In "Facts about ACS" (2012, http://www.cancer.org/AboutUs/WhoWeAre/acs-fact-sheet), the ACS states that it has invested over $3.6 billion in cancer research at leading centers throughout the United States and has funded 46 Nobel Prize winners early in their careers. It also supports epidemiological research to provide cancer surveillance information about occurrence rates, risk factors, mortality, and availability of treatment services. The ACS publishes an array of patient information brochures and four clinical journals for health professionals: *Cancer, Cancer Cytopathology, CA: A Cancer Journal for Clinicians*, and *Cancer Practice*. The ACS also maintains a 24-hour consumer telephone line that is staffed by trained cancer information specialists and a website with information for professionals, patients and families, and the media.

Besides education, prevention, and patient services, the ACS advocates for cancer survivors, their families, and every potential cancer patient. The ACS seeks to obtain support and passage of laws, policies, and regulations that benefit people who are affected by cancer. The ACS is especially concerned with developing strategies to better serve the poor and people with little formal education, who historically have been disproportionately affected by cancer.

March of Dimes

The March of Dimes was founded in 1938 by President Franklin D. Roosevelt (1882–1945) to help protect American children from polio. Besides supporting the research that produced the polio vaccine, it has advocated birth defects research and the fortification of food supplies with folic acid to prevent neural tube defects. It has also supported increasing access to quality prenatal care and the growth of neonatal intensive care units to help improve the chances of survival for babies born prematurely or those with serious medical conditions.

The March of Dimes continues to partner with volunteers, scientific researchers, educators, and community outreach workers to help prevent birth defects. It funds genetic research, investigates the causes and treatment of premature birth, educates pregnant women, and provides health care services for women and children, such as immunizations, checkups, and treatment for childhood illnesses.

In *2011 Annual Report* (April 2012, http://www .marchofdimes.com/downloads/2011Annual_ReportOnline .pdf), the March of Dimes notes that in 2011 it provided support to more than 80,000 families with infants in newborn intensive care units, supported research to improve understanding of birth defects, took action to prevent premature births, and raised $211 million to fund research and programs to prevent birth defects, premature birth, and infant deaths.

CHAPTER 5
THE INCREASING COST OF HEALTH CARE

HOW MUCH DOES HEALTH CARE COST?

American society places a high value on human life and generally wants—and expects—quality medical care. However, quality care comes with an increasingly high cost. In 1970 the United States spent 7.2% of its gross domestic product (GDP; the total market value of final goods and services produced within an economy in a given year) on health care. By 2009 health care expenditures reached 17.6% of the GDP. Table 5.1 shows the growth in health care expenditures, the growth in the GDP, and the annual percent change for select years between 1960 and 2009.

For many years the consumer price index (CPI; a measure of the average change in prices paid by consumers) increased at a greater rate for medical care than for any other commodity. In 1990 the average annual increase in the overall CPI was 4.7%, whereas the average annual increase in the medical care index stood at 8.1%. (See Table 5.2.) In 2000 the average annual growth in the medical care index fell to 3.4%, but in 2005 it rose again to 4.4%, outpacing overall inflation, which was 2.5%. In 2010 the medical care index was 3.4%, more than twice overall inflation of 1.6%. The medical care index has consistently outpaced the CPI in each decade. Of all the components of health care delivery, the sharpest price increase in 2010 was in hospital services at 7.8%.

The Centers for Medicare and Medicaid Services (CMS) projects that by 2021 the national health expenditure will grow to nearly $4.8 trillion—19.6% of the GDP, from 17.9% in 2012. (See Table 5.3.) (Because the numbers in Table 5.3 are projections, they may differ from the actual numbers presented in some other tables and figures that appear in this chapter.) In *National Health Expenditures Projections 2011–2021* (2012, https://www.cms.gov/Research-Statistics-Data-and-Systems/Statistics-Trends-and-Reports/NationalHealthExpendData/Downloads/Proj2011PDF.pdf), the CMS indicates that Medicare accounted for a staggering 21.3% of national care expenditures in 2012.

Generally, projections are most accurate for the near future and less accurate for the distant future. For example, predictions for 2030 should be viewed more warily than predictions for 2014, because it is unlikely that the conditions on which the projections are based will remain the same. As a result, the CMS cautions that its projections should not be viewed as predictions for the future. Rather, they are intended to help policy makers evaluate the costs or savings of proposed legislative or regulatory changes.

Total Health Care Spending

The CMS, along with the Centers for Disease Control and Prevention and the U.S. Government Accountability Office, maintain most of the nation's statistics on health care costs. The CMS reports that the United States spent $2.8 trillion for health care in 2012, up 4.2% from $2.7 trillion in 2011. (See Table 5.3.) This rate has decreased since the 6.2% increase in 2007 and is projected to rise in 2014 and then remain relatively constant, although it will likely be as high as three times the rate of inflation through 2021.

Over $1.2 trillion of the 2012 health care expenditures came from private funds (out-of-pocket payments and private health insurance), and the balance was paid with public money. (See Table 5.4.) The 2012 per capita cost for health care (the average per individual if spending was divided equally among all people in the country) was $8,953.

Of the $2.8 trillion that was spent on health care in 2012, nearly $2.4 trillion was spent on personal health services (expenses incurred by individuals as opposed to institutions). (See Table 5.5.) Some of the services included hospital care, physician and dental services, nursing and home health care, prescription drugs, and durable medical equipment.

TABLE 5.1

Gross domestic product (GDP), national health expenditures, per capita amounts, and average annual percent change, selected years 1960–2009

Gross domestic product and national health expenditures	1960	1970	1980	1990	2000	2005	2008	2009
					Amount in billions			
Gross domestic product (GDP)	$526	$1,038	$2,788	$5,801	$9,952	$12,638	$14,369	$14,119
					Deflator (2005 = 100.0)			
Implicit price deflator for GDP[a]	18.6	24.3	47.8	72.2	88.6	100.0	108.6	109.6
					Amount in billions			
National health expenditures	$27.3	$74.8	$255.7	$724.0	$1,378.0	$2,021.0	$2,391.4	$2,486.3
Health consumption expenditures	24.8	67.0	235.6	675.3	1,288.5	1,890.3	2,234.2	2,330.1
Personal health care	23.3	63.1	217.1	616.6	1,164.4	1,692.6	1,997.2	2,089.9
Administration and net cost of private health insurance	1.1	2.6	12.0	38.7	81.1	141.6	164.0	163.0
Public health	0.4	1.4	6.4	20.0	43.0	56.2	72.9	77.2
Investment[b]	2.6	7.8	20.1	48.7	89.6	130.7	157.2	156.2
					Per capita amount in dollars			
National health expenditures	$147	$356	$1,110	$2,853	$4,878	$6,827	$7,845	$8,086
Health consumption expenditures	133	319	1,022	2,661	4,561	6,385	7,329	7,578
Personal health care	125	300	942	2,430	4,122	5,717	6,552	6,797
Administration and net cost of private health insurance	6	12	52	153	287	478	538	530
Public health	2	6	28	79	152	190	239	251
Investment[b]	14	37	87	192	317	441	516	508
					Percent			
National health expenditures as percent of GDP	5.2	7.2	9.2	12.5	13.8	16.0	16.6	17.6
					Percent distribution			
National health expenditures	100.0	100.0	100.0	100.0	100.0	100.0	100.0	100.0
Health consumption expenditures	90.6	89.6	92.1	93.3	93.5	93.5	93.4	93.7
Personal health care	85.4	84.3	84.9	85.2	84.5	83.7	83.5	84.1
Administration and net cost of private health insurance	3.9	3.5	4.7	5.4	5.9	7.0	6.9	6.6
Public health	1.4	1.8	2.5	2.8	3.1	2.8	3.1	3.1
Investment[b]	9.4	10.4	7.9	6.7	6.5	6.5	6.6	6.3
					Average annual percent change from previous year shown			
GDP	—	7.0	10.4	7.6	5.5	4.9	4.4	−1.7
National health expenditures	—	10.6	13.1	11.0	6.6	8.0	5.8	4.0
Health consumption expenditures	—	10.5	13.4	11.1	6.7	8.0	5.7	4.3
Personal health care	—	10.4	13.2	11.0	6.6	7.8	5.7	4.6
Administration and net cost of private health insurance	—	9.4	16.4	12.4	7.7	11.8	5.0	−0.6
Public health	—	13.8	16.9	12.0	8.0	5.5	9.1	5.9
Investment[b]	—	11.7	10.0	9.2	6.3	7.9	6.3	−0.6
National health expenditures, per capita	—	9.3	12.0	9.9	5.5	7.0	4.7	3.1
Health consumption expenditures	—	9.1	12.4	10.0	5.5	7.0	4.7	3.4
Personal health care	—	9.1	12.1	9.9	5.4	6.8	4.6	3.7
Administration and net cost of private health insurance	—	8.1	15.4	11.3	6.5	10.8	4.0	−1.5
Public health	—	12.5	15.8	10.9	6.8	4.5	8.0	4.9
Investment[b]	—	10.4	8.9	8.2	5.2	6.8	5.3	−1.5

—Category not applicable.
[a]Year 2005 = 100. Last revised July 30, 2010, by the Bureau of Economic Analysis.
[b]Investment consists of research and structures and equipment.
Notes: Dollar amounts shown are in current dollars. The data reflect U.S. Census Bureau resident population estimates as of July 1, 2009, excluding the Armed Forces overseas. Percents are calculated using unrounded data. Estimates may not add to totals because of rounding. Starting with *Health, United States, 2010,* estimates are based on a revised methodology that incorporates available source data and various methodological and definitional changes. These revisions are due to a comprehensive change in the classification structure of how estimates are defined and presented. Data have been revised and differ from previous editions of *Health, United States.*

SOURCE: "Table 125. Gross Domestic Product, National Health Expenditures, per Capita Amounts, Percent Distribution, and Average Annual Percent Change: United States, Selected Years 1960–2009," in *Health, United States, 2011: With Special Feature on Socioeconomic Status and Health,* U.S. Department of Health and Human Services, Centers for Disease Control and Prevention, National Center for Health Statistics, May 2012, http://www.cdc.gov/nchs/data/hus/hus11.pdf (accessed June 13, 2012)

Table 5.5 shows the trends and annual percent changes in personal health care expenditures by category. In 2012 the nation spent $884.7 billion on hospital care, by far the largest amount of personal health care spending, followed by $735.4 billion on professional services. This expense was followed by $549.6 billion on physician and clinical services, $367.4 billion on retail outlet sales of medical products, $277.1 billion on prescription drugs, and $155.2 billion on nursing home and continuing care.

WHO PAYS THE BILL?

In general, the government is the fastest-growing payer of health care expenses. In 2010 the public share (Medicare, Medicaid, and other health insurance

TABLE 5.2

Consumer price index and average annual percent change for all items, selected items, and medical care costs, selected years 1960–2009

Items and medical care components	1960	1970	1980	1990	1995	2000	2005	2009	2010
					Consumer Price Index (CPI)				
All items	29.6	38.8	82.4	130.7	152.4	172.2	195.3	214.5	218.1
All items less medical care	30.2	39.2	82.8	128.8	148.6	167.3	188.7	206.6	209.7
Services	24.1	35.0	77.9	139.2	168.7	195.3	230.1	259.2	261.3
Food	30.0	39.2	86.8	132.4	148.4	167.8	190.7	218.0	219.6
Apparel	45.7	59.2	90.9	124.1	132.0	129.6	119.5	120.1	119.5
Housing	—	36.4	81.1	128.5	148.5	169.6	195.7	217.1	216.3
Energy	22.4	25.5	86.0	102.1	105.2	124.6	177.1	193.1	211.4
Medical care	22.3	34.0	74.9	162.8	220.5	260.8	323.2	375.6	388.4
Components of medical care									
Medical care services	19.5	32.3	74.8	162.7	224.2	266.0	336.7	397.3	411.2
Professional services	—	37.0	77.9	156.1	201.0	237.7	281.7	319.4	328.2
Physicians' services	21.9	34.5	76.5	160.8	208.8	244.7	287.5	320.8	331.3
Dental services	27.0	39.2	78.9	155.8	206.8	258.5	324.0	388.1	398.8
Eyeglasses and eye care[a]	—	—	—	117.3	137.0	149.7	163.2	175.5	176.7
Services by other medical professionals[a]	—	—	—	120.2	143.9	161.9	186.8	209.8	214.4
Hospital and related services	—	—	69.2	178.0	257.8	317.3	439.9	567.9	607.7
Hospital services[b]	—	—	—	—	—	115.9	161.6	210.7	227.2
Inpatient hospital services[b,c]	—	—	—	—	—	113.8	156.6	203.6	221.5
Outpatient hospital services[a,c]	—	—	—	138.7	204.6	263.8	373.0	490.6	520.6
Hospital rooms	9.3	23.6	68.0	175.4	251.2	—	—	—	—
Other inpatient services[a]	—	—	—	142.7	206.8	—	—	—	—
Nursing homes and adult day care[b]	—	—	—	—	—	117.0	145.0	171.6	177.0
Health insurance[d]	—	—	—	—	—	—	—	110.5	106.6
Medical care commodities	46.9	46.5	75.4	163.4	204.5	238.1	276.0	305.1	314.7
Medicinal drugs[e]	—	—	—	—	—	—	—	—	102.3
Prescription drugs[f]	54.0	47.4	72.5	181.7	235.0	285.4	349.0	391.1	407.8
Nonprescription drugs[e]	—	—	—	—	—	—	—	—	100.0
Medical equipment and supplies[e]	—	—	—	—	—	—	—	—	99.1
Nonprescription drugs and medical supplies[a,g]	—	—	—	120.6	140.5	149.5	151.7	161.4	—
Internal and respiratory over-the-counter drugs[h]	—	42.3	74.9	145.9	167.0	176.9	179.7	193.0	—
Nonprescription medical equipment and supplies[i]	—	—	79.2	138.0	166.3	178.1	180.6	188.2	—
					Average annual percent change from previous year shown				
All items	. . .	2.7	7.8	4.7	3.1	2.5	2.5	2.4	1.6
All items less medical care	. . .	2.6	7.8	4.5	2.9	2.4	2.4	2.3	1.5
Services	. . .	3.8	8.3	6.0	3.9	3.0	3.3	3.0	0.8
Food	. . .	2.7	8.3	4.3	2.3	2.5	2.6	3.4	0.8
Apparel	. . .	2.6	4.4	3.2	1.2	−0.4	−1.6	0.1	−0.5
Housing	. . .	—	8.3	4.7	2.9	2.7	2.9	2.6	−0.4
Energy	. . .	1.3	12.9	1.7	0.6	3.4	7.3	2.2	9.5
Medical care	. . .	4.3	8.2	8.1	6.3	3.4	4.4	3.8	3.4
Components of medical care									
Medical care services	. . .	5.2	8.8	8.1	6.6	3.5	4.8	4.2	3.5
Professional services	. . .	—	7.7	7.2	5.2	3.4	3.5	3.2	2.8
Physicians' services	. . .	4.6	8.3	7.7	5.4	3.2	3.3	2.8	3.3
Dental services	. . .	3.8	7.2	7.0	5.8	4.6	4.6	4.6	2.7
Eyeglasses and eye care[a]	. . .	—	—	—	3.2	1.8	1.7	1.8	0.7
Services by other medical professionals[a]	. . .	—	—	—	3.7	2.4	2.9	2.9	2.2
Hospital and related services	. . .	—	—	9.9	7.7	4.2	6.8	6.6	7.0
Hospital services[b]	. . .	—	—	—	—	—	6.9	6.9	7.8
Inpatient hospital services[b,c]	. . .	—	—	—	—	—	6.6	6.8	8.8
Outpatient hospital services[a,c]	. . .	—	—	—	8.1	5.2	7.2	7.1	6.1
Hospital rooms	. . .	9.8	11.2	9.9	7.4	—	—	—	—
Other inpatient services[a]	. . .	—	—	—	7.7	—	—	—	—
Nursing homes and adult day care[b]	. . .	—	—	—	—	—	4.4	4.3	3.1
Health insurance[d]	. . .	—	—	—	—	—	—	—	−3.5
Medical care commodities	. . .	−0.1	5.0	8.0	4.6	3.1	3.0	2.5	3.1
Medicinal drugs[e]	. . .	—	—	—	—	—	—	—	. . .
Prescription drugs[f]	. . .	−1.3	4.3	9.6	5.3	4.0	4.1	2.9	4.3
Nonprescription drugs[e]	. . .	—	—	—	—	—	—	—	. . .
Medical equipment and supplies[e]	. . .	—	—	—	—	—	—	—	. . .
Nonprescription drugs and medical supplies[a,g]	. . .	—	—	—	3.1	1.2	0.3	1.6	—
Internal and respiratory over-the-counter drugs[h]	. . .	—	5.9	6.9	2.7	1.2	0.3	1.8	—
Nonprescription medical equipment and supplies[i]	. . .	—	—	5.7	3.8	1.4	0.3	1.0	—

programs and third-party payers) of the nation's total health care bill was 55.7%, and it is projected to rise to 59.3% by 2021. (See Table 5.4.) In 2010 private health insurance, the major nongovernmental payer of health care costs, paid 32.7% of all health expenditures. The share of health care spending from private,

TABLE 5.2

Consumer price index and average annual percent change for all items, selected items, and medical care costs, selected years 1960–2009 [CONTINUED]

—Data not available.
. . .Category not applicable.
ªDecember 1986 = 100.
ᵇDecember 1996 = 100.
ᶜSpecial index based on a substantially smaller sample.
ᵈDecember 2005 = 100.
ᵉDecember 2009 = 100.
ᶠPrior to 2006, this category included medical supplies.
ᵍStarting with 2010 updates, this index series will no longer be published.
ʰStarting with 2010 updates, replaced by the series, Nonprescription drugs.
ⁱStarting with 2010 updates, replaced by the series, Medical equipment and supplies.
Notes: CPI for all urban consumers (CPI-U) U.S. city average, detailed expenditure categories. 1982–1984 = 100, except where noted. Data are not seasonally adjusted. Data for additional years are available.

SOURCE: "Table 126. Consumer Price Index and Average Annual Percent Change for All Items, Selected Items, and Medical Care Components: United States, Selected Years 1960–2009," in *Health, United States, 2011: With Special Feature on Socioeconomic Status and Health*, U.S. Department of Health and Human Services, Centers for Disease Control and Prevention, National Center for Health Statistics, May 2012, http://www.cdc.gov/nchs/data/hus/hus11.pdf (accessed June 13, 2012)

out-of-pocket (paid by the patient) funds declined from 12.2% in 2008 to 11.6% in 2011.

The Patient Protection and Affordable Care Act and the Health Care and Education Reconciliation Act (which are now commonly known as the ACA) authorize and fund programs that are aimed at slowing health care spending increases, such as funding comparative effectiveness research and care delivered via patient-centered medical homes. The ACA also evaluates the ability of accountable care organizations (ACOs; groups of health care providers that offer coordinated care and chronic disease management in an effort to improve the quality of care patients receive; an ACO's payment is tied to achieving health care quality goals and outcomes that result in cost savings) to control health care costs.

The Congressional Budget Office (CBO) indicates in *Estimates for the Insurance Coverage Provisions of the Affordable Care Act Updated for the Recent Supreme Court Decision* (July 2012, http://www.cbo.gov/sites/default/files/cbofiles/attachments/43472-07-24-2012-CoverageEstimates.pdf) that the ACA, with its limit on Medicaid expansion, will leave 6 million fewer people insured than previously projected. Approximately half of these people will be covered by the insurance exchanges. Per capita (per head), these people will be more expensive to the government, but there will be far fewer of them. The remaining 3 million people will go without any insurance, and this decrease in coverage will save the federal government $84 billion by 2022.

In *America under the Affordable Care Act* (December 2010, http://www.rwjf.org/files/research/71555.pdf), Matthew Buettgens, Bowen Garrett, and John Holahan predict that costs of uncompensated care for people who are uninsured will decline 60.9%, from $69.6 billion to $27.3 billion. Total spending on acute health care for all people except older adults by the government, employers,

and individuals will increase 4.5%, or $53.1 billion. This estimate does not, however, consider the cost-savings that are likely to result from multiyear provisions such as Medicare and Medicaid savings and cost-containment programs, nor does it take into account savings that result from the limited expansion of Medicaid.

Personal Health Care Bill

Much of the increase in government spending has occurred in the area of personal health care. In 2006 government sources paid 49.4% of personal health care expenditures; by 2010 they covered 52.2% of the $2.2 trillion spent on personal health care services. (See Table 5.6.) Some of the federal increase was attributed to Medicare spending, which grew from 21.1% of all personal health care expenditures in 2006 to 22.6% in 2010.

WHY HAVE HEALTH CARE COSTS AND SPENDING INCREASED?

The increase in the cost of medical care is challenging to analyze because the methods and quality of health care change constantly and as a result are often not comparable. A hospital stay in 1970 did not include the same services offered in 2012. Furthermore, the care received in a physician's office in 2012 is not comparable to that received a generation ago. One contributing factor to the rising cost of health care is the increase in biomedical technology, much of which is now available for use outside of a hospital.

Many other factors also contribute to the increase in health care costs. These include population growth, high salaries for physicians and some other health care workers, and the expense of malpractice insurance. Escalating malpractice insurance costs and professional liability premiums have prompted some physicians and other health

TABLE 5.3

National health expenditures and annual percent change, 2006–21

Item	2006	2007	2008	2009	2011	2012	Projected 2013	2014	2015	2016	2017	2018	2019	2020	2021
National health expenditures (billions)	$2,162.4	$2,297.1	$2,403.9	$2,495.8	$2,695.0	$2,809.0	$2,915.5	$3,130.2	$3,307.6	$3,514.4	$3,723.3	$3,952.3	$4,207.3	$4,487.2	$4,781.0
National health expenditures as a percent of gross domestic product	16.2%	16.4%	16.8%	17.9%	17.9%	17.9%	17.8%	18.2%	18.2%	18.3%	18.4%	18.6%	18.9%	19.2%	19.6%
National health expenditures per capita	$7,250.6	$7,627.7	$7,910.9	$8,148.6	$8,660.5	$8,952.8	$9,214.2	$9,807.5	$10,272.0	$10,817.6	$11,360.2	$11,955.0	$12,618.3	$13,345.6	$14,102.6
Gross domestic product (billions)	$13,377.2	$14,028.7	$14,291.5	$13,939.0	$15,093.0	$15,696.8	$16,387.4	$17,223.2	$18,204.9	$19,224.4	$20,243.3	$21,295.9	$22,318.1	$23,344.7	$24,395.3
Gross domestic product (billions of 2005 $)	$12,958.5	$13,206.4	$13,161.9	$12,703.1	$13,323.6	$13,616.7	$13,998.0	$14,487.9	$15,067.4	$15,640.0	$16,156.1	$16,640.8	$17,040.2	$17,415.0	$17,780.8
Gross domestic product implicit price deflator (chain weighted 2005 base year)	1.032	1.062	1.086	1.097	1.133	1.154	1.171	1.190	1.210	1.232	1.256	1.284	1.315	1.346	1.379
Consumer price index (CPI-W)—1982–1984 base	2.016	2.073	2.153	2.145	2.207	2.244	2.287	2.333	2.379	2.427	2.480	2.545	2.616	2.689	2.765
U.S. Population*	298.2	301.2	303.9	306.3	311.2	313.8	316.4	319.2	322.0	324.9	327.7	330.6	333.4	336.2	339.0
Population age less than 65 years	261.2	263.4	265.2	266.8	270.4	271.7	272.9	274.3	275.8	277.2	278.6	279.8	281.0	282.1	283.1
Population age 65 years and older	37.1	37.8	38.7	39.5	40.8	42.1	43.5	44.9	46.2	47.7	49.2	50.8	52.4	54.1	55.9
Private health insurance—NHE (billions)	$740.2	$776.2	$807.6	$828.8	$864.4	$888.6	$925.2	$997.8	$1,060.4	$1,130.5	$1,191.0	$1,252.5	$1,329.2	$1,412.0	$1,495.4
Private health insurance—PHC (billions)	640.6	673.5	707.5	734.0	758.5	775.9	799.6	863.5	919.7	981.6	1,039.2	1,096.1	1,166.2	1,239.3	1,313.7
National health expenditures (billions)	—	6.2%	4.7%	3.8%	3.9%	4.2%	3.8%	7.4%	5.7%	6.3%	5.9%	6.2%	6.5%	6.7%	6.5%
National health expenditures as a percent of gross domestic product (change)	—	1.3	2.7	6.4	0.0	0.2	-0.6	2.2	0.0	0.6	0.6	0.9	1.6	2.0	2.0
National health expenditures per capita	—	5.2	3.7	3.0	3.1	3.4	2.9	6.4	4.7	5.3	5.0	5.2	5.5	5.8	5.7
Gross domestic product (billions)	—	4.9	1.9	-2.5	3.9	4.0	4.4	5.1	5.7	5.6	5.3	5.2	4.8	4.6	4.5
Gross domestic product (billions of 2005 $)	—	1.9	-0.3	-3.5	1.8	2.2	2.8	3.5	4.0	3.8	3.3	3.0	2.4	2.2	2.1
Gross domestic product implicit price deflator (chain weighted 2005 base year)	—	2.9	2.2	1.1	2.1	1.8	1.5	1.6	1.7	1.8	2.0	2.2	2.4	2.4	2.4
Consumer price index (CPI-W)—1982–1984 base	—	2.8	3.8	-0.4	1.2	1.7	1.9	2.0	2.0	2.0	2.2	2.6	2.8	2.8	2.8
U.S. population*	—	1.0	0.9	0.8	0.8	0.8	0.8	0.9	0.9	0.9	0.9	0.9	0.9	0.8	0.8
Population age less than 65 years	—	0.9	0.7	0.6	0.6	0.5	0.5	0.5	0.5	0.5	0.5	0.5	0.4	0.4	0.4
Population age 65 years and older	—	1.9	2.5	2.0	2.4	3.2	3.4	3.1	3.1	3.1	3.1	3.2	3.3	3.3	3.2
Private health insurance—NHE	—	4.9	4.0	2.6	1.8	2.8	4.1	7.9	6.3	6.6	5.4	5.2	6.1	6.2	5.9
Private health insurance—PHC	—	5.1	5.1	3.7	1.7	2.3	3.1	8.0	6.5	6.7	5.9	5.5	6.4	6.3	6.0

*July 1 Census resident based population estimates.

Note: The health spending projections were based on the National Health Expenditures released in January 2012. The projections include impacts of the Affordable Care Act. Numbers and percents may not add to totals because of rounding.

SOURCE: "Table 1. National Health Expenditures and Selected Economic Indicators, Levels and Annual Percent Change: Calendar Years 2006–2021," in *National Health Expenditures Projections 2011–2021*, U.S. Department of Health and Human Services, Centers for Medicare and Medicaid Services, 2012, http://www.cms.gov/Research-Statistics-Data-and-Systems/Statistics-Trends-and-Reports/NationalHealthExpendData/Downloads/Proj2011PDF.pdf (accessed June 24, 2012)

TABLE 5.4

National health expenditures, by source of funds, 2006–21

Year	Total	Out-of-pocket payments	Health insurance[a]					Other third party payers[c]
			Total	Private health insurance	Medicare	Medicaid	Other health insurance programs[b]	
Historical estimates			Amount in billions					
2006	$2,162.4	$271.9	$1,520.2	$740.2	$403.1	$306.8	$70.1	$370.3
2007	2,297.1	287.3	1,610.2	776.2	432.3	326.4	75.4	399.6
2008	2,403.9	294.0	1,700.7	807.6	466.9	343.8	82.4	409.2
2009	2,495.8	294.4	1,793.3	828.8	499.8	374.4	90.3	408.1
2010	2,593.6	299.7	1,870.8	848.7	524.6	401.4	96.1	423.2
Projected								
2011	2,695.0	304.4	1,953.4	864.4	557.8	428.7	102.5	437.2
2012	2,809.0	312.1	2,046.1	888.6	590.8	458.9	107.7	450.8
2013	2,915.5	322.7	2,127.5	925.2	598.4	491.0	113.0	465.3
2014	3,130.2	317.7	2,331.6	997.8	635.0	579.2	119.5	480.8
2015	3,307.6	328.9	2,474.6	1,060.4	666.5	621.0	126.8	504.1
2016	3,514.4	340.0	2,642.7	1,130.5	707.0	672.4	132.7	531.7
2017	3,723.3	359.4	2,799.3	1,191.0	754.8	719.4	134.1	564.6
2018	3,952.3	381.6	2,971.8	1,252.5	809.1	769.9	140.3	598.8
2019	4,207.3	402.9	3,172.1	1,329.2	867.9	825.8	149.1	632.2
2020	4,487.2	426.0	3,394.3	1,412.0	934.9	888.6	158.8	667.0
2021	4,781.0	449.2	3,628.5	1,495.4	1,006.9	957.4	168.9	703.2
Historical estimates			Per capita amount					
2006	$7,251	$912	d	d	d	d	d	d
2007	7,628	954	d	d	d	d	d	d
2008	7,911	967	d	d	d	d	d	d
2009	8,149	961	d	d	d	d	d	d
2010	8,402	971	d	d	d	d	d	d
Projected								
2011	8,661	978	d	d	d	d	d	d
2012	8,953	995	d	d	d	d	d	d
2013	9,214	1,020	d	d	d	d	d	d
2014	9,807	996	d	d	d	d	d	d
2015	10,272	1,022	d	d	d	d	d	d
2016	10,818	1,046	d	d	d	d	d	d
2017	11,360	1,097	d	d	d	d	d	d
2018	11,955	1,154	d	d	d	d	d	d
2019	12,618	1,209	d	d	d	d	d	d
2020	13,346	1,267	d	d	d	d	d	d
2021	14,103	1,325	d	d	d	d	d	d
Historical estimates			Percent distribution					
2006	100.0	12.6	70.3	34.2	18.6	14.2	3.2	17.1
2007	100.0	12.5	70.1	33.8	18.8	14.2	3.3	17.4
2008	100.0	12.2	70.7	33.6	19.4	14.3	3.4	17.0
2009	100.0	11.8	71.9	33.2	20.0	15.0	3.6	16.4
2010	100.0	11.6	72.1	32.7	20.2	15.5	3.7	16.3
Projected								
2011	100.0	11.3	72.5	32.1	20.7	15.9	3.8	16.2
2012	100.0	11.1	72.8	31.6	21.0	16.3	3.8	16.0
2013	100.0	11.1	73.0	31.7	20.5	16.8	3.9	16.0
2014	100.0	10.2	74.5	31.9	20.3	18.5	3.8	15.4
2015	100.0	9.9	74.8	32.1	20.1	18.8	3.8	15.2
2016	100.0	9.7	75.2	32.2	20.1	19.1	3.8	15.1
2017	100.0	9.7	75.2	32.0	20.3	19.3	3.6	15.2
2018	100.0	9.7	75.2	31.7	20.5	19.5	3.6	15.2
2019	100.0	9.6	75.4	31.6	20.6	19.6	3.5	15.0
2020	100.0	9.5	75.6	31.5	20.8	19.8	3.5	14.9
2021	100.0	9.4	75.9	31.3	21.1	20.0	3.5	14.7
Historical estimates			Annual percent change from previous year shown					
2006	—	—	—	—	—	—	—	—
2007	6.2	5.6	5.9	4.9	7.2	6.4	7.6	7.9
2008	4.7	2.3	5.6	4.0	8.0	5.3	9.3	2.4
2009	3.8	0.2	5.4	2.6	7.0	8.9	9.6	−0.3
2010	3.9	1.8	4.3	2.4	5.0	7.2	6.5	3.7

care practitioners to refrain from performing high-risk procedures that increase their vulnerability or have caused them to relocate to states where malpractice pre-miums are lower. Furthermore, to protect themselves from malpractice suits, many health care practitioners routinely order diagnostic tests and prescribe treatments

TABLE 5.4

National health expenditures, by source of funds, 2006–21 [CONTINUED]

| Year | Total | Out-of-pocket payments | Health insurance[a] | | | | | Other third party payers[c] |
			Total	Private health insurance	Medicare	Medicaid	Other health insurance programs[b]	
Projected								
2011	3.9	1.6	4.4	1.8	6.3	6.8	6.6	3.3
2012	4.2	2.5	4.7	2.8	5.9	7.0	5.1	3.1
2013	3.8	3.4	4.0	4.1	1.3	7.0	4.9	3.2
2014	7.4	−1.5	9.6	7.9	6.1	18.0	5.8	3.3
2015	5.7	3.5	6.1	6.3	4.9	7.2	6.1	4.8
2016	6.3	3.4	6.8	6.6	6.1	8.3	4.7	5.5
2017	5.9	5.7	5.9	5.4	6.8	7.0	1.0	6.2
2018	6.2	6.2	6.2	5.2	7.2	7.0	4.6	6.1
2019	6.5	5.6	6.7	6.1	7.3	7.3	6.3	5.6
2020	6.7	5.7	7.0	6.2	7.7	7.6	6.4	5.5
2021	6.5	5.5	6.9	5.9	7.7	7.7	6.4	5.4

[a]Includes private health insurance (employer sponsored insurance, state health insurance exchanges, and other private insurance), Medicare, Medicaid, children's health insurance program (Titles XIX and XXI), Department of Defense, and Department of Veterans' Affairs.
[b]Children's health insurance program (Titles XIX and XXI), Department of Defense, and Department of Veterans' Affairs.
[c]Includes worksite health care, other private revenues, Indian Health Service, workers' compensation, general assistance, maternal and child health, vocational rehabilitation, other federal programs, Substance Abuse and Mental Health Services Administration, other state and local programs, and school health.
[d]Calculation of per capita estimates is not applicable.
Notes: The health spending projections were based on the National Health Expenditures (NHE) released in January 2012. The projections include impacts from the Affordable Care Act. Per capita amounts based on July 1 Census resident based population estimates. Numbers and percents may not add to totals because of rounding.

SOURCE: "Table 3. National Health Expenditures; Aggregate and per Capita Amounts, Percent Distribution and Annual Percent Change by Source of Funds: Calendar Years 2006–2021," in *National Health Expenditures Projections 2011–2021*, U.S. Department of Health and Human Services, Centers for Medicare and Medicaid Services, 2012, http://www.cms.gov/Research-Statistics-Data-and-Systems/Statistics-Trends-and-Reports/NationalHealthExpendData/Downloads/Proj2011PDF.pdf (accessed June 24, 2012)

that are not medically necessary and do not serve to improve their patients' health. This practice is known as defensive medicine, and even though its precise contribution to rising health care costs is difficult to gauge, industry observers agree that it is a significant factor.

In "National and Surgical Health Care Expenditures, 2005–2025" (*Annals of Surgery*, vol. 251, no. 2, February 2010), Eric Muñoz et al. attribute unabated health care spending in part to defensive medicine. However, other industry observers, such as Tom Baker in "Liability = Responsibility" (*New York Times*, July 11, 2009) and Daphne Eviatar in "Tort Reform Unlikely to Cut Health Care Costs" (*Washington Independent*, August 19, 2009), assert that defensive medicine makes a very small contribution to health care expenditures. They also suggest that malpractice liability costs are just a scant 1.5% of U.S. health care system costs and that the medical errors that malpractice liability tries to prevent pose greater costs—to injured patients and to the health care system.

Steven A. Schroeder of the University of California, San Francisco, attributes in "Personal Reflections on the High Cost of American Medical Care: Many Causes but Few Politically Sustainable Solutions" (*Archives of Internal Medicine*, vol. 171, no, 8, April 2011) escalating costs to unexplained variations in the use of medical services such as diagnostic laboratory testing, a protechnology payment bias (medical practices that perform and

bill for a greater number and more frequent diagnostic tests, which generate higher physician incomes even when they see far fewer patients than practices that do not), increased use of medical technologies such as advanced imaging, escalating hospital expenditures, expanded number and use of intensive care units, more intensive end-of-life care, and overreliance on expensive medical specialists.

In "Overuse of Health Care Services in the United States: An Understudied Problem" (*Archives of Internal Medicine*, vol. 172, no. 2, January 23, 2012), Deborah Korenstein et al. researched overuse (the provision of health care services for which harms outweigh the benefits). The researchers conclude that overuse of diagnostic tests, therapeutic procedures, and medications may not only harm patients but may also contribute to as much as 30% of health care expenditures in the United States.

Other factors for the increase in health care costs include advanced biomedical procedures that require high-technology expertise and equipment, redundant (excessive and unnecessary) technology in hospitals, cumbersome medical insurance programs and consumer demand for less restrictive insurance plans (ones that offer more choices, benefits, and coverage, but usually mean higher premiums), and consumer demand for the latest and most comprehensive testing and treatment. Legislation that increased Medicare spending and the

TABLE 5.5

National health expenditures, by type of expenditures, 2006–21

Type of expenditure	2006	2007	2008	2009	2010	2011	2012	2013	2014	Projected 2015	2016	2017	2018	2019	2020	2021
National health expenditures	$2,162.4	$2,297.1	$2,403.9	$2,495.8	$2,593.6	$2,695.0	$2,809.0	$2,915.5	$3,130.2	$3,307.6	$3,514.4	$3,723.3	$3,952.3	$4,207.3	$4,487.2	$4,781.0
Health consumption expenditures	2,031.5	2,153.4	2,250.1	2,349.5	2,444.6	2,543.2	2,655.3	2,757.8	2,964.9	3,132.7	3,329.2	3,526.5	3,743.0	3,985.3	4,252.4	4,532.7
Personal health care	1,804.9	1,914.6	2,010.2	2,109.0	2,186.0	2,270.4	2,364.1	2,441.8	2,622.7	2,774.1	2,948.9	3,130.4	3,326.1	3,544.2	3,782.6	4,034.0
Hospital care	651.9	692.5	729.3	776.1	814.0	848.9	884.7	920.7	982.7	1,038.3	1,106.6	1,170.7	1,240.0	1,317.7	1,404.1	1,495.7
Professional services	585.6	618.6	652.6	671.2	688.6	708.0	735.4	745.9	805.6	849.9	900.6	956.5	1,016.4	1,084.3	1,156.1	1,229.1
Physician and clinical services	438.8	461.8	486.6	502.7	515.5	529.2	549.6	554.5	601.5	633.4	670.6	712.4	757.0	807.3	860.5	914.9
Other professional services	55.4	59.5	63.6	66.0	68.4	70.9	74.5	76.1	83.8	89.7	96.5	103.1	109.7	117.6	125.9	134.5
Dental services	91.4	97.3	102.4	102.5	104.8	107.9	111.4	115.2	120.3	126.8	133.6	141.1	149.6	159.5	169.7	179.8
Other health, residential, and personal care	101.7	107.7	113.3	122.0	128.5	134.3	143.9	152.8	163.7	175.3	188.1	201.8	216.9	233.1	250.8	269.9
Home health care	52.6	57.8	61.5	66.1	70.2	72.9	77.5	81.9	88.3	94.5	101.2	108.4	117.1	126.6	137.0	148.3
Nursing care facilities and continuing care retirement communities	117.3	126.4	132.7	138.7	143.1	151.3	155.2	163.2	172.0	181.1	191.0	201.7	213.6	226.2	239.9	255.0
Retail outlet sales of medical products	295.8	311.5	321.0	334.9	341.6	355.0	367.4	377.4	410.4	435.0	461.4	491.2	522.1	556.3	594.7	635.9
Prescription drugs	224.2	236.2	243.6	256.1	259.1	269.2	277.1	283.7	308.7	327.3	347.8	371.1	394.9	420.9	450.7	483.2
Other medical products	71.6	75.3	77.4	78.8	82.5	85.8	90.3	93.7	101.7	107.6	113.6	120.1	127.2	135.4	144.0	152.7
Durable medical equipment	32.9	34.3	34.9	35.2	37.7	39.7	42.5	44.7	47.3	50.1	52.2	55.2	58.6	62.4	66.5	70.7
Other non-durable medical products	38.7	41.0	42.5	43.6	44.8	46.1	47.8	49.0	54.4	57.5	61.4	64.9	68.6	73.0	77.5	82.0
Government administration	29.5	30.2	29.5	29.6	30.1	33.8	37.5	39.8	44.5	47.4	51.0	52.9	56.3	59.9	63.8	68.0
Net cost of private health insurance	134.5	139.7	137.8	134.7	146.0	152.3	162.6	180.8	197.4	205.6	217.7	225.1	235.3	248.4	265.2	281.3
Government public health activities	62.5	69.0	72.7	76.2	82.5	86.7	91.0	95.3	100.3	105.7	111.6	118.1	125.2	132.7	140.8	149.4
Investment	130.9	143.7	153.8	146.3	149.0	151.9	153.7	157.7	165.3	174.9	185.2	196.8	209.3	221.9	234.9	248.2
Research*	41.4	41.9	43.4	45.7	49.3	50.2	48.7	48.6	50.8	53.7	57.1	60.9	64.8	68.9	73.3	77.8
Structures & equipment	89.6	101.7	110.4	100.6	99.8	101.7	105.0	109.1	114.5	121.2	128.1	136.0	144.5	153.0	161.6	170.4
National health expenditures	—	6.2%	4.7%	3.8%	3.9%	3.9%	4.2%	3.8%	7.4%	5.7%	6.3%	5.9%	6.2%	6.5%	6.7%	6.5%
Health consumption expenditures	—	6.0	4.5	4.4	4.0	4.0	4.4	3.9	7.5	5.7	6.3	5.9	6.1	6.5	6.7	6.6
Personal health care	—	6.1	5.0	4.9	3.7	3.9	4.1	3.3	7.4	5.8	6.3	6.2	6.3	6.6	6.7	6.6
Hospital care	—	6.2	5.3	6.4	4.9	4.3	4.2	4.1	6.7	5.7	6.6	5.8	5.9	6.3	6.6	6.5
Professional services	—	5.6	5.5	2.9	2.6	2.8	3.9	1.4	8.0	5.5	6.0	6.2	6.3	6.7	6.6	6.3
Physician and clinical services	—	5.2	5.4	3.3	2.5	2.7	3.8	0.9	8.5	5.3	5.9	6.2	6.3	6.6	6.6	6.3
Other professional services	—	7.4	6.9	3.8	3.6	3.7	5.0	2.1	10.1	7.1	7.5	6.8	6.5	7.1	7.1	6.8
Dental services	—	6.4	5.2	0.1	2.3	2.9	3.3	3.5	4.4	5.4	5.4	5.6	6.1	6.6	6.4	6.0
Other health, residential, and personal care	—	5.9	5.2	7.7	5.3	4.5	7.1	6.2	7.1	7.1	7.3	7.3	7.5	7.5	7.6	7.6
Home health care	—	9.9	6.4	7.5	6.2	3.9	6.4	5.7	7.8	6.9	7.1	7.1	8.1	8.1	8.2	8.3
Nursing care facilities and continuing care retirement communities	—	7.8	4.9	4.5	3.2	5.8	2.6	5.1	5.4	5.3	5.5	5.6	5.9	5.9	6.0	6.3
Retail outlet sales of medical products	—	5.3	3.0	4.3	2.0	3.9	3.5	2.7	8.7	6.0	6.1	6.5	6.3	6.5	6.9	6.9
Prescription drugs	—	5.3	3.1	5.1	1.2	3.9	2.9	2.4	8.8	6.0	6.2	6.7	6.4	6.6	7.1	7.2
Other medical products	—	5.2	2.8	1.8	4.7	4.0	5.3	3.8	8.5	5.8	5.6	5.7	5.9	6.5	6.3	6.0
Durable medical equipment	—	4.4	1.7	0.8	7.3	5.1	7.2	5.0	6.0	5.8	4.2	5.8	6.1	6.5	6.5	6.3
Other non-durable medical products	—	5.9	3.7	2.6	2.6	3.0	3.6	2.7	10.8	5.9	6.7	5.7	5.7	6.4	6.2	5.8
Government administration	—	2.3	-2.5	0.4	1.7	12.3	11.0	6.3	11.7	6.5	7.6	3.7	6.4	6.5	6.5	6.5
Net cost of private health insurance	—	3.8	-1.4	-2.2	8.4	4.3	6.8	11.2	9.2	4.1	5.9	3.4	4.5	5.6	6.7	6.1
Government public health activities	—	10.4	5.3	4.9	8.2	5.1	5.0	4.6	5.3	5.4	5.6	5.8	6.1	6.0	6.2	6.1

TABLE 5.5

National health expenditures, by type of expenditures, 2006–21 [CONTINUED]

Type of expenditure	2006	2007	2008	2009	2010	2011	2012	2013	2014	Projected						
										2015	2016	2017	2018	2019	2020	2021
Investment	—	9.7	7.1	−4.9	1.9	1.9	1.2	2.6	4.8	5.8	5.9	6.3	6.3	6.0	5.8	5.7
Research*	—	1.3	3.4	5.3	7.9	1.8	−3.0	−0.1	4.4	5.7	6.4	6.6	6.5	6.3	6.3	6.2
Structures & equipment	—	13.6	8.6	−8.9	−0.8	1.9	3.3	3.8	5.0	5.8	5.7	6.2	6.3	5.9	5.6	5.4

Notes: The health spending projections were based on the National Health Expenditures released in January 2012. The projections include impacts from the Affordable Care Act. Numbers may not add to totals due to rounding.
*Research and development expenditures of drug companies and other manufacturers and providers of medical equipment and supplies are excluded from research expenditures. These research expenditures are implicitly included in the expenditure class in which the product falls, in that they are covered by the payment received for that product.

SOURCE: "Table 2. National Health Expenditure Amounts, and Annual Percent Change by Type of Expenditure: Calendar Years 2006–2011," in *National Health Expenditures Projections 2011–2021*, U.S. Department of Health and Human Services, Centers for Medicare and Medicaid Services, 2012, http://www.cms.gov/Research-Statistics-Data-and-Systems/Statistics-Trends-and-Reports/NationalHealthExpendData/Downloads/Proj2011PDF.pdf (accessed June 24, 2012)

TABLE 5.6

Personal health expenditures, by source of funds, 2006–21

Year	Total	Out-of-pocket payments	Health insurance[a] Total	Private health insurance	Medicare	Medicaid	Other health insurance programs[b]	Other third party payers[c]
Historical estimates				Amount in billions				
2006	$1,804.9	$271.9	$1,372.0	$640.6	$381.7	$283.4	$66.3	$161.0
2007	1,914.6	287.3	1,455.0	673.5	408.2	301.9	71.4	172.2
2008	2,010.2	294.0	1,544.9	707.5	442.0	317.1	78.3	171.4
2009	2,109.0	294.4	1,637.1	734.0	471.2	345.9	86.1	177.4
2010	2,186.0	299.7	1,703.0	746.0	493.8	371.6	91.6	183.3
Projected								
2011	2,270.4	304.4	1,777.4	758.5	525.0	396.3	97.7	188.6
2012	2,364.1	312.1	1,857.9	775.9	555.8	423.7	102.5	194.1
2013	2,441.8	322.7	1,918.7	799.6	560.1	451.6	107.4	200.4
2014	2,622.7	317.7	2,103.3	863.5	595.3	530.8	113.6	201.7
2015	2,774.1	328.9	2,235.0	919.7	626.9	568.0	120.5	210.1
2016	2,948.9	340.0	2,388.8	981.6	666.5	614.3	126.3	220.2
2017	3,130.4	359.4	2,536.7	1,039.2	712.2	656.7	128.5	234.4
2018	3,326.1	381.6	2,696.8	1,096.1	763.5	702.3	134.8	247.7
2019	3,544.2	402.9	2,881.3	1,166.2	818.6	753.1	143.4	260.0
2020	3,782.6	426.0	3,083.8	1,239.3	881.2	810.6	152.7	272.8
2021	4,034.0	449.2	3,298.9	1,313.7	948.9	873.7	162.6	286.0
Historical estimates				Per capita amount				
2006	$6,052	$912	d	d	d	d	d	d
2007	6,357	954	d	d	d	d	d	d
2008	6,615	967	d	d	d	d	d	d
2009	6,886	961	d	d	d	d	d	d
2010	7,082	971	d	d	d	d	d	d
Projected								
2011	7,296	978	d	d	d	d	d	d
2012	7,535	995	d	d	d	d	d	d
2013	7,717	1,020	d	d	d	d	d	d
2014	8,217	996	d	d	d	d	d	d
2015	8,615	1,022	d	d	d	d	d	d
2016	9,077	1,046	d	d	d	d	d	d
2017	9,551	1,097	d	d	d	d	d	d
2018	10,061	1,154	d	d	d	d	d	d
2019	10,630	1,209	d	d	d	d	d	d
2020	11,250	1,267	d	d	d	d	d	d
2021	11,899	1,325	d	d	d	d	d	d
Historical estimates				Percent distribution				
2006	100.0	15.1	76.0	35.5	21.1	15.7	3.7	8.9
2007	100.0	15.0	76.0	35.2	21.3	15.8	3.7	9.0
2008	100.0	14.6	76.8	35.2	22.0	15.8	3.9	8.5
2009	100.0	14.0	77.6	34.8	22.3	16.4	4.1	8.4
2010	100.0	13.7	77.9	34.1	22.6	17.0	4.2	8.4
Projected								
2011	100.0	13.4	78.3	33.4	23.1	17.5	4.3	8.3
2012	100.0	13.2	78.6	32.8	23.5	17.9	4.3	8.2
2013	100.0	13.2	78.6	32.7	22.9	18.5	4.4	8.2
2014	100.0	12.1	80.2	32.9	22.7	20.2	4.3	7.7
2015	100.0	11.9	80.6	33.2	22.6	20.5	4.3	7.6
2016	100.0	11.5	81.0	33.3	22.6	20.8	4.3	7.5
2017	100.0	11.5	81.0	33.2	22.8	21.0	4.1	7.5
2018	100.0	11.5	81.1	33.0	23.0	21.1	4.1	7.4
2019	100.0	11.4	81.3	32.9	23.1	21.2	4.0	7.3
2020	100.0	11.3	81.5	32.8	23.3	21.4	4.0	7.2
2021	100.0	11.1	81.8	32.6	23.5	21.7	4.0	7.1
Historical estimates				Annual percent change from previous year shown				
2006	—	—	—	—	—	—	—	—
2007	6.1	5.6	6.1	5.1	6.9	6.6	7.6	7.0
2008	5.0	2.3	6.2	5.1	8.3	5.0	9.7	−0.5
2009	4.9	0.2	6.0	3.7	6.6	9.1	9.9	3.5
2010	3.7	1.8	4.0	1.6	4.8	7.4	6.5	3.3

growing number of older adults who use a disproportionate amount of health care services have also accelerated health care spending.

David Morgan reports in "Healthcare Costs to Rise 7.5 Percent in 2013: Report" (Reuters, May 31, 2012) that according to PricewaterhouseCoopers, national

Year	Total	Out-of-pocket payments	Health insurance[a]				Other health insurance programs[b]	Other third party payers[c]
			Total	Private health insurance	Medicare	Medicaid		
Projected			Annual percent change from previous year shown					
2011	3.9	1.6	4.4	1.7	6.3	6.7	6.6	2.9
2012	4.1	2.5	4.5	2.3	5.9	6.9	5.0	3.0
2013	3.3	3.4	3.3	3.1	0.8	6.6	4.8	3.2
2014	7.4	−1.5	9.6	8.0	6.3	17.5	5.8	0.6
2015	5.8	3.5	6.3	6.5	5.3	7.0	6.0	4.2
2016	6.3	3.4	6.9	6.7	6.3	8.1	4.9	4.8
2017	6.2	5.7	6.2	5.9	6.9	6.9	1.7	6.4
2018	6.3	6.2	6.3	5.5	7.2	6.9	4.9	5.7
2019	6.6	5.6	6.8	6.4	7.2	7.2	6.4	5.0
2020	6.7	5.7	7.0	6.3	7.7	7.6	6.5	4.9
2021	6.6	5.5	7.0	6.0	7.7	7.8	6.4	4.8

[a]Includes private health insurance (employer sponsored insurance, state health insurance exchanges, and other private insurance), Medicare, Medicaid, Children's Health Insurance Program (Titles XIX and XXI), Department of Defense, and Department of Veterans' Affairs.
[b]Children's Health Insurance Program (Titles XIX and XXI), Department of Defense, and Department of Veterans' Affairs.
[c]Includes worksite health care, other private revenues, Indian Health Service, workers' compensation, general assistance, maternal and child health, vocational rehabilitation, other federal programs, Substance Abuse and Mental Health Services Administration, other state and local programs, and school health.
[d]Calculation of per capita estimates is not applicable.
Notes: The health spending projections were based on the National Health Expenditures (NHE) released in January 2012. The projections include impacts from the Affordable Care Act. Per capita amounts based on July 1 Census resident based population estimates. Numbers and percents may not add to totals because of rounding.

SOURCE: "Table 5. Personal Health Care Expenditures; Aggregate and per Capita Amounts, Percent Distribution and Annual Percent Change by Source of Funds: Calendar Years 2006–2021," in *National Health Expenditures Projections 2011–2021*, U.S. Department of Health and Human Services, Centers for Medicare and Medicaid Services, 2012, http://www.cms.gov/Research-Statistics-Data-and-Systems/Statistics-Trends-and-Reports/NationalHealthExpendData/Downloads/Proj2011PDF.pdf (accessed June 24, 2012)

health spending is anticipated to increase 7.5% in 2013, outpacing the projected rates of inflation and economic growth three times over and nearly twice the 3.9% increase in health care spending in 2010. A Reuters economic survey forecasts a 2.4% increase in the GDP and a 2% rise in consumer prices in 2013.

In "Government Health Spending Seen Hitting $1.8 Trillion" (Reuters, February 7, 2012), Morgan indicates that the CBO expects government spending on health care to more than double between 2012 and 2022, growing to $1.8 trillion, or 7.3% of the nation's total economic output. A significant proportion of this increase is attributable to the enormous baby-boom generation (people born between 1946 and 1964), which is only now becoming eligible for government-sponsored health care. The first wave of baby boomers became eligible for Medicare in 2011.

CONTROLLING HEALTH CARE SPENDING

In an effort to control health expenditures, the nation's health care system underwent some dramatic changes. Beginning in the late 1980s employers began looking for new ways to contain health benefit costs for their employees. Many enrolled their employees in managed care programs as alternatives to traditional, fee-for-service insurance. Managed care programs offered lower premiums by keeping a tighter control on costs and utilization and by emphasizing the importance of preventive care. Insurers negotiated discounts with providers (physicians, hospitals, clinical laboratories, and others) in exchange for guaranteed access to employer-insured groups. In 2010 private insurance paid for 32.7% of the nation's health costs. (See Table 5.4.) Public sources covered 55.7% of the nation's costs, and 11.6% of the costs came directly from consumers' pockets.

One approach some employers use to control health care costs is offering their employees consumer-driven health plans (CDHPs). CDHPs provide the same coverage as traditional preferred provider organization (PPO) plans, including 100% coverage of preventive services, and the premiums are less expensive than traditional PPOs. CDHPs also offer the option of opening a health savings account (HSA) to help pay out-of-pocket expenses. The CDHP enrollee pays the cost of all approved medical services until the deductible is met. The CDHP then pays 80% of medical care costs and the enrollee pays the remaining 20%. After the enrollee pays the maximum out-of-pocket, the CDHP pays 100% of all medical care costs for the remainder of the year.

In "Growth of Consumer-Directed Health Plans to One-Half of All Employer-Sponsored Insurance Could Save $57 Billion Annually" (*Health Affairs*, vol. 31, no. 5, May 2012), Amelia M. Haviland et al. observe that "enrollment is increasing in consumer-directed health insurance plans, which feature high deductibles and a personal health care savings account." The researchers conclude that an increase in market share of these plans—from 13% of employer-sponsored coverage in 2010 to half the people with employer-based plans—has the potential to reduce annual health care spending by an estimated $57 billion, which represents a 4% decline in the total health care spending for working-age Americans. The savings would not be limited to just employers, for consumers' costs would decline by as much as 20%.

How Will the ACA Influence Health Care Spending?

Even though many aspects of the ACA spark fiery debate, few are as divisive as the question of whether its implementation will reduce health care costs. Proponents of the legislation claim that it will lower the federal budget deficit over time, whereas critics assert that it will inflate the deficit and national debt. As many of the key provisions of the ACA take effect in 2014, industry observers will assess how new provisions such as permitting the purchase of health insurance across state lines and malpractice reform affect U.S. expenditures for health care.

Phil Galewitz explains in "Consumers Guide to Health Reform" (April 13, 2010, http://www.kaiserhealth news.org/stories/2010/march/22/consumers-guide-health-reform.aspx) that the ACA is projected to cost $938 billion over 10 years. Furthermore, the CBO (March 20, 2010, http://www.cbo.gov/sites/default/files/cbofiles/ftpdocs/113xx/doc11379/amendreconprop.pdf) anticipates that the legislation will produce a net reduction in federal deficits of $143 billion between 2010 and 2019 in response to changes in spending and revenues.

According to the Robert Wood Johnson Foundation, in the issue brief "How Does the ACA Control Health Care Costs?" (July 2011, http://www.rwjf.org/files/resea rch/howdoestheacaattempttocontrolhealthcarecosts.pdf), several of the provisions of the ACA—spurring competition between health plans, taxing high-priced insurance coverage (a 40% excise tax on enrollees in plans with individual premiums above $10,200 or family premiums above $27,500), and taking action to eliminate fraud and abuses—have the potential to control health care costs. However, the foundation notes that even though the CBO forecasts cost savings resulting from implementation of the ACA, it is not yet known which provisions will be most effective in controlling costs.

Revenues will be generated through higher taxes and fees and cost savings will be realized as a result of reduced Medicare payments to health care providers. For example, Galewitz notes that beginning in 2013 individuals and couples with an income between $200,000 and $250,000 will pay a Medicare payroll tax of 2.3%, which is an increase from the 2010 rate of 1.4%. High-income taxpayers will also be required to pay a 3.8% tax on unearned income over the earning limits. The CBO estimates that the 40% excise tax (often referred to as a Cadillac tax because it applies to higher cost plans) starting in 2018 on richer, more costly health coverage will raise $32 billion over a decade.

According to Galewitz, the act also raises the threshold for deducting out-of-pocket unreimbursed medical expenses from 7.5% of a taxpayer's adjusted gross income to 10%. Beginning in 2013 it also limits contributions to flexible spending accounts, which may be used to pay medical expenses up to $2,500, and charges tanning salon users a 10% tax.

Prescription Drug Prices Continue to Rise

One of the fastest-growing components of health care is the market for prescription drugs. In 2010 Americans spent $259.1 billion on prescription medication—this was a 1.2% increase from $256.1 billion in 2009. (See Table 5.5.) A large part of the increase was financed by private insurers, who paid $117 billion of the drug costs in 2010, more than the $110.1 billion they paid for prescription drugs in 2008. (See Table 5.7.) The health needs and chronic conditions of the aging population have fueled growth in this sector of health services.

In *Trends in Retail Prices of Prescription Drugs Widely Used by Medicare Beneficiaries 2005 to 2009* (March 2012, http://www.aarp.org/content/dam/aarp/research/public_policy_institute/health/rx-pricewatch-march-2012-AARP-ppi-health.pdf), Stephen W. Schondelmeyer and Leigh Purvis note that the average annual increase in manufacturer prices for selected drugs that are widely used by Medicare beneficiaries consistently surpasses the general inflation rate. For example, in 2009 the average rate of increase for these widely used drugs was 4.8%, which was higher than the general inflation rate of −0.3%. The researchers note that "the average annual cost of therapy for the most widely used drugs used for treating chronic conditions increased by 46.7 percent between 2005 and 2009."

The Medicare drug benefit, which was implemented in 2006 to provide prescription drug savings for older Americans and people with disabilities, increased government spending for prescription drugs. The voluntary program allows Medicare beneficiaries to choose from dozens of plans that are offered by health insurers and health plans called pharmacy benefit managers. The ACA reduced Medicare Part D enrollees' out-of-pocket drug costs when they reach the coverage gap, known as the so-called donut hole. Most Medicare Part D basic drug benefit plans require enrollees to pay all their prescription drug costs after their drug spending exceeds the predesignated dollar amount that is their initial coverage limit until they satisfy the dollar amount that qualifies them for catastrophic coverage.

TABLE 5.7

Prescription drug expenditures, by source of funds, 2006–21

Year	Total	Out-of-pocket payments	Health insurance[a]					Other third party payers[c]
			Total	Private health insurance	Medicare	Medicaid	Other health insurance programs[b]	
Historical estimates			Amount in billions					
2006	$224.2	$51.3	$168.9	$102.2	$39.6	$18.9	$8.2	$4.0
2007	236.2	53.0	179.4	106.8	45.9	18.1	8.6	3.8
2008	243.6	51.0	188.9	110.1	50.6	18.9	9.2	3.6
2009	256.1	50.8	201.7	117.2	54.5	20.1	9.9	3.5
2010	259.1	48.8	206.9	117.0	59.5	20.2	10.3	3.4
Projected								
2011	269.2	49.6	216.0	121.0	64.3	20.0	10.8	3.7
2012	277.1	49.7	223.2	121.5	69.4	21.1	11.2	4.2
2013	283.7	50.0	229.4	122.3	73.4	22.1	11.7	4.3
2014	308.7	49.5	254.3	132.0	77.9	32.0	12.4	4.9
2015	327.3	50.3	271.9	140.6	83.3	34.7	13.3	5.1
2016	347.8	50.7	291.5	150.6	89.3	37.6	14.0	5.5
2017	371.1	53.5	311.3	160.2	96.7	40.5	14.0	6.2
2018	394.9	56.7	331.5	168.3	105.0	43.6	14.6	6.8
2019	420.9	59.5	354.2	177.9	114.2	46.4	15.6	7.2
2020	450.7	63.1	379.9	189.4	124.4	49.3	16.8	7.8
2021	483.2	67.0	407.8	201.9	135.7	52.2	18.1	8.5
Historical estimates			Per capita amount					
2006	$752	$172	d	d	d	d	d	d
2007	784	176	d	d	d	d	d	d
2008	802	168	d	d	d	d	d	d
2009	836	166	d	d	d	d	d	d
2010	839	158	d	d	d	d	d	d
Projected								
2011	865	159	d	d	d	d	d	d
2012	883	158	d	d	d	d	d	d
2013	897	158	d	d	d	d	d	d
2014	967	155	d	d	d	d	d	d
2015	1,017	156	d	d	d	d	d	d
2016	1,070	156	d	d	d	d	d	d
2017	1,132	163	d	d	d	d	d	d
2018	1,195	171	d	d	d	d	d	d
2019	1,262	178	d	d	d	d	d	d
2020	1,341	188	d	d	d	d	d	d
2021	1,425	198	d	d	d	d	d	d
Historical estimates			Percent distribution					
2006	100.0	22.9	75.3	45.6	17.7	8.4	3.6	1.8
2007	100.0	22.5	76.0	45.2	19.5	7.7	3.6	1.6
2008	100.0	21.0	77.6	45.2	20.8	7.8	3.8	1.5
2009	100.0	19.9	78.8	45.8	21.3	7.8	3.9	1.4
2010	100.0	18.8	79.9	45.2	23.0	7.8	4.0	1.3
Projected								
2011	100.0	18.4	80.2	44.9	23.9	7.4	4.0	1.4
2012	100.0	17.9	80.6	43.9	25.1	7.6	4.0	1.5
2013	100.0	17.6	80.9	43.1	25.9	7.8	4.1	1.5
2014	100.0	16.0	82.4	42.8	25.2	10.4	4.0	1.6
2015	100.0	15.4	83.1	42.9	25.4	10.6	4.1	1.6
2016	100.0	14.6	83.8	43.3	25.7	10.8	4.0	1.6
2017	100.0	14.4	83.9	43.2	26.1	10.9	3.8	1.7
2018	100.0	14.4	83.9	42.6	26.6	11.0	3.7	1.7
2019	100.0	14.1	84.1	42.3	27.1	11.0	3.7	1.7
2020	100.0	14.0	84.3	42.0	27.6	10.9	3.7	1.7
2021	100.0	13.9	84.4	41.8	28.1	10.8	3.7	1.7
Historical estimates			Annual percent change from previous year shown					
2006	—	—	—	—	—	—	—	—
2007	5.3	3.4	6.2	4.5	15.9	−4.2	4.7	−7.0
2008	3.1	−3.8	5.3	3.2	10.2	4.5	7.5	−3.6
2009	5.1	−0.4	6.8	6.4	7.7	6.1	7.5	−2.7
2010	1.2	−4.1	2.6	−0.2	9.0	0.3	3.7	−3.4

As part of the ACA, starting in 2011 non-low-income Medicare Part D enrollees received a 50% discount on brand-name prescription drugs and a 7% discount on generic prescription drugs while they were in the coverage gap. In 2012 the coverage gap began after an individual had $2,930 in total drug costs and continued until out-of-pocket

TABLE 5.7

Prescription drug expenditures, by source of funds, 2006–21 [CONTINUED]

Year	Total	Out-of-pocket payments	Health insurance[a]						Other third party payers[c]
			Total	Private health insurance	Medicare	Medicaid	Other health insurance programs[b]	
Projected			Annual percent change from previous year shown					
2011	3.9	1.6	4.4	3.4	8.1	−0.9	5.2	8.2
2012	2.9	0.3	3.3	0.5	8.0	5.7	3.6	12.8
2013	2.4	0.7	2.8	0.7	5.7	4.5	4.4	2.7
2014	8.8	−1.0	10.9	7.9	6.2	45.2	5.8	14.8
2015	6.0	1.7	6.9	6.5	6.9	8.3	7.6	4.6
2016	6.2	0.8	7.2	7.2	7.3	8.2	5.1	7.7
2017	6.7	5.5	6.8	6.4	8.2	7.7	−0.2	12.6
2018	6.4	5.9	6.5	5.0	8.7	7.6	4.6	8.7
2019	6.6	5.0	6.8	5.7	8.7	6.4	7.1	7.1
2020	7.1	6.0	7.3	6.4	8.9	6.2	7.4	7.8
2021	7.2	6.2	7.4	6.6	9.0	5.9	7.5	8.4

[a]Includes private health insurance (employer sponsored insurance, state health insurance exchanges, and other private insurance), Medicare, Medicaid, Children's Health Insurance Program (Titles XIX and XXI), Department of Defense, and Department of Veterans' Affairs.
[b]Children's health insurance program (Titles XIX and XXI), Department of Defense, and Department of Veterans' Affairs.
[c]Includes worksite health care, other private revenues, Indian Health Service, workers' compensation, general assistance, maternal and child health, vocational rehabilitation, other federal programs, Substance Abuse and Mental Health Services Administration, other state and local programs, and school health.
[d]Calculation of per capita estimates is not applicable.
Notes: The health spending projections were based on the National Health Expenditures (NHE) released in January 2012. The projections include impacts from the Affordable Care Act. Per capita amounts based on July 1 Census resident based population estimates. Numbers and percents may not add to totals because of rounding.

SOURCE: "Table 11. Prescription Drug Expenditures; Aggregate and per Capita Amounts, Percent Distribution and Annual Percent Change by Source of Funds: Calendar Years 2006–2021," in *National Health Expenditures Projections 2011–2021*, U.S. Department of Health and Human Services, Centers for Medicare and Medicaid Services, 2011, http://www.cms.gov/Research-Statistics-Data-and-Systems/Statistics-Trends-and-Reports/NationalHealthExpendData/Downloads/Proj2011PDF.pdf (accessed June 24, 2012)

drug costs totaled $4,700. These discounts will continue growing until 2020, when the ACA's provisions are fully implemented and the beneficiary coinsurance rate will drop to 25%. The ACA also reduces the out-of-pocket spending required for enrollees' eligibility for catastrophic coverage, which further reduces out-of-pocket costs for people with high prescription drug expenses.

Schondelmeyer and Purvis observe that manufacturers' drug price increases produce higher pharmacy prices and higher out-of-pocket costs for Medicare beneficiaries who pay a percentage of their drug costs as opposed to fixed co-payment per prescription. The higher prices also result in higher costs for drug plans, which in turn may serve to increase the plans' premiums or cause them to reduce benefits.

HEALTH CARE FOR OLDER ADULTS, PEOPLE WITH DISABILITIES, AND THE POOR

Despite passage of the groundbreaking ACA, which promises to expand health care coverage, the United States remains one of the few industrialized nations that does not have a government-funded national health care program that provides coverage for all of its citizens. Government-funded health care exists, and it forms a major part of the health care system, but it is available only to specific segments of the U.S. population. In other developed countries government-funded national medical care programs cover almost all their citizens' health-related costs, from maternity care to long-term care.

In the United States the major government health care entitlement programs are Medicare and Medicaid. They provide financial assistance for people aged 65 years and older, the poor, and people with disabilities. Before the existence of these programs, many older Americans could not afford adequate medical care. For older adults who are beneficiaries, the Medicare program provides reimbursement for hospital and physician care, whereas Medicaid pays for the cost of nursing home care.

Medicare

The Medicare program, which was enacted under Title XVIII (Health Insurance for the Aged) of the Social Security Act, was approved in 1965. The program consists of four parts:

- Part A provides hospital insurance. Coverage includes physicians' fees, nursing services, meals, semiprivate rooms, special-care units, operating room costs, laboratory tests, and some drugs and supplies. Part A also covers rehabilitation services, limited posthospital care in a skilled nursing facility, home health care, and hospice care for the terminally ill.

- Part B (Supplemental Medical Insurance [SMI]) is elective medical insurance; that is, enrollees must pay premiums to obtain coverage. SMI covers outpatient physicians' services, diagnostic tests, outpatient hospital services, outpatient physical therapy, speech pathology services, home health services, and medical equipment and supplies.

- Part C is the Medicare+Choice program, which was established by the Balanced Budget Act of 1997 to expand beneficiaries' options and allow them to participate in private-sector health plans.

- Part D is also elective and provides voluntary, subsidized access to prescription drug insurance coverage, for a premium, to individuals who are entitled to Part A or who are enrolled in Part B. Part D also has provisions (premium and cost-sharing subsidies) for low-income enrollees. Part D coverage began in 2006 and includes most of the prescription drugs that are approved by the U.S. Food and Drug Administration (FDA).

In general, Medicare reimburses physicians on a fee-for-service basis (paid for each visit, procedure, or treatment that is delivered), as opposed to per capita or per member per month. In response to the increasing administrative burden of paperwork, reduced compensation, and delays in reimbursements, some physicians opt out of Medicare participation—they do not provide services under the Medicare program and choose not to accept Medicare patients into their practice. Others still provide services to Medicare beneficiaries but do not "accept assignment," meaning that patients must pay out of pocket for services and then seek reimbursement from Medicare.

Because of these problems, the Tax Equity and Fiscal Responsibility Act of 1982 authorized a risk managed care option for Medicare, based on agreed-on prepayments. Beginning in 1985 the Health Care Financing Administration (now known as the CMS) could contract to pay health care providers, such as health maintenance organizations (HMOs) or health care prepayment plans, to serve Medicare and Medicaid patients. These groups are paid a predetermined cost per patient for their services.

Medicare-Risk HMOs Control Costs, but Some Senior Health Plans Do Not Survive

During the 1980s and 1990s the federal government, employers that provided health coverage for retiring employees, and many states sought to control costs by encouraging Medicare and Medicaid beneficiaries to enroll in HMOs. From the early 1980s through the late 1990s Medicare-risk HMOs did contain costs because, essentially, the federal government paid the health plans that operated them with fixed fees—a predetermined dollar amount per member per month (PMPM). For this fixed fee, Medicare recipients were to receive a fairly comprehensive, preset array of benefits. PMPM payment provided financial incentives for Medicare-risk HMO physicians to control costs, unlike physicians who were reimbursed on a fee-for-service basis.

Even though Medicare recipients were generally pleased with these HMOs (even when enrolling meant they had to change physicians and thereby end long-standing relationships with their family doctors), many of the health plans did not fare well financially. The health plans suffered for a variety of reasons: some had underestimated the service utilization rates of older adults, and some were unable to provide the stipulated range of services as cost effectively as they had believed possible. Other plans found that the PMPM payment was simply not sufficient to enable them to cover all the clinical services and their administrative overhead.

Still, the health plans providing these senior HMOs competed fiercely to enroll older adults. Some health plans feared that closing their Medicare-risk programs would be viewed negatively by employer groups, which, when faced with the choice of plans that offered coverage for both younger workers and retirees or one that only covered younger workers, would choose the plans that covered both. Despite losing money, most health plans maintained their Medicare-risk programs to avoid alienating the employers they depended on to enroll workers who were younger, healthier, and less expensive to serve than the older adults.

By the mid-1990s some of the Medicare-risk plans faced a challenge that proved daunting. Their enrollees had aged and required even more health care services than they had previously. For example, a senior HMO member who had joined as a healthy 65-year-old could now be a frail 75-year-old with multiple chronic health conditions requiring many costly health services. Even though the PMPM had increased over the years, for some plans it was insufficient to cover their costs. Some Medicare-risk plans, especially those operated by smaller health plans, were forced to end their programs abruptly, leaving thousands of older adults scrambling to join other health plans. Others endured by offering older adults comprehensive care and generating substantial cost savings for employers and the federal government.

The Balanced Budget Act of 1997 produced another plan for Medicare recipients called Medicare+Choice. This plan offers Medicare beneficiaries a wider range of managed care plan options than just HMOs—older adults may join PPOs and provider-sponsored organizations that generally offer greater freedom of choice of providers (physicians and hospitals) than what is available through HMO membership. These plans (as well as those formerly called Medicare-risk plans), are known as Medicare Advantage (MA) plans. MA plans include HMOs, PPOs, private fee-for-service plans, and medical savings account plans (which deposit money from Medicare into an account that can be used to pay medical expenses). According to the Kaiser Family Foundation, in *Medicare Advantage 2012 Data Spotlight: Enrollment Market*

Update (June 2012, http://www.kff.org/medicare/upload/8323.pdf), in 2012 these plans had 13 million members—27% of all Medicare beneficiaries.

Medicare Faces Challenges

For 45 years, Medicare has successfully provided access to health care services for the elderly ages 65 and over and many nonelderly people with disabilities, and currently covers 47 million Americans. Persistently high rates of growth in national health expenditures combined with demographic trends, however, pose a serious challenge to the financing of Medicare in the 21st century.

—Lisa Potetz, Juliette Cubanski, and Tricia Neuman, *Medicare Spending and Financing: A Primer* (February 2011)

The Medicare program's continuing financial viability is in jeopardy. In 1995, for the first time since 1972, the Medicare trust fund lost money, a sign that the financial condition of Medicare was worse than previously assumed. The CMS did not expect a deficit until 1997; however, income to the trust fund, primarily from payroll taxes, was less than expected and spending was higher. The deficit is significant because losses are anticipated to grow from year to year. Lisa Potetz, Juliette Cubanski, and Tricia Neuman explain in *Medicare Spending and Financing: A Primer* (February 2011, http://www.kff.org/medicare/upload/7731-03.pdf) that ensuring Medicare's long-term financial viability is a continuing and increasingly urgent challenge for policy makers. Medicare provides health coverage for 47 million beneficiaries, many of whom have multiple chronic conditions and significant health needs.

A NATIONAL BIPARTISAN COMMISSION CONSIDERS THE FUTURE OF MEDICARE. The National Bipartisan Commission on the Future of Medicare was created by Congress in the Balanced Budget Act of 1997. The commission was charged with examining the Medicare program and drafting recommendations to avert a future financial crisis and reinforce the program in anticipation of the retirement of the baby boomers.

The commission observed that much like Social Security, Medicare would suffer because there would be fewer workers per retiree to fund it. Furthermore, it predicted that beneficiaries' out-of-pocket costs would rise and forecast soaring Medicare enrollment.

When the commission disbanded in March 1999, it was unable to forward an official recommendation to Congress because its plan fell one vote short of the required majority needed to authorize an official recommendation. The plan would have changed Medicare into a premium system, where instead of Medicare directly covering beneficiaries, the beneficiaries would be given a fixed amount of money to purchase private health insurance. The plan would have also raised the age of eligibility from 65 to 67 (as had already been done with

Social Security in 1983) and provided prescription drug coverage for low-income beneficiaries, much like the Medicare Prescription Drug, Improvement, and Modernization Act of 2003.

In February 2010 President Barack Obama (1961–) established the National Commission on Fiscal Responsibility and Reform to suggest strategies to reduce the federal budget deficit. Among the commission's tasks was to recommend ways to slow the growth in entitlement program spending. The 18-member commission issued its final report in January 2011, which contained a variety of controversial recommendations that were designed to balance the budget by 2015. Lori Montgomery explains in "Deficit Panel Leaders Propose Curbs on Social Security, Major Cuts in Spending, Tax Breaks" (*Washington Post*, November 11, 2010) that the report proposed a $200 billion reduction in discretionary spending to be achieved by reducing defense spending and decreasing the federal workforce by 10%. The report called for tax reforms including a $0.15-per-gallon gasoline tax and eliminating or restricting a variety of tax deductions, such as the home mortgage interest deduction and the deduction for employer-provided health care benefits, as well as reducing entitlements, such as farm subsidies, civilian and military federal pensions, and student loan subsidies. It also recommended increasing the payroll tax and raising the retirement age to 69.

The report was criticized by Republicans and Democrats alike. Republicans were displeased with the increased taxes and Democrats decried the recommendations that might reduce retiree benefits. President Obama indicated his support for the commission's work, but he initially chose not to endorse its recommendations. However, by April 2011 the president appeared to concur with most of the major tenets supported by a majority of the commission's members, though his proposals were not as drastic as the commission's. In "Obama's Deficit Dilemma" (*New York Times*, February 27, 2012), Jackie Calmes reports that President Obama has "called for cutting deficits more than $4 trillion over 10 years by shaving all spending, including for the military, Medicare and Social Security; overhauling the tax code to raise revenues and lower rates; and writing rules to lock in savings."

MEDICARE PRESCRIPTION DRUG, IMPROVEMENT, AND MODERNIZATION ACT AIMS TO REFORM MEDICARE. The Medicare Prescription Drug, Improvement, and Modernization Act of 2003 was a measure intended to introduce private-sector enterprise into a Medicare model in urgent need of reform.

According to the CMS, in "Medicare Premiums: Rules for Higher Income Beneficiaries" (March 2012, http://www.ssa.gov/pubs/10536.pdf), one of the reforms introduced by the act is that older adults with substantial incomes face increasing Part B premium costs. Table 5.8

TABLE 5.8

Monthly Medicare premiums, 2012

Modified Adjusted Gross Income (MAGI)	Part B monthly premium amount	Prescription drug coverage monthly premium amount
Individuals with a MAGI of $85,000 or less Married couples with a MAGI of $170,000 or less	2012 standard premium = $99.90	Your plan premium
Individuals with a MAGI above $85,000 up to $107,000 Married couples with a MAGI above $170,000 up to $214,000	Standard premium + $40.00	Your plan premium + $11.60
Individuals with a MAGI above $107,000 up to $160,000 Married couples with a MAGI above $214,000 up to $320,000	Standard premium + $99.90	Your plan premium + $29.90
Individuals with a MAGI above $160,000 up to $214,000 Married couples with a MAGI above $320,000 up to $428,000	Standard premium + $159.80	Your plan premium + $48.10
Individuals with a MAGI above $214,000 Married couples with a MAGI above $428,000	Standard premium + $219.80	Your plan premium + $66.40
Individuals with a MAGI of $85,000 or less	2012 standard premium = $99.90	Your plan premium
Individuals with a MAGI above $85,000 up to $129,000	Standard premium + $159.80	Your plan premium + $48.10
Individuals with a MAGI above $129,000	Standard premium + $219.80	Your plan premium + $66.40

SOURCE: "Monthly Medicare Premiums for 2012," in *Medicare Premiums: Rules For Higher-Income Beneficiaries*, Social Security Administration, March 2012, http://www.ssa.gov/pubs/10536.pdf (accessed June 25, 2012)

shows the standard Part B premium of $99 per month and monthly premiums for high-income individuals and couples. It also shows the premium amounts (paid in addition to the prescription drug plan premiums) that must be paid to obtain prescription drug coverage.

The act expanded coverage of preventive medical services. According to the CMS, new beneficiaries receive a free physical examination along with laboratory tests to screen for heart disease and diabetes. The act also provides employers with $89 billion in subsidies and tax breaks to help offset the costs associated with maintaining retiree health benefits.

IMPACT OF THE ACA ON MEDICARE. Potetz, Cubanski, and Neuman explain that the majority of the Medicare provisions in the ACA reduce spending, and between 2010 and 2019 total expenditures will be reduced by an estimated $424 billion, which is a 6% reduction from spending that had been projected for the decade. Besides higher monthly premiums for higher-income older adults, actions to reduce spending include:

- Reducing payments to providers and Medicare Advantage Plans

- Reforming the delivery system—incentivizing providers to improve quality and coordination of care rather than to increase volume to boost reimbursement

- Creating the Independent Payment Advisory Board, which will recommend Medicare program changes should spending growth exceed predesignated targets, beginning in 2015

In *Summary of New Health Reform Law* (July 2012, http://www.kff.org/healthreform/upload/8061.pdf), the Kaiser Family Foundation indicates that besides changes in the prescription drug benefit (Part D) between 2014 and 2019, the ACA reduces the out-of-pocket expenditures an individual must incur to become eligible for catastrophic coverage. It immediately extends Medicare coverage to individuals who have been exposed to environmental health hazards and have developed certain health conditions as a result of these exposures. For example, being exposed to asbestos (a group of minerals that are heat resistant and have been used in many industries) is considered to be an environmental health hazard because it is linked to the development of lung cancer, mesothelioma (a noncancerous tumor in the lining of the chest or abdomen), and other cancers. The act also gives a 10% bonus payment to primary care physicians practicing in underserved areas between 2011 and 2015 and in fiscal years (FYs) 2011 and 2012 it provided additional payments to hospitals with the lowest Medicare spending.

Medicaid

Medicaid was enacted by Congress in 1965 under Title XIX (Grants to States for Medical Assistance Programs) of the Social Security Act. It is a joint federal-state program that provides medical assistance to selected categories of low-income Americans: the aged, people who are blind or disabled, and financially struggling families with dependent children. Medicaid covers hospitalization, physicians' fees, laboratory and radiology fees, and long-term care in nursing homes. It is the largest source of funds for medical and health-related services for the poorest Americans and the second-largest public payer of health care costs, after Medicare.

The Deficit Reduction Act (DRA) was signed into law by President George W. Bush (1946–) in 2006. The DRA changed many aspects of the Medicaid program.

Some of the changes are mandatory provisions that the states must enact, such as proof of citizenship and other criteria that will make it more difficult for people to qualify for or enroll in Medicaid. Other changes are optional; they allow the states to make drastic changes to the Medicaid program through state plan amendments. For example, states can choose to require anyone with a family income more than 150% of the poverty level to pay a premium of as much as 5% of their income. Before the DRA, the states had to provide a mandatory set of services to Medicaid recipients. As of March 31, 2006, the states could modify their Medicaid benefits such that they were comparable to those offered to federal and state employees, the benefits provided by the HMO with the largest non-Medicaid enrollment, or coverage approved by the U.S. secretary of health and human services.

The Kaiser Commission on Medicaid and the Uninsured reports in "Quick Take: Who Benefits from the ACA Medicaid Expansion?" (June 20, 2012, http://www.kff.org//medicaid/quicktake_aca_medicaid.cfm) that in 2012 Medicaid covered more than 60 million people, including 25% of children. The ACA expands coverage by establishing national Medicaid eligibility criteria. In 2014 people with incomes below 133% of the poverty level will be eligible for Medicaid coverage. By 2016 the CBO estimates that Medicaid, along with the Children's Health Insurance Program, will cover an additional 17 million people, mostly low-income adults, which will significantly reduce the number of uninsured Americans. The expansion of Medicaid between 2014 and 2016 will be financed by the federal government. In view of the June 2012 U.S. Supreme Court decision enabling states to opt out of Medicaid expansion, these numbers are estimates and are subject to change depending on how many states choose not to expand Medicaid eligibility.

According to the article "How the Health Care Overhaul Could Affect You" (*New York Times*, March 21, 2010), the ACA prevents a state from dropping Medicaid coverage for beneficiaries until 2014, when insurance exchanges will be available, unless the state has a budget shortfall. States are prohibited from dropping children from Medicaid or the Children's Health Insurance Program until 2019. Medicaid coverage will include preventive services at no cost, and payments to physicians will be increased to spur physicians to accept Medicaid patients into their practice.

LONG-TERM HEALTH CARE

One of the most urgent health care problems facing Americans in the 21st century is the growing need for long-term care. Long-term care refers to health and social services for people with chronic illnesses or mental or physical conditions so disabling that they cannot live independently without assistance—they require care daily. Longer life spans and improved life-sustaining technologies are increasing the likelihood that more people than ever before may eventually require costly, long-term care.

Limited and Expensive Options

Caring for chronically ill or elderly patients presents difficult and expensive choices for Americans: they must either provide long-term care at home or rely on a nursing home. Home health care was the fastest-growing segment of the health care industry during the first half of the 1990s. Even though the rate of growth slowed during the late 1990s, the CMS projects that the home health care sector will more than double, from $70.2 billion in 2010 to $148.3 billion in 2021. (See Table 5.5.)

High Cost of Long-Term Care

The options for quality, affordable long-term care in the United States are limited but improving. Nursing home costs average about $80,000 per year, depending on services and location. According to MetLife, in *2011 Market Survey of Long-Term Care Costs* (October 2011, http: //www.metlife.com/assets/cao/mmi/publications/studies/2011/mmi-market-survey-nursing-home-assisted-living-adult-day-services-costs.pdf), in 2011 nursing home care cost an average of $239 per day for a private room, or $83,585 per year. Many nursing home residents rely on Medicaid to pay these fees. In 2011 Medicaid covered an estimated 45.3% of nursing home costs for older Americans. (See Table 5.9.) The most common sources of payment at admission were Medicare (which pays only for short-term stays after hospitalization), private insurance, and other private funds. The primary source of payment changes as a stay lengthens. After their funds are exhausted, nursing home residents on Medicare shift to Medicaid.

To be eligible for long-term-care coverage by Medicaid, an individual must have an income that is less than the cost of care in the facility at the Medicaid rate and must meet income and resource limits. Many older adults must "spend down" to deplete their life savings to qualify for Medicaid assistance. This term refers to a provision in Medicaid coverage that provides care for seniors whose income exceeds eligibility requirements. For example, if their monthly income is $100 over the state Medicaid eligibility line, they can spend $100 per month on their medical care, and Medicaid will cover the remainder.

Nursing home care may seem cost-prohibitive, but even an unskilled caregiver who makes home visits earned an average of $20 per hour in 2011; skilled care costs much more, and most older adults cannot afford this expense. In *2011 Market Survey of Long-Term Care Costs* MetLife reports that in 2011 the average hourly rates were $19 for homemaker services and $21 for home health aide services.

TABLE 5.9

Nursing home and continuing care expenditures, by source of funds, 2006–21

Year	Total	Out-of-pocket payments	Health insurance[a] Total	Private health insurance	Medicare	Medicaid	Other health insurance programs[b]	Other third party payers[c]
Historical estimates			Amount in billions					
2006	$117.3	$33.9	$75.8	$9.4	$22.4	$41.3	$2.8	$7.6
2007	126.4	37.2	80.3	10.2	24.8	42.1	3.3	8.9
2008	132.7	38.6	85.9	10.9	27.6	43.8	3.7	8.2
2009	138.7	39.5	90.6	11.8	29.9	44.9	4.0	8.6
2010	143.1	40.4	93.7	12.7	31.9	45.1	4.0	8.9
Projected								
2011	151.3	41.2	100.9	13.6	37.5	45.3	4.5	9.2
2012	155.2	42.2	103.7	14.6	37.6	46.8	4.7	9.4
2013	163.2	43.6	109.8	15.8	40.8	48.3	4.9	9.7
2014	172.0	44.8	117.2	17.0	44.6	50.4	5.2	10.0
2015	181.1	46.0	124.9	18.3	48.6	52.5	5.5	10.2
2016	191.0	47.2	133.5	19.5	53.2	55.0	5.8	10.4
2017	201.7	48.6	142.5	20.9	57.7	57.9	6.0	10.7
2018	213.6	50.2	152.4	22.3	62.4	61.5	6.3	11.0
2019	226.2	52.0	162.9	23.7	67.3	65.2	6.7	11.4
2020	239.9	53.9	174.2	25.2	72.7	69.2	7.0	11.7
2021	255.0	56.3	186.6	26.9	78.6	73.7	7.5	12.2
Historical estimates			Per capita amount					
2006	$393	$114	d	d	d	d	d	d
2007	420	123	d	d	d	d	d	d
2008	437	127	d	d	d	d	d	d
2009	453	129	d	d	d	d	d	d
2010	464	131	d	d	d	d	d	d
Projected								
2011	486	133	d	d	d	d	d	d
2012	495	134	d	d	d	d	d	d
2013	516	138	d	d	d	d	d	d
2014	539	140	d	d	d	d	d	d
2015	562	143	d	d	d	d	d	d
2016	588	145	d	d	d	d	d	d
2017	616	148	d	d	d	d	d	d
2018	646	152	d	d	d	d	d	d
2019	679	156	d	d	d	d	d	d
2020	713	160	d	d	d	d	d	d
2021	752	166	d	d	d	d	d	d
Historical estimates			Percent distribution					
2006	100.0	28.9	64.7	8.0	19.1	35.2	2.4	6.4
2007	100.0	29.4	63.5	8.0	19.6	33.3	2.6	7.1
2008	100.0	29.1	64.7	8.2	20.8	33.0	2.8	6.2
2009	100.0	28.5	65.3	8.5	21.6	32.4	2.9	6.2
2010	100.0	28.3	65.5	8.9	22.3	31.5	2.8	6.3
Projected								
2011	100.0	27.3	66.7	9.0	24.8	29.9	3.0	6.1
2012	100.0	27.2	66.8	9.4	24.2	30.1	3.0	6.1
2013	100.0	26.7	67.3	9.7	25.0	29.6	3.0	6.0
2014	100.0	26.1	68.2	9.9	25.9	29.3	3.0	5.8
2015	100.0	25.4	69.0	10.1	26.9	29.0	3.0	5.6
2016	100.0	24.7	69.9	10.2	27.8	28.8	3.0	5.5
2017	100.0	24.1	70.6	10.3	28.6	28.7	3.0	5.3
2018	100.0	23.5	71.4	10.4	29.2	28.8	3.0	5.2
2019	100.0	23.0	72.0	10.5	29.8	28.8	3.0	5.0
2020	100.0	22.5	72.6	10.5	30.3	28.9	2.9	4.9
2021	100.0	22.1	73.2	10.5	30.8	28.9	2.9	4.8
Historical estimates			Annual percent change from previous year shown					
2006	—	—	—	—	—	—	—	—
2007	7.8	9.7	5.9	8.5	11.1	1.9	15.8	18.2
2008	4.9	3.9	6.9	6.9	11.1	4.0	12.2	−8.5
2009	4.5	2.4	5.5	8.3	8.5	2.6	8.3	4.9
2010	3.2	2.3	3.5	8.2	6.5	0.4	1.7	4.2

It should be noted that lifetime savings may be exhausted long before the need for care ends. The National Health Policy Forum estimates in "National Spending for Long-Term Services and Supports (LTSS)" (February 23, 2012, http://www.nhpf.org/library/the-basics/Basics_LongTermServicesSupports_02-23-12.pdf) that the

TABLE 5.9

Nursing home and continuing care expenditures, by source of funds, 2006–21 [CONTINUED]

| | | | Health insurance[a] | | | | | |
| | | | Private | | | | Other health | Other |
Year	Total	Out-of-pocket payments	Total	health insurance	Medicare	Medicaid	insurance programs[b]	third party payers[c]
Projected			Annual percent change from previous year shown					
2011	5.8	2.0	7.7	7.1	17.8	0.4	10.9	2.5
2012	2.6	2.2	2.7	7.2	0.3	3.3	4.1	2.7
2013	5.1	3.5	5.9	8.2	8.4	3.3	5.8	3.3
2014	5.4	2.7	6.7	7.7	9.3	4.3	5.9	2.5
2015	5.3	2.6	6.6	7.3	9.1	4.3	5.3	2.2
2016	5.5	2.6	6.8	6.8	9.3	4.7	4.9	2.3
2017	5.6	3.0	6.8	6.8	8.4	5.3	4.8	2.7
2018	5.9	3.3	7.0	6.8	8.2	6.1	5.1	2.9
2019	5.9	3.6	6.9	6.6	7.9	6.1	5.3	3.1
2020	6.0	3.8	6.9	6.3	8.0	6.2	5.4	3.3
2021	6.3	4.4	7.1	6.4	8.1	6.4	5.8	3.8

[a]Includes private health insurance (employer sponsored insurance, state health insurance exchanges, and other private insurance), Medicare, Medicaid, Children's Health Insurance Program (Titles XIX and XXI), Department of Defense, and Department of Veterans' Affairs.
[b]Children's Health Insurance Program (Titles XIX and XXI), Department of Defense, and Department of Veterans' Affairs.
[c]Includes worksite health care, other private revenues, Indian Health Service, workers' compensation, general assistance, maternal and child health, vocational rehabilitation, other federal programs, Substance Abuse and Mental Health Services Administration, other state and local programs, and school health.
[d]Calculation of per capita estimates is not applicable.
Notes: The health spending projections were based on the National Health Expenditures (NHE) released in January 2012. The projections include impacts from the Affordable Care Act. Per capita amounts based on July 1 Census resident based population estimates. Numbers and percents may not add to totals because of rounding.

SOURCE: "Table 13. Nursing Care Facilities and Continuing Care Retirement Communities; Aggregate and per Capita Amounts, Percent Distribution and Annual Percent Change by Source of Funds: Calendar Years 2006–2021," in *National Health Expenditures Projections 2011–2021*, U.S. Department of Health and Human Services, Centers for Medicare and Medicaid Services, 2012, http://www.cms.gov/Research-Statistics-Data-and-Systems/Statistics-Trends-and-Reports/NationalHealthExpendData/Downloads/Proj2011PDF.pdf (accessed June 24, 2012)

total expenditure for long-term-care services in 2010 (excluding the value of donated care from relatives and friends) was $207.9 billion—8% of total U.S. personal health care spending. Approximately 6% of people who turned 65 in 2005 are likely to incur out-of-pocket long-term-care expenses in excess of $100,000 over their remaining lifetime, and about 12% are likely to spend between $25,000 and $100,000.

In *The Next Four Decades: The Older Population in the United States, 2010 to 2050* (May 2010, http://www.census.gov/prod/2010pubs/p25-1138.pdf), Grayson K. Vincent and Victoria A. Velkoff of the U.S. Census Bureau project that the population over the age of 85 years (those most likely to require long-term care) will nearly quadruple by 2050. Even though disability rates among older adults have declined in recent years, reducing somewhat the need for long-term care, the CBO anticipates that the growing population of people likely to require long-term care will no doubt increase spending commensurate with this growth.

MENTAL HEALTH SPENDING

In *Projections of National Expenditures for Mental Health Services and Substance Abuse Treatment, 2004–2014* (2008, http://www.samhsa.gov/), a study funded by the Substance Abuse and Mental Health Services Administration (SAMHSA), Katharine R. Levit et al. predict that spending for mental health and substance abuse (alcohol and chemical dependency) treatment in the United States will reach $239 billion in 2014, up from $121 billion in 2003, representing 6.9% of all health care spending. Even though mental health and substance abuse spending is projected to increase fourfold between 1986 and 2014, the rate of increase is less than the sixfold increase that is forecast for total health care spending. This is in part because mental health treatment does not involve the costly technology that drives overall health care costs. Figure 5.1 shows how mental health and substance abuse spending will account for a smaller share of total health care spending by 2014.

Levit et al. also report that:

- Mental health spending rose from an average of $136 per person in 1986 to $339 per person in 2003 and is forecast to reach $626 per person in 2014

- In 2014 Medicaid will pay 27% of mental health expenditures, private payers will pay 26%, and out-of-pocket costs will be 12%

- Prescription drug costs will increase from 23% of mental health expenditures in 2003 to 30% in 2014

- The largest contributors to the increase in mental health spending between 2003 and 2014 will be prescription drugs (37%), physician services (18%), and hospitals (17%) (see Figure 5.2)

FIGURE 5.1

FIGURE 5.2

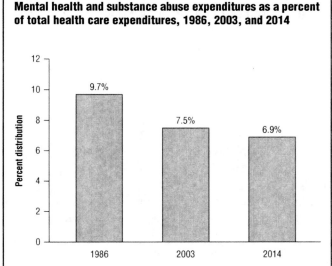

Mental health and substance abuse expenditures as a percent of total health care expenditures, 1986, 2003, and 2014

SOURCE: Katharine R. Levit et al., "Figure 2.1. MHSA Expenditures As a Percent of Total Health Care Expenditures: 1986, 2003, and 2014," in *Projections of National Expenditures for Mental Health and Substance Abuse Treatment 2004–2014*, Substance Abuse and Mental Health Services Administration, 2008, http://www.samhsa.gov/Financing/file .axd?file=2009%2F6%2FProjections+of+National+Expenditures+for+ Mental+Health+Services+and+Substance+Abuse+Treatment%2C+ 2004-2014.pdf (accessed June 25, 2012)

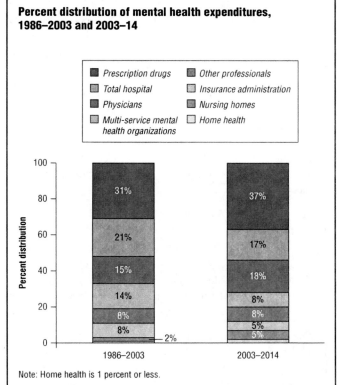

Percent distribution of mental health expenditures, 1986–2003 and 2003–14

Note: Home health is 1 percent or less.

SOURCE: Katharine R. Levit et al., "Figure 3.8. Contribution of MH Provider Expenditures to Increases in MH Expenditures: 1986–2003 and 2003–2014," in *Projections of National Expenditures for Mental Health and Substance Abuse Treatment 2004–2014*, Substance Abuse and Mental Health Services Administration, 2008, http://www.samhsa .gov/Financing/file.axd?file=2009%2F6%2FProjections+of+National+ Expenditures+for+Mental+Health+Services+and+Substance+Abuse+ Treatment%2C+2004-2014.pdf (accessed June 25, 2012)

Health care industry observers attribute the decrease in mental health inpatient services to the increased emphasis on drug treatment of mental health disorders, the increasing frequency of outpatient treatment, the closure of psychiatric hospitals, and the cost containment efforts of managed care. Figure 5.2 shows an increasing share of mental health spending for prescription drugs. Levit et al. indicate that spending for prescription drugs increased from 7% in 1986 to 23% in 2003 and is projected to reach 30% in 2014. Despite the higher spending for these psychoactive prescription drugs, some industry observers believe the increased availability of effective drug therapy actually served to contain mental health spending by enabling providers to offer drug therapy instead of more costly inpatient treatment.

SAMHSA Spending

According to the U.S. Department of Health and Human Services (HHS), in *U.S. Department of Health and Human Services Budget in Brief, Fiscal Year 2013: Advancing the Health, Safety, and Well-Being of Our Nation* (February 2012, http://www.hhs.gov/budget/ budget-brief-fy2013.pdf), the FY 2013 budget for SAMHSA was $3.4 billion, $142 million less than the FY 2012 budget. The funds were used to continue to prevent youth violence and reduce youth drug use, promote emotional health and prevent substance abuse disorders and mental illnesses, improve children's mental health, and help people with mental illness who face homelessness.

State Mental Health Agency Expenditures

A number of court rulings during the 1970s and an evolution in professional thinking prompted the release of many people with serious mental illness from institutions to community treatment programs. The census (the number of patients or occupants, which is frequently referred to as a rate) of public mental hospitals sharply declined, and there was increasing pressure on the states to deliver community-based treatment.

State mental health agencies (SMHAs) operate the public mental health system that acts as a safety net for poor, uninsured, and otherwise indigent people suffering from mental illness. In *Mental Health Financing in the United States: A Primer* (April 2011, http://www.kff.org/ medicaid/upload/8182.pdf), the Kaiser Commission on Medicaid and the Uninsured explains that these public mental health systems are heavily dependent on Medicaid and "in many states, the two are jointly budgeted, with states attributing their matching funds for Medicaid to the budget of state mental health agencies." The SMHAs vary from state to state—some purchase, regulate, administer, manage, and provide care and treatment, whereas others simply purchase care using public funds that include general state revenues and federal funds. Medicaid is also the fastest-growing component of SMHA spending; however, the share of Medicaid mental health spending that is controlled by the SMHAs varies widely by state.

Increased Medicaid financing of the SMHAs has had several beneficial effects on state systems. For example, it increased the amount of funds that are available for mental health services, catalyzed the shift to community-based treatment over institutional care, and improved access to insurance coverage and treatment for low-income people with mental health needs.

Similar to the movement of privately insured people into managed care, during the 1990s state Medicaid programs turned to managed care organizations (MCOs) and behavioral health services in an effort to contain costs. More than half the states have separated the administration and financing of physical health and mental health in their MCO contracts.

The SMHAs manage funds from the SAMHSA Mental Health Block Grant (MHBG) program. The MHBG was created in 1982 and its flexible funding enables states to innovate, develop, and expand successful community-based programs. Block grants (lump sums of money) are awarded based on a formula that considers each state's population, service costs, income, and taxable resources, and the funds enable the states to finance community mental health treatment programs.

HIGH COSTS OF RESEARCH

Medical and pharmaceutical research, disease prevention research, and the work to develop and conduct clinical trials of new drugs are expensive. The National Institutes of Health (NIH) reports in "Estimates of Funding for Various Research, Condition, and Disease Categories (RCDC)" (February 13, 2012, http://report.nih.gov/catego rical_spending.aspx) that its FY 2013 budget allocated an estimated $3.1 billion for human immunodeficiency virus (HIV) and acquired immunodeficiency syndrome (AIDS) research, compared with $827 million to investigate obesity prevention and treatment. Pharmaceutical manufacturers also spend billions of dollars every year researching and developing new medicines. For example, according to the Pharmaceutical Research and Manufacturers of America (PhRMA; 2012 http://www.phrma.org/about/phrma) U.S. pharmaceutical companies spent $49.5 billion in 2011. By contrast, the entire NIH FY 2011 budget was $30.7 billion. (See Table 4.3 in Chapter 4.)

Decisions about how much is spent to research a particular disease are not based solely on how many people develop the disease or die from it. Rightly or wrongly, economists base the societal value of an individual on his or her earning potential and productivity (the ability to contribute to society as a worker). The bulk of the people who die from heart disease, stroke, and cancer are older adults. Many have retired from the workforce, and their potential economic productivity is usually low or nonexistent. (This is not an observation about how society values older adults; instead, it is simply an economic measure of present and future financial productivity.)

In contrast, AIDS patients are often much younger and die in their 20s, 30s, and 40s. Until they develop AIDS, their potential productivity, measured in economic terms, is high. The number of work years lost when they die is considerable. Using this economic equation to determine how disease research should be funded, it may be considered economically wise to invest more money to research AIDS because the losses, which are measured in potential work years rather than in lives, are so much greater.

Once a new drug receives FDA approval, its manufacturer is ordinarily allowed to hold the patent on the drug to recoup its investment. During the life of the patent the drug is priced much higher than if other manufacturers were allowed to compete by producing generic versions of the same drug. After the patent expires, competition between pharmaceutical manufacturers generally lowers the price. For example, HIV/AIDS drugs are granted only seven years of exclusivity under legislation to encourage research and promote development of new treatments.

In *PhRMA 2012 Profile* (2012, http://www.phrma .org/sites/default/files/159/phrma_industry_profile.pdf), PhRMA explains that the pharmaceutical manufacturer must cover the cost not only of research and development for the approximately three out of 10 drugs that succeed but also for many that fail. PhRMA observes that "for every 5,000 to 10,000 compounds that enter the discovery pipeline, only five make it to clinical trials, and only one receives approval from the FDA." On average, manufacturers spend over $1.2 billion to bring brand-name drugs to market, including the expense of 10 to 15 years of product development.

HARDSHIP OF HIGH HEALTH CARE COSTS ON FAMILIES

The Families USA Foundation is a national health care advocacy organization that is dedicated to achieving affordable, quality health care and long-term care for all American families. The organization contends that American families pay about two-thirds of the nation's health care bill, whereas American businesses pay the other one-third. This ratio is based on the premise that families and businesses pay for health care in several ways:

- Directly, through out-of-pocket payments and insurance expenses. These include premiums, deductibles (annual amounts that must be paid by the employee before the insurance plan begins paying), and co-payments.

- Indirectly, through Medicare payroll, income, and other federal, state, and local taxes that support public health programs. These include veterans' health benefits, military health benefits, the Medicaid program, and a variety of smaller public health programs.

As a result, Families USA Foundation estimates of per capita health care spending differ from other reports, such as those from the CMS and the Census Bureau, which take into account only direct payments.

Families also purchase insurance themselves when they work for employers that do not offer group health insurance or when insurers refuse to insure certain groups they consider to be at high risk (such as people with chronic diseases). Workers who retire before reaching age 65 and are not yet eligible for Medicare coverage must also purchase insurance on their own. Furthermore, many Medicare beneficiaries pay insurance premiums for supplemental (Medigap) insurance to cover the difference in charges that Medicare does not pay.

High Cost of Prescription Drugs

Even though it has slowed somewhat in recent years, spending for prescription drugs remains the fastest-growing component of health care spending. In 2010 prescription drug expenditures reached an estimated $259.1 billion and were projected to more than double to $483.2 billion by 2021. (See Table 5.7.) Tauren Dyson observes in "Prices for Brand-Name Drugs Most Used by Medicare Patients Jump Almost 10 Percent: It's the Biggest Hike in Eight Years" (*AARP Bulletin*, May 18, 2010) that the cost of brand-name prescription drugs most commonly used by those in Medicare rose 9.7% between March 2009 and March 2010 (the most recent years for which data are available).

To control prescription drug expenditures, many hospitals, health plans, employers, and other group purchasers have attempted to obtain discounts and rebates for bulk purchases from pharmaceutical companies. Some have developed programs to encourage health care practitioners and consumers to use less costly generic drugs, and others have limited, reduced, or even eliminated prescription drug coverage.

In "Medicare: Seniors Saved $3.7 Billion on Medicine" (CNNMoney, June 25, 2012), Parija Kavilanz reports that by June 2012 the ACA had already provided much needed relief from prescription drug costs for Medicare beneficiaries, saving them a total of $3.7 billion. Kavilanz explains that the ACA not only gave Medicare beneficiaries a one-time tax-free $250 rebate to defray the cost of prescription drugs in 2010 but also gave those

with high prescription drug costs a 50% discount on brand-name drugs and a 7% discount on generic drugs.

Generic Drugs Promise Cost Savings

When patents expire on popular brand-name drugs, the entry of generic versions of these drugs to the market promises cost savings for consumers and payers. Generic drugs usually cost 10% to 30% less when they first enter the market and even less once additional generic manufacturers join in the competition. According to Fred Gebhart, in "Generics Continue to Roll up Medication Markets" (*Drug Topics*, vol. 155, no. 8, August 15, 2011), among the drugs with patents that were set to expire in 2012 were Plavix (to prevent strokes and heart attacks), Viagra (to treat erectile dysfunction), Seroquel (to treat schizophrenia, a serious mental illness that causes disturbed thinking and behavior), Crestor (a cholesterol-lowering drug), Singulair (to prevent asthma attacks), and Lexapro (an antidepressant). Industry observers predict that consumers can expect to pay $5 to $20 less per prescription when they opt for generic drugs rather than for brand-name drugs. Several major chain stores, such as Wal-Mart, Target, Walgreens, and Kroger, sell 30-day supplies of various generic drugs for a flat $4, and 90-day supplies for $10.

How Will the ACA Affect Drug Costs?

The ACA authorizes the FDA to approve generic versions of biologic drugs (drugs derived from living organisms that are used to prevent, diagnose, or treat diseases) and grant biologics manufacturers 12 years of exclusive use before generics can be developed. In "In Health Care Overhaul, Boons for Hospitals and Drug Makers" (*New York Times*, March 21, 2010), Reed Abelson asserts that because the legislation will provide insurance coverage for an additional 32 million Americans, there will be more customers for health services including prescription drugs. Abelson observes that even though pharmaceutical companies have been asked to "contribute $85 billion toward the cost of the bill in the form of industry fees and lower prices paid under government programs over 10 years," this will be more than offset by the revenues generated by millions of additional prescription drug purchases. Furthermore, because the legislation closes the Medicare coverage gap, older adults who may have delayed or deferred filling their prescriptions when they exhausted coverage will no longer have to do so, which will generate even more prescription sales.

Abelson reports that consumers are unlikely to realize prescription drug savings as a result of the legislation and quotes Jon Leibowitz, the chairman of the Federal Trade Commission, who said, "The big loser is the American consumer, who is going to have to pay an extra $3.5 billion a year in much-needed drugs." Nearly four out of 10 American consumers appear to understand that prescription drug prices will rise. According to Rasmussen

Reports, in "43% Say Cost of Prescription Drugs Will Go up If Health Plan Becomes Law" (March 22, 2010, http://www.rasmussenreports.com/public_content/politics/current_events/healthcare/march_2010/), 43% of Americans anticipate a rise in drug costs and 23% believe prescription drug costs will decrease. Over one-third (36%) of respondents said they were paying more for prescription drugs than they had six months prior to the survey, whereas 52% said they were not paying more.

RATIONING HEALTH CARE

When health care rationing (allocating medical resources) is defined as "all care that is expected to be beneficial is not always available to all patients," most health care practitioners, policy makers, and consumers accept that rationing has been, and will continue to be, a feature of the U.S. health care system. Most American opinion leaders and industry observers accept that even a country as wealthy as the United States cannot afford all the care that is likely to benefit its citizens. The practical considerations of allocating health care resources involve establishing priorities and determining how these resources should be rationed.

Opponents of Rationing

There is widespread agreement among Americans that rationing according to patients' ability to pay for health care services or insurance is unfair. Ideally, health care should be equitably allocated on the basis of need and the potential benefit derived from the care. Those who argue against rationing fear that society's most vulnerable populations—older adults, the poor, and people with chronic illnesses—suffer most from the rationing of health care.

Many observers believe improving the efficiency of the U.S. health care system will save enough money to supply basic health care services to all Americans. They suggest that because expenditures for the same medical procedures vary greatly in different areas of the country, standardizing fees and costs could realize great savings. They also believe money could be saved if greater emphasis is placed on preventive care and on effective strategies to prevent or reduce behaviors that increase health risk such as smoking, alcohol and drug abuse, and unsafe sexual practices. Furthermore, they insist that the high cost of administering the U.S. health care system could be streamlined with a single payer for health care—as in the Canadian system.

Supporters of Rationing

Those who endorse rationing argue that the spiraling cost of the U.S. health care system stems from more than simple inefficiency. They attribute escalating costs to the aging population, rapid technological innovation, and the increasing costs for labor and supplies.

Not everyone who supports rationing thinks the U.S. health care system is working well. Some rationing supporters believe that the nation's health care system charges too much for the services it delivers and that it fails altogether to deliver to the millions of the uninsured. In fact, they point out that the United States already rations health care by not covering the uninsured. Other health care–rationing advocates argue that the problem is one of basic cultural assumptions, not the economics of the health care industry. Americans value human life, believe in the promise of health and quality health care for all, and insist that diseases can be cured. They contend the issue is not whether health care should be rationed but how care is rationed. They believe the United States spends too much on health compared with other societal needs, too much on the old rather than on the young, more on curing and not enough on caring, and too much on extending the length of life and not enough on enhancing the quality of life. Supporters of rationing argue instead for a system that guarantees a minimally acceptable level of health care for all, while reining in the expensive excesses of the current system, which often acts to prolong life at any cost.

The Oregon Health Plan: An Experiment in Rationing

In 1987 Oregon designed a new, universal health care plan that would simultaneously expand coverage and contain costs by limiting services. Unlike other states, which trimmed budgets by eliminating people from Medicaid eligibility, Oregon chose to eliminate low-priority services. Michael Janofsky reports in "Oregon Starts to Extend Health Care" (*New York Times*, February 19, 1994) that the Oregon Health Plan, which was approved in August 1993, aimed to provide Medicaid to 120,000 additional residents living below the federal poverty level. The plan also established a high-risk insurance pool for people who were refused health insurance coverage because of preexisting medical conditions, offered more insurance options for small businesses, and improved employees' abilities to retain their health insurance benefits when they changed jobs. A gradual increase in the state cigarette tax was expected to provide $45 million annually, which would help fund the additional estimated $200 million needed over the next several years.

Oregon developed a table of health care services and performed a cost-benefit analysis to rank them. It was decided that Oregon Medicaid would cover the top 565 services on a list of 696 medical procedures. Janofsky notes that services that fell below the cutoff point were "not deemed to be serious enough to require treatment, like common colds, flu, mild food poisoning, sprains, cosmetic procedures and experimental treatments for diseases in advanced stages."

As the Oregon Health Services Commission (HSC) prepared to establish the priorities, it decided that disease prevention and quality of well-being (QWB) were the factors that most influenced the ranking of the treatments. QWB drew fire from those who felt that such judgments could not be decided subjectively. Active medical or surgical treatment of terminally ill patients also ranked low on the QWB scale, whereas comfort and hospice care ranked high. The HSC emphasized that its QWB judgments were not based on an individual's quality of life at a given time; such judgments were considered ethically questionable. Instead, it focused on the potential for change in an individual's life, posing questions such as: "After treatment, how much better or worse off would the patient be?"

Critics countered that the plan obtained its funding by reducing services that were currently offered to Medicaid recipients (often poor women and children) rather than by emphasizing cost control. Others objected to the ranking and the ethical questions raised by choosing to support some treatments over others.

According to Jonathan Oberlander of the University of North Carolina, Chapel Hill, in "Health Reform Interrupted: The Unraveling of the Oregon Health Plan" (*Health Affairs*, vol. 26, no. 1, January 2007), the Oregon Health Plan initially did serve to reduce the percentage of uninsured Oregonians from 18% in 1992 to 11% in 1996, but its early success proved difficult to sustain. By 2003 the Oregon plan was not even close to achieving its goal of having no uninsured people in the state. In fact, the ranks of the uninsured were growing, so much so that by 2003 they reached 17%. An economic downturn in the state and the state's strategy of explicit rationing are cited by Oberlander as reasons for the ambitious plan's failure to achieve its goals.

The Oregon HSC continued to modify the plan's covered benefits. In January 2002 the HSC began refining the list of covered services. The HSC sought to reduce the overall costs of the plan by eliminating less effective treatments and determining if any covered medical conditions could be more effectively treated using standardized clinical practice guidelines (step-by-step instructions for diagnosis and treatment of specific illnesses or disorders) while preserving basic coverage. The benefit review process will be ongoing with the HSC submitting a new prioritized list of benefits on July 1 of each even-numbered year for review by the legislative assembly.

Oregon is credited with initiating health care reform earlier than other states. Jonathan J. Cooper reports in "Feds to Put up $1.9B for Oregon Health Overhaul" (Associated Press, May 3, 2012) that in 2012 Oregon launched another initiative that was aimed at generating Medicaid saving without sacrificing quality of care. The new initiative, which will be funded by the federal government, creates "coordinated care organizations" to manage all mental, physical, and dental care for 600,000 low-income patients in the state's Medicaid program. It achieves cost savings by targeting the sickest patients with the highest costs (e.g., people with chronic diseases such as diabetes and asthma) with preventive services. For example, when caseworkers ensure that patients schedule and attend medical appointments and take their medications as prescribed, they can potentially avert expensive emergency department visits and costly hospitalizations.

Rationing by HMOs

Until 2000 steadily increasing numbers of Americans received their health care from HMOs or other managed care systems. According to the Kaiser Family Foundation, in "Health Insurance & Managed Care" (http://www. state healthfacts.org/comparemaptable.jsp?cat=7&ind=348), by July 2011 national enrollment in HMOs was 70.2 million, which was more than four times the enrollment rate two decades earlier (15.1 million). By contrast, the number of HMOs operating in the United States had risen slightly, from 564 in July 2000 to 452 in July 2011.

Managed care programs have sought to control costs by limiting coverage for experimental, duplicative, and unnecessary treatments. Before physicians can perform experimental procedures or prescribe new treatment plans, they must obtain prior authorization (approval from the patient's managed care plan) to ensure that the expenses will be covered.

Increasingly, patients and physicians are battling HMOs for approval to use and receive reimbursement for new technology and experimental treatments. Judges and juries, moved by the desperate situations of patients, have frequently decided cases against HMOs, regardless of whether the new treatment has been shown to be effective.

"SILENT RATIONING." Physicians and health care consumers are concerned that limiting coverage for new, high-cost technology will discourage research and development for new treatments before they have even been developed. This is called "silent rationing," because patients will never know what they have missed.

In an effort to control costs, some HMOs have discouraged physicians from informing patients about certain treatment options—those that are extremely expensive or not covered by the HMO. This has proved to be a highly controversial issue, both politically and ethically. In December 1996 the HHS ruled that HMOs and other health plans cannot prevent physicians from telling Medicare patients about all available treatment options.

Could Less Health Care Be Better Than More?

Even though health care providers and consumers fear that rationing sharply limits access to medical care and will ultimately result in poorer health among affected Americans, researchers are also concerned about the effects of too much care on the health of the nation. Several studies suggest that an oversupply of medical care may be as harmful as an undersupply.

In the landmark study *Geography and the Debate over Medicare Reform* (February 13, 2002, http://content .healthaffairs.org/cgi/reprint/hlthaff.w2.96v1), John E. Wennberg, Elliott S. Fisher, and Jonathan S. Skinner of Dartmouth Medical School find tremendous regional variation in both the utilization and the cost of health care that they believe is explained, at least in part, by the distribution of health care providers. Variations in physicians' practice styles—whether they favor outpatient treatment over hospitalization for specific procedures such as biopsies (surgical procedures to examine tissue to detect cancer cells)—greatly affect demand for hospital care.

Variation in demand for health care services in turn produces variation in health care expenditures. Wennberg, Fisher, and Skinner report wide geographic variation in Medicare spending. Medicare paid more than twice as much to care for a 65-year-old in Miami, Florida, where the supply of health care providers is overabundant, than it spent on care for a 65-year-old in Minneapolis, Minnesota, a city with an average supply of health care providers. To be certain that the differences were not simply higher fees and charges in Miami, the researchers also compared rates of utilization. They find that older adults in Miami visited physicians and hospitals much more often than their counterparts in Minneapolis.

Wennberg, Fisher, and Skinner also wanted to be sure that the differences were not caused by the severity of illness, so they compared care during the last six months of life to control for any underlying regional differences in the health of the population. Remarkably, the widest variations were observed in care during the last six months of life, when older adults in Miami saw physician specialists six times as often as those in Minneapolis. The researchers assert that higher expenditures, particularly at the end of life, do not purchase better care. Instead, they finance generally unpleasant and futile interventions that are intended to prolong life rather than to improve the quality of patients' lives. Wennberg, Fisher, and Skinner conclude that areas with more medical care, higher utilization, and higher costs fared no better in terms of life expectancy, morbidity (illness), or mortality (death), and that the care that people received was no different in quality from care received by people in areas with average supplies of health care providers.

In *The Care of Patients with Severe Chronic Illness: An Online Report on the Medicare Program by the Dartmouth Atlas Project* (2006, http://www.dartmouthatlas.org/ downloads/atlases/2006_Chronic_Care_Atlas.pdf), John E. Wennberg et al. of Dartmouth Medical School detail differences in the management of Medicare enrollees with severe chronic illnesses. The researchers find that average utilization and health care spending varied by state, region, and even by hospital in the same region. Expenditures were not linked with rates of illness in different parts of the country;

instead, they reflected how intensively selected resources (e.g., acute care hospital beds, specialist physician visits, tests, and other services) were used to care for patients who were very ill but could not be cured. Because other research demonstrates that, for these chronically ill Americans, receiving more services does not result in improved health outcomes, and because most Americans say they prefer to avoid excessively high-tech end-of-life care, the researchers conclude that Medicare spending for the care of the chronically ill could be reduced by as much as 30%, while improving quality, patient satisfaction, and outcomes. Wennberg et al.'s research and similar studies pose two important and as yet unanswered questions: How much health care is needed to deliver the best health to a population? Are Americans getting the best value for the dollars spent on health care?

Elliot S. Fisher, Julie P. Bynum, and Jonathan S. Skinner of Dartmouth Medical School assert in "Slowing the Growth of Health Care Costs—Lessons from Regional Variation" (*New England Journal of Medicine*, vol. 360, no. 9, February 26, 2009) that "by learning from regions that have attained sustainable growth rates and building on successful models of delivery-system and payment-system reform, we might, with adequate physician leadership, manage to 'bend the cost curve.'" The researchers also suggest that "such a change would not solve the country's long-term fiscal challenges. But it suggests that if we focus reform efforts on current areas of overspending—overuse of hospitals and unnecessary visits, consultations, tests, and minor procedures—we may be able to bend the cost curve while continuing to enjoy the benefits of technological advances."

In "Stemming the Tide of Overtreatment in U.S. Healthcare" (Reuters, February 16, 2012), Debra Sherman reports that in an effort to prevent increased government intervention, medical professional societies such as the American College of Physicians (the largest medical specialty group in the United States) are disseminating guidelines to help physicians refine screening procedures to prevent excessive testing and procedures. Industry observers also believe that economic incentives must be realigned to support this effort. Otis Brawley, the chief medical officer of the American Cancer Society, explains that patients are often given expensive tests, even though cheaper ones are better, because "no one can make money off of" the less costly tests.

Economic Impact of the ACA

According to the CBO, in *Updated Estimates for the Insurance Coverage Provisions of the Affordable Care Act* (March 20, 2012, http://www.cbo.gov/sites/default/files/ cbofiles/attachments/03-13-Coverage%20Estimates.pdf), the ACA has the capacity to reduce the budget deficit by half a percent of the GDP—more than a trillion dollars— between 2010 and 2019. The bill also serves to reduce the total cost of health care via changes in Medicare and Medicaid eligibility and in reimbursement, such as by reducing payments to insurance plans under the Medicare Advantage program. Furthermore, the bill funds comparative effectiveness research to identify the most cost-effective medical procedures.

The ACA will have a net cost of nearly $1.1 trillion from 2012 through 2021, $50 billion less than the CBO's March 2011 forecast. The revision reflects changes in the U.S. economy, primarily a slower economic recovery than had been anticipated, slower growth in private health insurance premiums, and legislative changes that affected insurance coverage. In *Estimates for the Insurance Coverage Provisions of the Affordable Care Act Updated for the Recent Supreme Court Decision*, the CBO provides a revised estimate—a net reduction of $84 billion over the 11-year period from 2012 through 2022—in response to the U.S. Supreme Court ruling, which is likely to reduce Medicaid enrollment.

The legislation generates revenues via new taxes and fees, including an excise tax on high-cost insurance plans, which the CBO estimates will raise $32 billion over 10 years. Additional tax changes that are slated to begin in 2013 and beyond include:

- Small companies with 25 or fewer employees will be eligible for tax credits up to 35% of the cost of premiums to help them purchase health insurance

- Companies with 50 employees or more that do not offer health care coverage will have to pay as much as $2,000 per full-time employee for each employee who obtains coverage from a government-subsidized insurance exchange

- People using indoor tanning salon services will pay a 10% tax

It is also anticipated that by enabling workers to seek new job opportunities without the fear of losing their employer-sponsored health care coverage, the legislation may stimulate business growth.

CHAPTER 6
INSURANCE: THOSE WITH AND THOSE WITHOUT

In 1798 Congress established the U.S. Marine Hospital Services for seamen. It was the first time an employer offered health insurance in the United States. Payments for hospital services were deducted from the sailors' salary.

In the 21st century many factors affect the availability of health insurance, including an economic recession, employment, income, personal health status, and age. As a result, an individual's or family's health insurance status often changes as circumstances change. Carmen DeNavas-Walt, Bernadette D. Proctor, and Jessica C. Smith of the U.S. Census Bureau report in *Income, Poverty, and Health Insurance Coverage in the United States: 2010* (September 2011, http://www.census.gov/prod/2011pubs/p60-239.pdf) that in 2010, 64% of Americans were covered during all or part of the year by private health insurance and 55.3% were covered by employment-based health insurance. (See Table 6.1.) The researchers note that the economic recession, which lasted from late 2007 to mid-2009, decreased the percentage of Americans who were covered by private and employment-based health insurance and that the percentage of people covered by government health insurance increased. Medicare (a federal health insurance program for people aged 65 years and older and people with disabilities) covered 14.5% of Americans in 2010, and Medicaid (a state and federal health insurance program for low-income people) covered 15.9%. Another 16.3% of Americans were without health coverage. DeNavas-Walt, Proctor, and Smith indicate that the percentage of the U.S. population without health coverage in 2010 was the highest it had been since 1997. (See Figure 6.1.)

According to Brian W. Ward et al. of the National Center for Health Statistics (NCHS), in *Early Release of Selected Estimates Based on Data from the 2011 National Health Interview Survey* (June 2012, http://www.cdc.gov/nchs/data/nhis/earlyrelease/earlyrelease201206_01.pdf),

the percentage of adults aged 18 to 64 years without health care coverage at the time of the interview was 15.1% in 2011, down slightly from 16% in 2010. (See Figure 6.2.) Robin A. Cohen and Michael E. Martinez of the NCHS indicate in *Health Insurance Coverage: Early Release of Estimates from the National Health Interview Survey, January–September 2011* (June 2012, http://www.cdc.gov/nchs/data/nhis/earlyrelease/earlyrelease201206_01.pdf) that in 2011 there were 58.7 million (19.2%) people who were uninsured for at least part of the 12 months preceding the interview and 34.2 million (11.2%) had been uninsured for more than a year. The overwhelming majority of the uninsured were adults aged 18 to 64 years. Figure 6.3 shows the percentages of children under the age of 18 years and adults aged 18 to 64 years that were uninsured at the time of the interview, by age group and sex. Figure 6.4 shows the percentages of people uninsured at the time of the interview, uninsured for at least part of the year, uninsured for more than a year, and those with public and private insurance.

WHO WAS UNINSURED IN 2011?

Not surprisingly, in 2011 poverty status was associated with a lack of health insurance coverage. Among people of all ages, those who were poor or near poor were more likely to be uninsured than the not poor. (The Census Bureau defines "poor" people as those below the poverty threshold; "near poor" people have incomes of 100% to less than 200% of the poverty threshold; and "not poor" people have incomes equal to or greater than 200% of the poverty threshold.) For example, among people aged 18 to 64 years, 40.1% of those who were poor and the same percentage of those who were near poor were uninsured at the time of the interview, compared with just 12% of those who were not poor in 2011. (See Table 6.2.)

The proportion of people who did not have health insurance in 2011 for at least part of the year preceding

TABLE 6.1

Coverage by type of health insurance, 2009 and 2010

Coverage type	2009	2010
Any private plan[a]	64.5	64.0
Any private plan alone[b]	53.3	52.7
Employment-based[a]	56.1	55.3
Employment-based alone[b]	46.6	45.8
Direct-purchase[a]	9.6	9.8
Direct-purchase alone[b]	3.7	3.7
Any government plan[a]	30.6	31.0
Any government plan alone[b]	19.4	19.7
Medicare[a]	14.3	14.5
Medicare alone[b]	4.5	4.7
Medicaid[a]	15.7	15.9
Medicaid alone[b]	11.2	11.2
Military health care[a, c]	4.1	4.2
Military health care alone[b, c]	1.3	1.3
Uninsured	16.1	16.3

[a]The estimates by type of coverage are not mutually exclusive; people can be covered by more than one type of health insurance during the year.
[b]The estimates by type of coverage are mutually exclusive; people did not have any other type of health insurance during the year.
[c]Military health care includes Tricare and CHAMPVA (Civilian Health and Medical Program of the Department of Veteran Affairs), as well as care provided by the Department of Veterans Affairs and the military.

SOURCE: Carmen DeNavas-Walt, Bernadette D. Proctor, and Jessica C. Smith, "Table 10. Coverage by Type of Health Insurance: 2009 and 2010," in *Income, Poverty, and Health Insurance Coverage in the United States: 2010*, U.S. Census Bureau, September 2011, http://www.census.gov/prod/2011pubs/p60-239.pdf (accessed June 26, 2012)

the interview varied by geography. It was greatest in the South (22%) and West (21.9%), and less in the Midwest (16.1%) and Northeast (13.9%). (See Table 6.3.) Hispanics (34.3%) and non-Hispanic African-Americans (22.2%) were more likely to be uninsured in 2011 than Asian-Americans (18.2%) and non-Hispanic whites (14.8%).

The Uninsured by Gender and Age

Among people under the age of 65 years in 2011, the percentage of people without insurance at the time of the interview was highest among adults aged 25 to 34 years (28.2%) and lowest among young people under the age of 18 years (7%). (See Figure 6.3.) Among adults of all ages, men were more likely than women to be uninsured.

LACK OF INSURANCE HAS SIGNIFICANT CONSEQUENCES

In *Sicker and Poorer: The Consequences of Being Uninsured* (May 2002, http://www.kff.org/uninsured/upload/Full-Report.pdf), a landmark report prepared for the Kaiser Commission on Medicaid and the Uninsured, Jack Hadley of the Urban Institute discusses an exhaustive review of the literature detailing the major findings

FIGURE 6.1

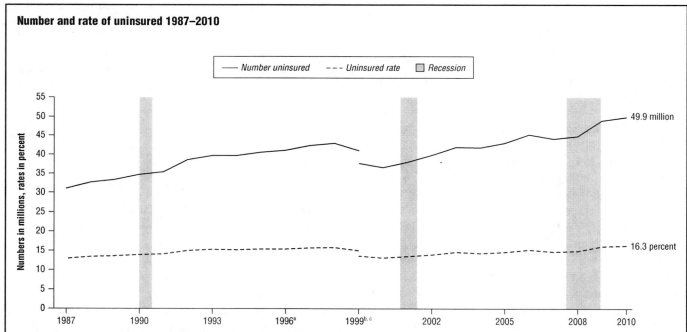

Number and rate of uninsured 1987–2010

[a]The data for 1996 through 1999 were revised using an approximation method for consistency with the revision to the 2004 and 2005 estimates.
[b]Implementation of Census 2000-based population controls occurred for the 2000 ASEC, which collected data for 1999. These estimates also reflect the results of follow-up verification questions, which were asked of people who responded "no" to all questions about specific types of health insurance coverage in order to verify whether they were actually uninsured. This change increased the number and percentage of people covered by health insurance, bringing the CPS more in line with estimates from other national surveys.
[c]The data for 1999 through 2009 were revised to reflect the results of enhancements to the editing process.
Note: Respondents were not asked detailed health insurance questions before the 1988 CPS.
The data points are placed at the midpoints of the respective years.

SOURCE: Carmen DeNavas-Walt, Bernadette D. Proctor, and Jessica C. Smith, "Figure 7. Number Uninsured and Uninsured Rate: 1987 to 2010," in *Income, Poverty, and Health Insurance Coverage in the United States: 2010*, U.S. Census Bureau, September 2011, http://www.census.gov/prod/2011pubs/p60-239.pdf (accessed June 26, 2012)

FIGURE 6.2

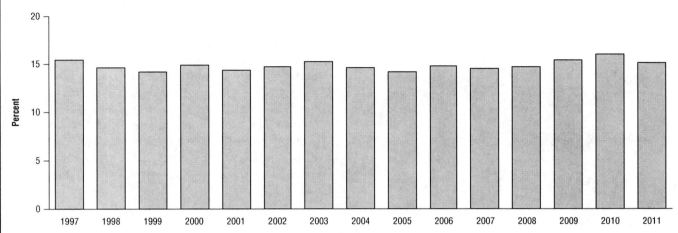

Percentage of persons of all ages without health insurance at the time of interview, for at least part of the past year, or for more than a year, 1997–2011

Notes: Data are based on household interviews of a sample of the civilian noninstitutionalized population. A person was defined as uninsured if he or she did not have any private health insurance, Medicare, Medicaid, Children's Health Insurance Program (CHIP), state-sponsored or other government-sponsored health plan, or military plan at the time of interview. A person was also defined as uninsured if he or she had only Indian Health Service coverage or had only a private plan that paid for one type of service, such as accidents or dental care. The data on health insurance status were edited using an automated system based on logic checks and keyword searches. For comparability, the estimates for all years were created using these same procedures. The resulting estimates of persons without health insurance coverage are generally 0.1–0.3 percentage point lower than those based on the editing procedures used for the final data files. Occasionally, due to decisions made for the final data editing and weighting, estimates based on preliminary editing procedures may differ by more than 0.3 percentage point. The analyses excluded persons with unknown health insurance status (about 1% of respondents each year).

SOURCE: B. W. Ward et al., "Figure 1.1. Percentage of Persons of All Ages without Health Insurance Coverage at the Time of Interview, United States, 1997–2011," in *Early Release of Selected Estimates Based on Data from the 2011 National Health Interview Survey*, National Center for Health Statistics, June 2012, http://www.cdc.gov/nchs/data/nhis/earlyrelease/earlyrelease201206_01.pdf (accessed June 26, 2012)

FIGURE 6.3

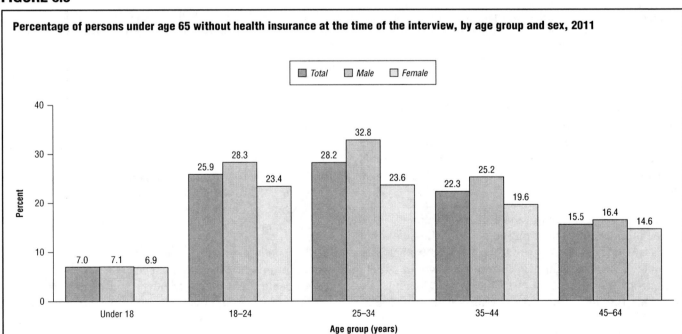

Percentage of persons under age 65 without health insurance at the time of the interview, by age group and sex, 2011

Note: Data are based on household interviews of a sample of the civilian noninstitutionalized population.

SOURCE: Robin A. Cohen and Michael E. Martinez, "Figure 2. Percentage of Persons under Age 65 without Health Insurance Coverage at the Time of Interview, by Age Group and Sex: United States, 2011," in *Health Insurance Coverage: Early Release of Estimates from the National Health Interview Survey, 2011*, National Center for Health Statistics, June 2012, http://www.cdc.gov/nchs/data/nhis/earlyrelease/insur201206.pdf (accessed June 26, 2012)

FIGURE 6.4

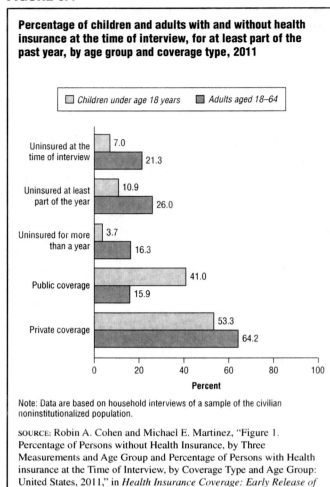

Percentage of children and adults with and without health insurance at the time of interview, for at least part of the past year, by age group and coverage type, 2011

☐ Children under age 18 years   ▨ Adults aged 18–64

Note: Data are based on household interviews of a sample of the civilian noninstitutionalized population.

SOURCE: Robin A. Cohen and Michael E. Martinez, "Figure 1. Percentage of Persons without Health Insurance, by Three Measurements and Age Group and Percentage of Persons with Health insurance at the Time of Interview, by Coverage Type and Age Group: United States, 2011," in *Health Insurance Coverage: Early Release of Estimates from the National Health Interview Survey, 2011*, National Center for Health Statistics, June 2012, http://www.cdc.gov/nchs/data/nhis/earlyrelease/insur201206.pdf (accessed June 26, 2012)

of more than 25 years of health services research on the effects of health insurance. Hadley notes that the uninsured receive less preventive care, are diagnosed at more advanced stages of disease, and receive less treatment as measured in terms of pharmaceutical and surgical interventions.

Hadley concludes that if the uninsured were provided with health insurance, their mortality rates (the number of deaths caused by disease) would be reduced by between 10% and 15%. The reduction in mortality would largely result from improved access to timely and appropriate care. This finding is supported by the Institute of Medicine (IOM), which observes in *America's Uninsured Crisis: Consequences for Health and Health Care* (February 2009, http://books.nap.edu/openbook.php?record_id =12511) that the economic downturn exacerbated Americans' health problems because more Americans are uninsured. The IOM explains that "fewer people have access to coverage at work, more people find the costs of private

coverage too expensive, and others lose public coverage because of changed personal circumstances, administrative barriers, and program cutbacks." The IOM also notes that rigorous research confirms that uninsurance has a profound negative affect on the health and mortality of adults and children.

One of the most dramatic conclusions of Families USA research is that having health insurance is literally a matter of life or death for some Americans. In *Dying for Coverage: The Deadly Consequences of Being Uninsured* (June 2012, http://familiesusa2.org/assets/pdfs/Dying-for-Coverage.pdf), Kim Bailey of Families USA reports that 26,100 people aged 25 to 64 years "died prematurely due to a lack of health coverage in 2010." Between 2005 and 2010, 134,120 deaths were attributable to the lack of health insurance.

SOURCES OF HEALTH INSURANCE
People under the Age of 65 Years

For people under the age of 65 years there are two principal sources of health insurance coverage: private insurance (from employer or private policies) and Medicaid. Between 1999 and 2009 the proportion of those covered by private insurance at the time of the interview declined and then increased in 2010 and 2011. (See Figure 6.5.) During this same period the percentage covered by public health plans grew.

DeNavas-Walt, Proctor, and Smith report that the percentage of people covered by employment-based health insurance dropped from 56.1% in 2009 to 55.3% in 2010. (See Table 6.1.) In contrast, during the 1980s close to 70% of workers obtained private health insurance through their employer. This decline is consistent with the continuing decline in all forms of private health coverage, which dropped from 75.5% in 1987 to 64% in 2010. For people under the age of 65 years, the overall decline in private health insurance coverage between 1997 and 2011 was just 9.6 percentage points, from 70.8% to 61.2%, but among people who were near poor the percentage covered by private insurance fell 20 percentage points, from 53.5% to 33.5%. (See Table 6.4.)

Two major factors contributed to the long-term decline in private health insurance. The first is the rising cost of health care, which frequently leads to greater cost sharing between employers and employees. Some workers simply cannot afford the higher premiums and co-payments (the share of the medical bill the employee pays for each health service). The second factor is the shift in U.S. commerce from the goods-producing sector, where health benefits have traditionally been provided, to the service sector, where many employers do not offer health insurance.

TABLE 6.2

Percentage of persons under age 65 who were uninsured at the time of interview, by age group and poverty status, 1997–2011

Age group and year	Poverty status[a]				
	Total	Poor	Near poor	Not poor	Unknown
Under 65 years			Percent uninsured[b]		
1997	17.4 (0.24)	32.7 (0.80)	30.4 (0.70)	8.9 (0.22)	21.6 (0.59)
1998	16.5 (0.26)	32.7 (0.84)	30.8 (0.79)	8.0 (0.22)	20.7 (0.59)
1999	16.0 (0.25)	32.1 (0.93)	30.7 (0.73)	7.8 (0.20)	20.1 (0.48)
2000	16.8 (0.24)	32.7 (0.89)	31.3 (0.69)	8.7 (0.22)	19.7 (0.51)
2001	16.2 (0.26)	31.0 (0.99)	28.6 (0.69)	8.4 (0.21)	20.3 (0.53)
2002	16.5 (0.24)	28.6 (0.80)	28.3 (0.70)	9.5 (0.24)	20.7 (0.55)
2003	17.2 (0.27)	29.4 (0.91)	30.2 (0.70)	9.1 (0.25)	21.3 (0.52)
2004 (Method 1)[c, d]	16.6 (0.23)	30.5 (0.93)	29.1 (0.67)	9.4 (0.23)	18.7 (0.48)
2004 (Method 2)[c, d]	16.4 (0.23)	30.1 (0.91)	28.9 (0.67)	9.4 (0.23)	18.6 (0.48)
2005[c]	16.0 (0.24)	28.4 (0.78)	28.6 (0.63)	9.1 (0.22)	18.5 (0.48)
2006[c, e]	16.8 (0.29)	29.2 (0.98)	30.8 (0.80)	9.7 (0.29)	17.5 (0.49)
2007[f]	16.4 (0.33)	28.0 (1.04)	30.2 (0.91)	9.8 (0.27)	20.8 (0.74)
2008[c]	16.7 (0.36)	27.9 (1.08)	30.6 (0.82)	10.2 (0.27)	21.0 (0.73)
2009[c]	17.5 (0.34)	30.2 (0.89)	29.4 (0.77)	10.7 (0.29)	22.3 (0.85)
2010[c]	18.2 (0.30)	29.5 (0.83)	32.3 (0.69)	10.7 (0.24)	22.7 (0.95)
2011[c, g]	17.3 (0.29)	28.2 (0.66)	30.4 (0.58)	10.1 (0.25)	21.0 (0.64)
0–17 years					
1997	13.9 (0.36)	22.4 (0.99)	22.8 (0.96)	6.1 (0.33)	18.3 (0.90)
1998	12.7 (0.34)	21.6 (1.02)	22.5 (0.97)	4.9 (0.29)	16.5 (0.75)
1999	11.8 (0.32)	21.4 (1.13)	21.6 (0.92)	4.4 (0.29)	14.9 (0.69)
2000	12.3 (0.32)	20.6 (1.04)	21.4 (0.93)	5.3 (0.30)	15.0 (0.72)
2001	11.0 (0.34)	18.8 (1.24)	17.0 (0.85)	4.4 (0.26)	15.5 (0.84)
2002	10.5 (0.32)	15.9 (0.97)	15.7 (0.84)	5.3 (0.36)	14.1 (0.76)
2003	10.1 (0.34)	15.4 (1.06)	14.7 (0.88)	4.8 (0.33)	13.5 (0.67)
2004 (Method 1)[c, d]	9.6 (0.29)	16.2 (1.23)	15.5 (0.81)	5.0 (0.30)	10.5 (0.56)
2004 (Method 2)[c, d]	9.4 (0.29)	15.3 (1.17)	15.1 (0.81)	5.0 (0.30)	10.3 (0.56)
2005[c]	8.9 (0.29)	13.0 (0.92)	14.7 (0.79)	4.6 (0.30)	11.0 (0.66)
2006[c, e]	9.3 (0.34)	12.7 (1.06)	16.5 (1.05)	4.8 (0.39)	10.0 (0.63)
2007[f]	8.9 (0.40)	11.4 (1.08)	15.5 (1.10)	4.9 (0.34)	11.8 (1.01)
2008[c]	8.9 (0.43)	12.4 (1.13)	15.6 (1.07)	4.8 (0.39)	11.0 (0.97)
2009[c]	8.2 (0.40)	11.8 (0.94)	12.1 (0.90)	5.0 (0.39)	9.8 (0.99)
2010[c]	7.8 (0.32)	10.2 (0.96)	12.6 (0.73)	4.6 (0.29)	8.8 (0.89)
2011[c, g]	7.0 (0.27)	8.1 (0.62)	11.5 (0.69)	4.0 (0.27)	10.4 (0.76)
18–64 years					
1997	18.9 (0.23)	40.2 (0.88)	34.9 (0.71)	9.9 (0.22)	22.9 (0.58)
1998	18.2 (0.27)	40.8 (1.02)	36.0 (0.83)	9.2 (0.23)	22.2 (0.60)
1999	17.8 (0.26)	39.9 (1.11)	36.3 (0.81)	9.0 (0.20)	22.2 (0.50)
2000	18.7 (0.27)	41.1 (1.05)	37.4 (0.77)	10.0 (0.24)	21.5 (0.53)
2001	18.3 (0.27)	39.5 (1.19)	35.6 (0.78)	9.9 (0.22)	22.1 (0.52)
2002	19.1 (0.26)	37.0 (1.09)	36.2 (0.77)	11.0 (0.25)	23.2 (0.56)
2003	20.1 (0.29)	38.2 (1.19)	39.5 (0.81)	10.6 (0.27)	24.2 (0.56)
2004 (Method 1)[c, d]	19.4 (0.26)	40.1 (1.10)	36.9 (0.72)	11.0 (0.26)	21.7 (0.54)
2004 (Method 2)[c, d]	19.3 (0.26)	39.9 (1.09)	36.8 (0.73)	11.0 (0.26)	21.6 (0.54)
2005[c]	18.9 (0.26)	38.5 (0.95)	36.6 (0.73)	10.7 (0.24)	21.2 (0.52)
2006[c, e]	19.8 (0.33)	40.0 (1.33)	38.6 (0.89)	11.4 (0.31)	20.3 (0.54)
2007[f]	19.4 (0.36)	38.6 (1.47)	39.3 (1.01)	11.4 (0.29)	23.8 (0.79)
2008[c]	19.7 (0.40)	37.7 (1.49)	39.9 (0.94)	11.9 (0.28)	24.4 (0.83)
2009[c]	21.1 (0.37)	42.5 (1.20)	39.1 (0.85)	12.5 (0.31)	26.7 (0.99)
2010[c]	22.3 (0.35)	42.2 (0.99)	43.0 (0.74)	12.6 (0.27)	27.1 (1.10)
2011[c, g]	21.3 (0.34)	40.1 (0.92)	40.1 (0.72)	12.0 (0.28)	25.6 (0.77)

Industry observers predict that the percentage of employers offering health benefits will continue to decrease. For example, Sarah Kliff reports in "Study: Fewer Employers Are Offering Health Insurance" (*Washington Post*, April 24, 2012) that under the Patient Protection and Affordable Care Act and the Health Care and Education Reconciliation Act (which are now commonly known as the ACA), this decrease will likely accelerate in 2014, when government-subsidized insurance is made available to people earning less than 400% of the federal poverty limit. Some employers may opt to save money by relying on the government to subsidize their workers' health insurance rather than doing so themselves.

People Aged 65 Years and Older

There are three sources of health insurance for people aged 65 years and older: private insurance, Medicare, and Medicaid. Medicare is the federal government's primary health program for people who are aged 65 years and older, and all people in this age group are eligible for certain basic benefits under Medicare. Medicaid is the federal program for the poor and people with disabilities. In 2011 a scant 2% of adults aged 65 years and older

TABLE 6.2

Percentage of persons under age 65 who were uninsured at the time of interview, by age group and poverty status, 1997–2011 [CONTINUED]

[a]Based on family income and family size, using the U.S. Census Bureau's poverty thresholds. "Poor" persons are defined as those below the poverty threshold; "Near poor" persons have incomes of 100% to less than 200% of the poverty threshold; and "Not poor" persons have incomes of 200% of the poverty threshold or greater. The percentages of respondents with unknown poverty status were 19.1% in 1997, 23.6% in 1998, 26.4% in 1999, 27.0% in 2000, 27.1% in 2001, 28.1% in 2002, 31.5% in 2003, 29.6% in 2004, 28.9% in 2005, 30.7% in 2006, 18.0% in 2007, 15.8% in 2008, 12.3% in 2009, 12.2% in 2010, and 11.5% in 2011.
[b]A person was defined as uninsured if he or she did not have any private health insurance, Medicare, Medicaid, Children's Health Insurance Program (CHIP), state-sponsored or other government-sponsored health plan, or military plan at the time of the interview. A person was also defined as uninsured if he or she had only Indian Health Service coverage or had only a private plan that paid for one type of service, such as accidents or dental care.
[c]Beginning in the third quarter of 2004, two additional questions were added to the NHIS insurance section to reduce potential errors in reporting Medicare and Medicaid status. Persons aged 65 and over not reporting Medicare coverage were asked explicitly about Medicare coverage, and persons under age 65 with no reported coverage were asked explicitly about Medicaid coverage. Estimates of uninsurance for 2004 were calculated both without the additional information from these questions (noted as Method 1) and with the responses to these questions (noted as Method 2). Respondents who were reclassified as "covered" by the additional questions received the appropriate follow-up questions concerning periods of noncoverage for insured respondents. Beginning in 2005, all estimates were calculated using Method 2.
[d]In 2004, a much larger than expected proportion of respondents reported a family income of "$2." Based on extensive review, these "$2" responses were coded to "not ascertained" for the final 2004 NHIS data files. Effective with the March 2006 Early Release report, the 2004 estimates were recalculated to reflect this editing decision. The problem with the "$2" income reports was fixed in the 2005 NHIS.
[e]In 2006, NHIS underwent a sample redesign. The impact of the new sample design on estimates presented in this report is minimal.
[f]In 2007, the income section of NHIS was redesigned, and estimates by poverty status may not be directly comparable with earlier years.
[g]In 2011, several new unfolding bracket income questions were added to the income section of NHIS.
Note: Data are based on household interviews of a sample of the civilian noninstitutionalized population.

SOURCE: Robin A. Cohen and Michael E. Martinez, "Table 7. Percentage of Persons under Age 65 Who Were Uninsured at the Time of Interview, by Age Group, and Poverty Status: United States, 1997–2011," in *Health Insurance Coverage: Early Release of Estimates from the National Health Interview Survey, 2011*, National Center for Health Statistics, June 2012, http://www.cdc.gov/nchs/data/nhis/earlyrelease/insur201206.pdf (accessed June 26, 2012)

went without some type of health insurance for at least part of the year preceding the interview. (See Table 6.3.)

Older adults may be covered by a combination of private health insurance and Medicare, or Medicare and Medicaid, depending on their income and level of disability. Nearly all adults over the age of 65 years are covered by Medicare. In *Health, United States, 2011: With Special Feature on Socioeconomic Status and Health* (May 2012, http://www.cdc.gov/nchs/data/hus/hus11.pdf), the NCHS reports that in 2008, 32.7% of older adults were covered by an employer-sponsored plan, 22.1% were covered by a Medicare-risk health maintenance organization (HMO), 21.5% had Medigap insurance to supplement their Medicare coverage, 14.9% used Medicare to obtain care on a fee-for-service basis, and 8.8% were covered by Medicaid.

MEDICARE C

Medicare C, also known as Medicare+Choice, became available to Medicare recipients on January 1, 1999. Medicare C came about as a result of the Balanced Budget Act of 1997 and was designed to supplement Medicare Parts A and B. Medicare C offers beneficiaries a wider variety of health plan options than previously available. These options include traditional (fee-for-service) Medicare, Medicare provider–sponsored organizations, preferred provider organizations (PPOs), Medicare HMOs, and medical savings accounts (MSAs).

Medicare provider–sponsored organizations are organized and operated the same way that HMOs are. However, they are administered by providers—physicians and hospitals. PPOs are similar to HMOs but permit patients to see providers outside the network and do not require their members to choose a network primary care

physician to coordinate their care. Patients in PPOs may seek care from any physician who is associated with the plan. Medicare HMOs are more like traditional Medicare, except patients may pay more out-of-pocket expenses. MSAs have two parts: an insurance policy and a savings account. Medicare pays the insurance premium and deposits a fixed amount into an MSA each year to pay for an individual's health care.

CHANGING MEDICARE REIMBURSEMENT

Medicare reimbursement varies in different parts of the country, although everyone pays the same amount to Medicare through taxes. As a result, older adults in some geographic regions have access to a more comprehensive range of services (e.g., coverage for nursing home care and eyeglasses) than older adults in other regions.

Describing this practice as unfair and outdated, legislators have repeatedly called for more equitable reimbursement formulas. For example, since 2002 the Medi-Fair Act (previously called the Medicare Fairness in Reimbursement Act; the act aimed to improve the provision of items and services provided to Medicare beneficiaries residing in rural areas in part by improving reimbursement) has repeatedly failed to pass. Senator Patty Murray (1950–; D-WA) and Representative Adam Smith (1965–; D-WA) reintroduced the legislation in May 2008 in an effort to raise the state of Washington's Medicare reimbursement rates to the national average and to ensure that all states receive at least the national average of per-patient spending. The Medicare Improvements for Patients and Providers Act of 2008 aimed to stem declining reimbursement by postponing a provision to reduce some Medicare reimbursement rates. The bill became law in July 2008.

TABLE 6.3

Percentage without health insurance, by selected characteristics, 2011

Selected characteristic	Uninsured[a] at the time of interview	Uninsured[a] for at least part of the past year[b]	Uninsured[a] for more than a year[b]
Age		Percent	
All ages	15.1	19.2	11.2
Under 65 years	17.3	21.8	12.7
0–17 years	7.0	10.9	3.7
18–64 years	21.3	26.0	16.3
18–24 years	25.9	33.2	18.2
25–34 years	28.2	35.3	21.7
35–44 years	22.3	26.8	17.4
45–64 years	15.5	18.2	12.3
65 years and over	1.1	2.0	0.9
0–18 years	7.5	11.4	4.0
19–25 years	27.9	36.1	20.1
Sex			
Male:			
All ages	16.8	20.8	13.0
Under 65 years	18.9	23.3	14.6
0–17 years	7.1	10.9	3.8
18–64 years	23.7	28.3	19.0
18–24 years	28.3	35.1	21.6
25–34 years	32.8	40.0	26.8
35–44 years	25.2	29.1	20.2
45–64 years	16.4	19.2	13.3
65 years and over	1.2	2.0	1.0
0–18 years	7.7	11.5	4.2
19–25 years	30.7	38.4	24.2
Female:			
All ages	13.5	17.6	9.4
Under 65 years	15.6	20.3	10.9
0–17 years	6.9	11.0	3.6
18–64 years	18.9	23.8	13.7
18–24 years	23.4	31.2	14.6
25–34 years	23.6	30.5	16.7
35–44 years	19.6	24.6	14.7
45–64 years	14.6	17.4	11.4
65 years and over	1.0	2.0	0.8
0–18 years	7.2	11.2	3.7
19–25 years	25.0	33.8	16.0
Race/ethnicity			
Hispanic or Latino	29.6	34.3	24.4
Non-Hispanic:			
White, single race	11.0	14.8	7.8
Black, single race	17.4	22.2	12.2
Asian, single race	14.6	18.2	10.8
Other races and multiple races	18.1	22.4	8.6
Region			
Northeast	10.2	13.9	7.4
Midwest	11.9	16.1	8.3
South	18.0	22.0	13.7
West	17.7	21.9	13.1
Education[c]			
Less than high school	31.5	35.5	26.8
High school diploma or GED[d]	22.4	26.5	17.2
More than high school	12.0	16.2	8.5
Employment status[e]			
Employed	18.5	23.1	14.5
Unemployed	49.0	55.6	34.7
Not in workforce	20.5	25.2	15.7

According to Patricia A. Davis et al. of the Congressional Research Service, in *Medicare Provisions in the Patient Protection and Affordable Care Act (PPACA)* (April 23, 2010, http://www.ncsl.org/documents/health/

Selected characteristic	Uninsured[a] at the time of interview	Uninsured[a] for at least part of the past year[b]	Uninsured[a] for more than a year[b]
Marital status[c]		Percent	
Married	12.8	16.0	9.8
Widowed	5.0	6.2	3.9
Divorced or separated	21.9	26.9	17.2
Living with partner	33.0	39.6	25.4
Never married	26.5	32.5	20.2

[a]A person was defined as uninsured if he or she did not have any private health insurance, Medicare, Medicaid, Children's Health Insurance Program (CHIP), state-sponsored or other government-sponsored health plan, or military plan. A person was also defined as uninsured if he or she had only Indian Health Service coverage or had only a private plan that paid for one type of service, such as accidents or dental care.
[b]A year is defined as the 12 months prior to interview.
[c]Shown only for persons aged 18 and over.
[d]GED is General Educational Development high school equivalency diploma.
[e]Shown only for persons aged 18–64.
Notes: Data are based on household interviews of a sample of the civilian noninstitutionalized population. Persons lacked health insurance coverage at the time of the interview, for at least part of the past year, and for more than a year.

SOURCE: Robin A. Cohen and Michael E. Martinez, "Table 7. Percentage of Persons Who Lacked Health Insurance Coverage at the Time of Interview, for at Least Part of the Past Year, and for More Than a Year, by Selected Demographic Characteristics: United States, 2011," in *Health Insurance Coverage: Early Release of Estimates from the National Health Interview Survey, 2011*, National Center for Health Statistics, June 2012, http://www.cdc.gov/nchs/data/nhis/earlyrelease/insur201206.pdf (accessed June 26, 2012)

MCProv.pdf), the ACA will further rectify persisting inequalities in Medicare reimbursement rates. The legislation created the Independent Payment Advisory Board to institute changes in Medicare payment rates. (The 15-member board is slated to begin operating in 2013 so that it can submit a proposal to control Medicare spending in January 2014 that can be implemented in 2015.) The ACA also permits some flexibility in the review and adjustment of Medicare payments for providers practicing in so-called frontier states (sparsely populated rural areas that are isolated from population centers and services).

Medicare Prescription Drug, Improvement, and Modernization Act

In December 2003 President George W. Bush (1946–) signed the Medicare Prescription Drug, Improvement, and Modernization Act into law. Heralded as landmark legislation, the act provides older adults and people with disabilities with a prescription drug benefit, more choices, and improved benefits under Medicare. On June 1, 2004, seniors and people with disabilities began using their Medicare-approved drug discount cards to obtain savings on prescription medicines. Low-income beneficiaries qualified for a $600 credit to help pay for their prescriptions. Besides providing coverage for prescription drugs, this legislation

FIGURE 6.5

Percentage without health insurance, by selected characteristics, 1997–2011

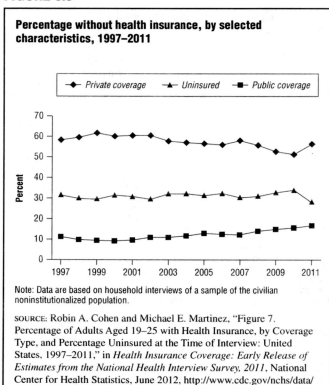

Note: Data are based on household interviews of a sample of the civilian noninstitutionalized population.

SOURCE: Robin A. Cohen and Michael E. Martinez, "Figure 7. Percentage of Adults Aged 19–25 with Health Insurance, by Coverage Type, and Percentage Uninsured at the Time of Interview: United States, 1997–2011," in *Health Insurance Coverage: Early Release of Estimates from the National Health Interview Survey, 2011*, National Center for Health Statistics, June 2012, http://www.cdc.gov/nchs/data/nhis/earlyrelease/insur201206.pdf (accessed June 26, 2012)

offers seniors the opportunity to choose the coverage and care that best meets their needs. For example, some older adults may opt for traditional Medicare coverage along with the new prescription benefit. Others may wish to obtain dental or eyeglass coverage or to enroll in managed care plans that reduce their out-of-pocket costs.

The legislation stipulated that as of 2005 all newly enrolled Medicare beneficiaries would be covered for a complete physical examination and other preventive services, such as blood tests to screen for diabetes. The new law also aimed to assist Americans in paying out-of-pocket health costs by enabling the creation of health savings accounts, which allow Americans to set aside up to $4,500 per year, tax free, to save for medical expenses.

Regardless, concerns about the solvency of the Medicare program and its capacity to meet the health care needs of growing numbers of Americans aging into eligibility have been increasing in recent years. The media have reported the ill effects of coverage gaps, with multiple stories of older adults opting to forgo prescription medication because they were unable to afford it. The ACA not only aims to extend the program's solvency for an additional 10 years but also fills the coverage gap (known as the donut hole) in prescription drug coverage by giving all Medicare beneficiaries who reach the gap a $250 rebate beginning in 2011 and completely closing the gap by 2020.

CHILDREN

In 2011, 7% of children under the age of 18 years were uninsured. (See Figure 6.4.) Approximately 10.9% had been uninsured for part of the year preceding the interview and 3.7% had been uninsured for more than a year. In 2011 poor children (8.1%) and near-poor children (11.5%) were much more likely to be uninsured at the time of the interview than not-poor children (4%). (See Table 6.2.) The percentage of children without health insurance at the time of the interview declined from 13.9% in 1997 to 7% in 2011.

Figure 6.6 shows that between 1997 and 2011 the percentage of poor and near-poor children who lacked health insurance coverage decreased. In 2011, 53.3% of American children were insured under private health insurance plans, either privately purchased or obtained through their parents' workplace. (See Table 6.4.) The rate of private coverage decreased from 66.2% in 1997 to 53.3% in 2011; during this period public coverage increased from 21.4% to 41%. (See Table 6.5.) Cohen and Martinez observe that 84.4% of poor children and 60.8% of near-poor children were covered by a public health plan in 2011.

Some health care industry observers believed the 1996 welfare reform law, the Personal Responsibility and Work Opportunity Reconciliation Act, would reduce enrollment in Medicaid. Under the 1996 law, federal money once dispensed through the Aid to Families with Dependent Children program was now given as a block grant (a lump sum of money) to states. In addition, the law no longer required that children who received cash assistance were automatically enrolled in the Medicaid program. The law gave states greater leeway in defining their requirements for aid, and in a few states some families were no longer eligible for Medicaid. Regardless, the NCHS shows in *Health, United States, 2011* that enrollment in Medicaid actually increased, rather than decreased, from 26.6 million in 1995 to 44.8 million in 2010. During this period the percentage of children covered by Medicaid also rose, from 21.1% to 35.7%.

Some industry analysts attributed the declining proportion of uninsured children and the increasing proportion of children covered by Medicaid during the late 1990s to expansion of the Children's Health Insurance Program (CHIP), which targeted children from low-income families and was instituted during the late 1990s. Others believed the economic boom of the late 1990s may have played a role in slowing or preventing even greater enrollment growth in Medicaid and predicted that the economic downturn and the uncertainty of the early years of the 21st century would reverse the downward trend in both the share of the population without health insurance and Medicaid enrollment. These industry observations were borne out as the economic

TABLE 6.4

Percentage of persons under age 65 with private health insurance at the time of interview, by age group and poverty status, 1997–2011

Age group and year	Poverty status[a]				
	Total	Poor	Near poor	Not poor	Unknown
Under 65 years		Percent of persons with private health insurance coverage[b]			
1997	70.8	22.9	53.5	87.6	66.7
1998	72.0	23.1	53.0	88.1	67.1
1999	73.1	26.1	50.9	88.9	68.0
2000	71.8	25.2	49.1	87.4	68.8
2001	71.6	25.5	48.4	87.2	67.8
2002	69.8	26.0	46.5	86.0	63.9
2003	68.2	23.4	42.3	85.8	64.1
2004[c]	68.6	20.0	44.9	85.0	66.3
2005	68.4	22.1	43.2	84.7	66.2
2006[d]	66.5	20.6	40.6	84.1	65.7
2007[e]	66.8	20.1	37.9	83.8	61.7
2008[c]	65.4	17.9	36.3	82.5	60.7
2009[c]	62.9	14.1	35.9	81.6	57.9
2010[c]	61.2	15.5	33.2	81.0	57.3
2011[c, f]	61.2	16.6	33.5	81.4	53.9
0–17 years					
1997	66.2	17.5	55.0	88.9	61.7
1998	68.5	19.3	56.3	89.9	62.1
1999	69.1	20.2	52.1	90.6	63.8
2000	67.1	19.5	48.8	88.4	64.2
2001	66.7	18.1	48.4	88.4	62.2
2002	63.9	17.2	44.9	86.9	56.3
2003	62.6	14.4	39.9	86.5	58.8
2004[c]	63.1	12.6	43.0	86.4	60.0
2005	62.4	15.0	40.0	85.6	59.3
2006[d]	59.7	13.1	36.9	85.9	57.8
2007[e]	59.9	11.9	34.0	85.1	54.8
2008[c]	58.3	10.4	32.9	83.1	54.8
2009[c]	55.7	8.2	32.8	82.4	55.3
2010[c]	53.8	9.2	30.5	81.4	53.7
2011[c, f]	53.3	8.9	29.9	82.1	44.5
18–64 years					
1997	72.8	26.8	52.6	87.1	68.6
1998	73.5	25.8	50.9	87.4	69.1
1999	74.7	30.4	50.2	88.2	69.7
2000	73.8	29.2	49.3	87.1	70.6
2001	73.7	31.7	48.4	86.8	69.9
2002	72.3	31.8	47.5	85.7	66.9
2003	70.6	29.0	43.7	85.5	66.0
2004[c]	70.9	24.9	46.0	84.6	68.6
2005	70.9	26.8	45.0	84.4	68.7
2006[d]	69.2	25.5	42.6	83.6	68.6
2007[e]	69.6	25.4	40.4	83.4	64.0
2008[c]	68.1	22.7	38.3	82.4	62.7
2009[c]	65.8	18.0	37.7	81.4	58.8
2010[c]	64.1	19.6	34.7	80.8	58.4
2011[c, f]	64.2	21.2	35.4	81.1	58.1

[a]Based on family income and family size, using the U.S. Census Bureau's poverty thresholds. "Poor" persons are defined as those below the poverty threshold; "Near poor" persons have incomes of 100% to less than 200% of the poverty threshold; and "Not poor" persons have incomes of 200% of the poverty threshold or greater. The percentages of respondents with unknown poverty status were 19.1% in 1997, 23.6% in 1998, 26.4% in 1999, 27.0% in 2000, 27.1% in 2001, 28.1% in 2002, 31.5% in 2003, 29.6% in 2004, 28.9% in 2005, 30.7% in 2006, 18.0% in 2007, 15.8% in 2008, 12.3% in 2009, 12.2% in 2010, and 11.5% in 2011.
[b]The category "Private health insurance" excludes plans that paid for only one type of service, such as accidents or dental care. A small number of persons were covered by both public and private plans and thus were included in both categories.
[c]In 2004, a much larger than expected proportion of respondents reported a family income of "$2." Based on extensive review, these "$2" responses were coded to "not ascertained" for the final 2004 NHIS data files. Effective with the March 2006 Early Release report the 2004 estimates were recalculated to reflect this editing decision.
[d]In 2006, NHIS underwent a sample redesign. The impact of the new sample design on estimates presented in this report is minimal.
[e]In 2007, the income section of NHIS was redesigned, and estimates by poverty status may not be directly comparable with earlier years.
[f]In 2011, several new unfolding bracket income questions were added to the income section of NHIS.
Note: Data are based on household interviews of a sample of the civilian noninstitutionalized population.

SOURCE: Robin A. Cohen and Michael E. Martinez, "Table 6. Percentage of Persons under Age 65 with Private Health Insurance Coverage at the Time of Interview, by Age Group and Poverty Status: United States, 1997–2011," in *Health Insurance Coverage: Early Release of Estimates from the National Health Interview Survey, 2011*, National Center for Health Statistics, June 2012, http://www.cdc.gov/nchs/data/nhis/earlyrelease/insur201206.pdf (accessed June 26, 2012)

FIGURE 6.6

Percentage of children under 18 without health insurance, by poverty status, 1997–2011

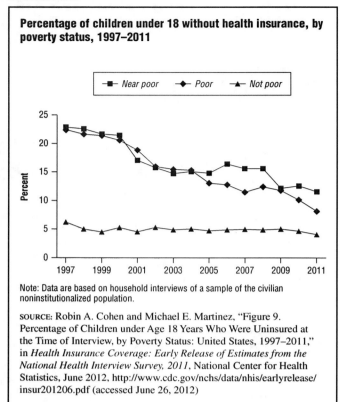

Note: Data are based on household interviews of a sample of the civilian noninstitutionalized population.

SOURCE: Robin A. Cohen and Michael E. Martinez, "Figure 9. Percentage of Children under Age 18 Years Who Were Uninsured at the Time of Interview, by Poverty Status: United States, 1997–2011," in *Health Insurance Coverage: Early Release of Estimates from the National Health Interview Survey, 2011*, National Center for Health Statistics, June 2012, http://www.cdc.gov/nchs/data/nhis/earlyrelease/insur201206.pdf (accessed June 26, 2012)

downturn spurred growth in the proportion of children covered by Medicaid.

The ACA increases health coverage, improves benefits, and provides new insurance protections for children. It eliminates preexisting coverage exclusions for children and improves health insurance coverage for children by expanding coverage through Medicaid and CHIP. It requires children's health insurance to provide coverage for basic dental and vision care. The legislation also guarantees children access to affordable child-only health insurance policies, regardless of whether their parents change or leave their jobs, relocate, or become ill or disabled.

HEALTH INSURANCE PORTABILITY AND ACCOUNTABILITY ACT

In August 1996 President Bill Clinton (1946–) signed the Health Insurance Portability and Accountability Act (HIPAA). This legislation aimed to provide better portability (transfer) of employer-sponsored insurance from one job to another. HIPAA ensured that people who had employer-sponsored health coverage would be able to maintain their health insurance even if they lost their job or moved to a different company. They would, of course, have to continue to pay for their insurance. However, they no longer had to fear that they would be denied coverage because of preexisting medical conditions or be forced to go without health insurance for prolonged waiting periods.

Industry observers and policy makers viewed HIPAA as an important first step in the federal initiative to significantly reduce the number of uninsured people in the United States. Besides its portability provisions, HIPAA changed tax laws to make it easier for Americans to pay for medical care and initiated a pilot program of MSAs that would grow into a significant new initiative in paying for health care.

HEALTH SAVINGS ACCOUNTS

HIPAA also authorized a pilot program: a five-year demonstration project designed to test the concept of MSAs, which are similar to individual retirement accounts. Beginning on January 1, 1997, approximately 750,000 people with high-deductible health plans (HDHPs; high-deductible plans were defined as those that carried a deductible of $1,600 to $2,400 for an individual or $3,200 to $4,800 for families) could make tax-deductible contributions into interest-bearing savings accounts. The funds deposited into these accounts could be used to purchase health insurance policies and pay co-payments and deductibles. People using MSAs could also deduct any employer contributions into the accounts as tax-deductible income. Any unspent money remaining in the MSA at the end of the year was carried over to the next year, thereby allowing the account to grow.

To be eligible to create an MSA, individuals had to be less than 65 years old, self-employed, and uninsured or had to work in firms with 50 or fewer employees that did not offer health care coverage. Withdrawals to cover out-of-pocket medical expenses were tax free and the money invested grew on a tax-deferred basis. Using MSA funds for any purpose unrelated to medical care or disability resulted in a 15% penalty. However, when MSA users reached age 65, the money could be withdrawn for any purpose and was taxed at the same rate as ordinary income.

Supporters of MSAs believed consumers would be less likely to seek unnecessary or duplicative medical care if they knew they could keep the money that was left in their accounts for themselves at the end of the year. Experience demonstrated that MSAs could simultaneously help contain health care costs, allow consumers greater control and freedom of choice of health care providers, enable consumers to save for future medical and long-term care expenses, and improve access to medical care.

In February 2001 President Bush advocated more liberal rules governing MSAs and proposed making them permanently available to all eligible Americans. Congress reviewed the president's proposed reforms and during its 2001–02 session lowered the minimum annual deductible to increase the number of eligible Americans, allowed annual MSA contributions up to 65% of the maximum deductible for individuals and 75% for families, and extended the availability of MSAs through December 31, 2003.

TABLE 6.5

Percentage of persons under age 65 with public health plan coverage at the time of interview, by age group and poverty status, 1997–2011

Age group and year	Poverty status[a]				
	Total	Poor	Near poor	Not poor	Unknown
Under 65 years			Percent of persons with public health plan coverage[b]		
1997	13.6	46.1	18.2	5.3	13.2
1998	12.7	44.7	17.5	5.1	13.4
1999	12.4	43.4	20.5	4.8	13.2
2000	12.9	43.7	21.7	5.3	12.8
2001	13.6	45.0	25.0	5.7	13.1
2002	15.2	47.0	27.5	6.1	16.6
2003	16.0	48.8	29.3	6.6	15.8
2004 (Method 1)[c, d]	16.1	50.7	27.6	6.9	16.0
2004 (Method 2)[c, d]	16.2	51.1	27.8	6.9	16.1
2005[c]	16.8	50.6	30.0	7.4	16.4
2006[c, e]	18.1	51.5	30.5	7.5	17.9
2007[f]	18.1	53.3	33.9	7.6	18.6
2008[c]	19.3	55.5	34.7	8.5	19.4
2009[c]	21.0	56.7	36.7	9.0	20.8
2010[c]	22.0	56.0	36.2	9.7	21.0
2011[c, g]	23.0	56.2	37.7	9.9	26.2
0–17 years					
1997	21.4	62.1	24.3	6.3	21.4
1998	20.0	61.1	22.9	6.0	22.1
1999	20.4	60.7	28.7	6.0	22.2
2000	22.0	61.8	32.4	7.4	22.1
2001	23.6	65.2	37.0	8.1	23.1
2002	27.1	69.0	42.2	8.9	30.7
2003	28.6	72.3	47.2	9.8	28.5
2004 (Method 1)[c, d]	28.5	72.5	43.4	9.7	30.4
2004 (Method 2)[c, d]	28.7	73.4	43.8	9.7	30.6
2005[c]	29.9	73.3	47.3	10.7	30.8
2006[c, e]	32.3	75.8	49.0	10.4	33.1
2007[f]	32.7	78.7	53.5	11.0	34.0
2008[c]	34.2	79.4	53.4	13.1	35.1
2009[c]	37.7	81.4	58.4	13.7	36.1
2010[c]	39.8	82.0	59.2	14.9	38.1
2011[c, g]	41.0	84.4	60.8	15.0	45.9
18–64 years					
1997	10.2	34.3	14.6	5.0	10.1
1998	9.5	32.9	14.1	4.8	10.0
1999	9.0	30.8	15.4	4.4	9.6
2000	9.1	31.1	15.2	4.5	9.1
2001	9.4	30.8	17.8	4.8	9.4
2002	10.3	32.5	18.3	5.1	11.2
2003	10.9	34.0	18.6	5.5	11.1
2004 (Method 1)[c, d]	11.1	36.1	18.5	5.9	10.8
2004 (Method 2)[c, d]	11.1	36.3	18.6	5.9	10.9
2005[c]	11.5	35.6	20.0	6.2	11.3
2006[c, e]	12.4	35.6	20.3	6.5	12.3
2007[f]	12.3	37.0	21.7	6.5	13.4
2008[c]	13.4	40.4	23.1	7.0	14.1
2009[c]	14.4	40.3	24.5	7.6	15.5
2010[c]	15.0	38.8	23.7	8.1	15.6
2011[c, g]	15.9	39.6	25.9	8.3	17.6

The Medicare Modernization Act of 2003 included provisions to establish health savings accounts (HSAs) for the general population. Like the MSA program it replaced, HSAs offer a variety of benefits, including more choice, greater control, and individual ownership. Specific features of HSAs include:

- Permanence and portability
- Availability to all individuals with a qualified HDHP
- Minimum deductible of $1,000 per individual plan and $2,000 per family plan
- Allowing annual contributions to equal 100% of the deductible
- Allowing both employer and employee contributions
- Not placing a cap on taxpayer participation
- Allowing tax-free rollover of up to $500 in unspent flexible spending accounts

As of 2012, HSAs enabled individuals to deposit up to $3,050 ($6,150 for families) per year in the accounts tax free and the funds were rolled over from one year to the

TABLE 6.5

ªBased on family income and family size, using the U.S. Census Bureau's poverty thresholds. "Poor" persons are defined as those below the poverty threshold; "Near poor" persons have incomes of 100% to less than 200% of the poverty threshold; and "Not poor" persons have incomes of 200% of the poverty threshold or greater. The percentages of respondents with unknown poverty status were 19.1% in 1997, 23.6% in 1998, 26.4% in 1999, 27.0% in 2000, 27.1% in 2001, 28.1% in 2002, 31.5% in 2003, 29.6% in 2004, 28.9% in 2005, 30.7% in 2006, 18.0% in 2007, 15.8% in 2008, 12.3% in 2009, 12.2% in 2010, and 11.5% in 2011. Estimates may differ from estimates that are based on both reported and imputed income.
ᵇThe category "Public health plan coverage" includes Medicaid, Children's Health Insurance Program (CHIP), state-sponsored or other government-sponsored health plans, Medicare (disability), and military plans. A small number of persons were covered by both public and private plans and were included in both categories.
ᶜBeginning in the third quarter of 2004, two additional questions were added to the NHIS insurance section to reduce potential errors in reporting Medicare and Medicaid status. Persons aged 65 and over not reporting Medicare coverage were asked explicitly about Medicare coverage, and persons under age 65 with no reported coverage were asked explicitly about Medicaid coverage. Estimates of uninsurance for 2004 were calculated both without the additional information from these questions (noted as Method 1) and with the responses to these questions (noted as Method 2). Respondents who were reclassified as "covered" by the additional questions received the appropriate follow-up questions concerning periods of noncoverage for insured respondents. Beginning in 2005, all estimates were calculated using Method 2.
ᵈIn 2004, a much larger than expected proportion of respondents reported a family income of "$2." Based on extensive review, these "$2" responses were coded to "not ascertained" for the final 2004 NHIS data files. Effective with the March 2006 Early Release report, the 2004 estimates were recalculated to reflect this editing decision.
ᵉIn 2006, NHIS underwent a sample redesign. The impact of the new sample design on estimates presented in this report is minimal.
ᶠIn 2007, the income section of NHIS was redesigned, and estimates by poverty status may not be directly comparable with earlier years.
ᵍIn 2011, several new unfolding bracket income questions were added to the income section of NHIS.
Note: Data are based on household interviews of a sample of the civilian noninstitutionalized population.

SOURCE: Robin A. Cohen and Michael E. Martinez, "Table 5. Percentage of Persons under Age 65 with Public Health Plan Coverage at the Time of Interview, by Age Group and Poverty Status: United States, 1997–2011," in *Health Insurance Coverage: Early Release of Estimates from the National Health Interview Survey, 2011*, National Center for Health Statistics, June 2012, http://www.cdc.gov/nchs/data/nhis/earlyrelease/insur201206.pdf (accessed June 26, 2012)

next. Also, funds could be withdrawn to pay for medical bills or saved for future needs, including retirement.

Pros and Cons of HSAs

John Goodman states in "Saving for Health Care: The Policy Pros and Cons of Different Vehicles" (April 17, 2012, http://healthaffairs.org/blog/2012/04/17/saving-for-heatlh-care-the-policy-pros-and-cons-of-different-vehicles/) that even though several different vehicles exist to enable consumers to save and pay for health care expenses, none are ideal. Goodman explains that "most families are not in the habit of saving while they are healthy for expenses that will arise with an unexpected illness." Furthermore, greater cost sharing may reduce health care use among people with low incomes, especially those with chronic conditions or disabilities and others with high-cost medical needs.

Nonetheless, America's Health Insurance Plans, a national association that represents companies providing health insurance coverage to more than 200 million Americans, reports in "Health Savings Account Enrollment Reaches 13.5 Million" (May 30, 2012, http://www.ahipcoverage.com/2012/05/30/health-savings-account-enrollment-reaches-13-5-million/) that as of January 2012, 13.5 million people had an HSA. This was an 18% increase of 2.1 million people since January 2011. HSA plan enrollment varied by geography, with the highest numbers in California (1,001,943 enrollees), Texas (755,432 enrollees), Illinois (717,384 enrollees), Ohio (662,999 enrollees), and Florida (539,778 enrollees).

Advocates of HSAs believe that by having consumers assume an increasing burden of escalating medical care costs, HSAs will stimulate both comparison shopping for health care providers and competition that will ultimately reduce the rate at which costs are rising. In "How Do Consumer-Directed Health Plans Affect Vulnerable Populations?" (*Forum for Health Economics and Policy*, vol. 14, no. 2, 2011), Amelia M. Haviland et al. report the results of their research comparing use of preventive services among people enrolled in consumer-directed health plans (CDHPs; HSAs, along with flexible spending accounts, are forms of CDHPs). This research was motivated by the observation that the ACA is likely to increase enrollment in CDHPs and that state Medicaid programs will employ similar designs to expand their Medicaid programs. Haviland et al. were especially eager to determine whether low-income and high-risk populations would be disadvantaged when using CDHPs.

The researchers find that spending was reduced for HDHPs for both low-income and high-risk enrollees and for higher-income enrollees. More specifically, HDHPs that were paired with HSAs generated reductions of nearly 30% in levels of total spending when compared with HDHPs that were not paired with HSAs. Haviland et al. also find that HSAs do not deter people at high risk from obtaining needed screening.

Despite Haviland et al.'s findings, other industry analysts question whether employer cost savings are the result of HSA enrollees' decisions to forgo needed medical care. For example, Physicians for a National Health Program argues in "Consumer Directed Health Care and Health Savings Accounts" (2012, http://www.pnhp.org/single_payer_resources/consumer_directed_health_care_and_health_savings_accounts.php) that "they offer no hope of controlling health costs, as the sickest 20 percent of the population responsible for 80 percent of health spending (people with tens or hundreds of thousands of dollars in health costs annually) has no incentive to change their spending. In reality, these plans add another complex layer of administration which will exacerbate wasteful health spending."

HEALTH INSURANCE COSTS CONTINUE TO SKYROCKET

According to the Kaiser Family Foundation, in *Employer Health Benefits: 2011 Annual Survey* (2011, http://ehbs.kff.org/pdf/2011/8225.pdf), health insurance premiums continued to increase much faster than inflation and wages, with the average family premium increasing 9% between 2010 and 2011. Premiums averaged $5,429 for individual coverage and $15,073 for family coverage. Workers paid an average of $921 per year toward the premium for individual coverage and $4,129 per year toward the premium for family coverage.

The Kaiser Family Foundation explains that the percentage of workers with deductibles for individual coverage of $1,000 or more increased, as did the average co-payments for primary or specialty physician office visits. Annual deductibles for individual coverage ranged from $675 for PPO members to $1,908 for those in HDHPs. The majority (77%) of covered workers incurred co-payments for office visits and prescription drugs. About three-quarters (74%) of workers were enrolled in plans with co-payments or another form of cost sharing for prescription drugs.

The Kaiser Family Foundation finds that 60% of employers offered health benefits in 2011, down from 69% from the previous year. In response to the ACA, "significant percentages of firms made changes in their preventive care benefits and enrolled adult children in their benefits plans in response to provisions in the new health reform law."

HEALTH INSURERS HAVE NEW AND HEIGHTENED OVERSIGHT

One of the consequences of the ACA was the establishment of the Office of Consumer Information and Insurance Oversight (OCIIO). The OCIIO is responsible for overseeing many of the provisions of the Health Care and Education Reconciliation Act, which was signed into law by President Barack Obama (1961–) in March 2010.

The OCIIO is responsible for ensuring compliance with the new insurance market rules, such as the elimination of the preexisting condition exclusions for children that took effect in 2010 and the development of a federally funded high-risk pool that will temporarily extend health insurance coverage to people with preexisting conditions who are currently uninsured. The high-risk pool program will operate until 2014, when state-based health insurance exchanges become available.

The OCIIO assists states to establish insurance rates and will offer guidance and oversight for the state-based insurance exchanges. It will administer several special programs, including temporary insurance options for early retirees, which will reimburse participating employment-based plans for some of the costs of health benefits for early retirees and their families. Furthermore, the OCIIO will create and regularly update an Internet portal that provides information about insurance options.

Impact of the ACA on Health Insurers

In "Health Insurance Companies Try to Shape Rules" (*New York Times*, May 15, 2010), Robert Pear reports that health insurance companies want to protect their ability to increase insurance premiums and spend a minimum percentage of premium dollars that are collected on direct patient care, as opposed to use it for administrative expenses or keep it as corporate profits. Of the legislation's 40 provisions affecting insurers, the provision that forbids insurers from an "'unreasonable' premium increase" and another that requires that premiums be used for "health care services and 'activities that improve health care quality' for patients" appear to be the requirements the insurance companies are most eager to redefine to their advantage. For example, insurers that offer coverage to large groups are expected to spend 85% of premiums on "'clinical services' and quality-enhancing activities." For health insurance coverage sold to individuals or small groups, the insurers must devote 80% of premiums to patient care and quality initiatives.

Health Insurers Must Comply with Many New Regulations

Roni Caryn Rabin reports in "In Health Law, a Clearer View of Coverage" (*New York Times*, May 17, 2010) that even though health insurers are likely to benefit from increasing numbers of subscribers, the ACA will require them to offer a package of basic health benefits comparable to the coverage offered by employer plans to individuals with preexisting conditions and will be prohibited from charging higher premiums to people with preexisting conditions. Insurers will have to present their plans in standardized formats that enable consumers to compare every aspect of them—coverage, cost sharing, provider networks, deductibles, and co-payments. Consumers will be able to select one of four standardized levels of coverage and benefits, with progressively increasing premiums associated with higher levels of coverage. Also standardized by the ACA is a cap on out-of-pocket expenses: after patients reach a limit of $5,950 a year for individuals and $11,900 for families, the plans must cover all additional health care costs. Furthermore, the law eliminates lifetime limits, which are commonly between $1 million and $2 million, amounts that are easily exceeded by some people with chronic, serious medical conditions such as acquired immunodeficiency syndrome (AIDS), some cancers, and organ transplants.

MENTAL HEALTH PARITY

In terms of mental health care, parity refers to the premise that the same range and scope of insurance benefits available for other illnesses should be provided for people with mental illness. Historically, private health insurance plans have provided less coverage for mental illness than for other medical conditions. Coverage for mental health was more restricted and often involved more cost sharing (higher co-payments and deductibles) than coverage for medical care. As a result, many patients with severe mental illness, who frequently required hospitalizations and other treatment, quickly depleted their mental health coverage.

During the 1990s there was growing interest in parity of mental health with other health services. The Mental Health Parity Act of 1996 sought to bring mental health benefits closer to other health benefits. The act amended the 1944 Public Health Service Act and the 1974 Employee Retirement Income Security Act by requiring parity for annual and lifetime dollar limits but did not place restrictions on other plan features such as hospital and office visit limits. It also imposed federal standards on the mental health coverage offered by employers through group health plans. By 2007 more than two-thirds of states had laws governing mental health parity that were more comprehensive in scope than the federal legislation, and one-third of the states required full parity.

Legislation Establishes Mental Health Parity

The Paul Wellstone and Pete Domenici Mental Health Parity and Addiction Equity Act of 2008 expands on the Mental Health Parity Act by prohibiting group health plans and group health insurance companies from imposing treatment limitations or financial requirements for coverage of mental health that are different from those used for medical and surgical benefits. In "New Rules Promise Better Mental Health Coverage" (*New York Times*, January 29, 2010), Robert Pear explains that eliminating disparities between physical health care and mental health care will make it easier for people to obtain care for conditions ranging from depression and anxiety to eating disorders and substance abuse. The Obama administration anticipates that the parity requirement will benefit "111 million people in 446,400 group health plans offered by private employers, and 29 million people in 20,000 plans sponsored by state and local governments." The act is projected to increase insurance premiums by 0.4%, which translates into $25.6 billion between 2010 and 2019.

Effects of the ACA on Mental Health Parity

According to Amanda K. Sarata of the Congressional Research Service, in *Mental Health Parity and the Patient Protection and Affordable Care Act of 2010* (December 28, 2011, http://www.ncsl.org/documents/health/MHpari ty&mandates.pdf), the ACA contains two main provisions that are aimed at improving mental health parity: expanding "the reach of the applicability of the federal mental health parity requirements" and establishing "a mandated benefit for the coverage of certain mental health and substance abuse disorder services." Furthermore, the legislation expands the reach of federal mental health parity requirements to qualified health plans as established by the ACA, to Medicaid nonmanaged care plans, and to plans offered to individuals.

Parity May Not Solve All Access Problems

According to Robert Pear, in "Fight Erupts over Rules Issued for 'Mental Health Parity' Insurance Law" (*New York Times*, May 9, 2010), health insurance companies believe that parity alone will not eliminate all obstacles to gaining access to mental health care. The insurers oppose some of the provisions of the parity legislation, especially the requirement to have a single deductible for all medical and mental health services combined, rather than the traditional practice of separate deductibles. Insurers contend that because the single deductible will be higher than the previous separate mental health deductible, it may serve to impede access to mental health care.

Pear explains that even though "the Obama administration praised the work of [managed behavioral health organizations (MBHOs)], saying they increased the use of mental health care while holding down costs," several of these MBHOs have taken aim at some of the provisions of the parity legislation. In particular, the MBHOs claim that the requirement to use a single deductible and the prohibition of nonquantitative treatment limitations (NQTLs are cost-control strategies that unlike annual and lifetime dollar limits or number of visit limits cannot be measured numerically) for mental health treatment will hinder their ability to offer parity coverage. The law states that NQTLs such as design of prescription drug formularies that limit drug coverage may not be applied to mental health coverage unless they are also used for medical and surgical insurance coverage. The article "APA Supports Provisions Being Challenged in Court" (*Psychiatric News*, vol. 45, no. 10, May 21, 2010) quotes James H. Scully Jr. of the American Psychiatric Association as saying, "NQTLs prevent patients from gaining access to adequate mental health and substance use disorder treatment, which is the very problem [the parity legislation] sought to rectify."

FINANCING THE ACA

In *Updated Estimates for the Insurance Coverage Provisions of the Affordable Care Act* (March 2012, http://cbo.gov/sites/default/files/cbofiles/attachments/03-13-Coverage%20Estimates.pdf), an analysis of the financial impact of the ACA, the Congressional Budget

TABLE 6.6

Estimate of the budgetary effects of the insurance coverage provisions in the Affordable Care Act, March 2012

Effects on the federal deficit[a, b]	2012	2013	2014	2015	2016	2017	2018	2019	2020	2021	2022	11-year total, 2012–2022
						(Billions of dollars, by fiscal year)						
Medicaid and CHIP outlays[c]	−1	1	48	81	98	103	107	113	118	127	136	931
Exchange subsidies and related spending[d, e]	2	4	16	46	74	92	102	109	114	121	127	808
Small employer tax credits[f]	1	2	3	4	2	1	2	2	2	2	2	23
Gross cost of coverage provisions	3	6	66	130	175	197	210	224	234	250	265	1,762
Penalty payments by uninsured individuals	0	0	0	−3	−6	−7	−7	−7	−8	−8	−9	−54
Penalty payments by employers[f]	0	0	−4	−9	−10	−12	−13	−15	−16	−16	−17	−113
Excise tax on high-premium insurance plans[f]	0	0	0	0	0	0	−11	−18	−22	−27	−32	−111
Other effects on tax revenues and outlays[g]	0	−1	−4	−8	−16	−24	−30	−35	−38	−37	−38	−231
Net cost of coverage provisions	3	5	58	110	143	154	150	149	151	161	169	1,252

Notes: The Affordable Care Act is comprised of the Patient Protection and Affordable Care Act (P.L. 111–148) and the health care provisions of the Health Care and Education Reconciliation Act of 2010 (P.L. 111–152). Numbers may not add up to totals because of rounding.

CHIP = Children's Health Insurance Program.

[a]Does not include federal administrative costs that are subject to appropriation.

[b]Positive numbers indicate increases in the deficit, and negative numbers indicate reductions in the deficit.

[c]Under current law, states have the flexibility to make programmatic and other budgetary changes to Medicaid and CHIP. CBO estimates that state spending on Medicaid and CHIP in the 2012–2022 period would increase by about $73 billion as a result of the coverage provisions.

[d]Includes spending for high-risk pools, premium review activities, loans to co-op plans, grants to states for the establishment of exchanges, and the net budgetary effects of proposed collections and payments for risk adjustment and transitional reinsurance.

[e]Figures may not equal the amounts shown in the table entitled "Health Insurance Exchanges: CBO's March 2012 Baseline" (posted on CBO's Web site) because different related items are included in the two tables.

[f]The effects on the deficit of this provision include the associated effects on tax revenues of changes in taxable compensation.

[g]The effects are almost entirely on tax revenues. CBO estimates that outlays for Social Security benefits would increase by about $7 billion over the 2012–2022 period, and that the coverage provisions would have negligible effects on outlays for other federal programs.

SOURCE: "Table 2. March 2012 Estimate of the Budgetary Effects of the Insurance Coverage Provisions Contained in the Affordable Care Act," in *Updated Estimates for the Insurance Coverage Provisions of the Affordable Care Act*, Congressional Budget Office, March 2012, http://cbo.gov/sites/default/files/cbofiles/attachments/03-13-Coverage%20Estimates.pdf (accessed June 27, 2012)

Office (CBO) reveals that from 2012 to 2021 the enactment of major components of the ACA will cost an estimated $1.1 trillion and reduce the federal deficit by an estimated $231 billion. (See Table 6.6.) The ACA's provisions related to insurance coverage are forecast to have a net cost of nearly $1.3 billion from 2012 to 2022.

The CBO estimates that the ACA will "reduce the number of nonelderly people without health insurance coverage by 30 million to 33 million in 2016 and subsequent years, leaving 26 million to 27 million nonelderly residents uninsured in those years." It also indicates that "fewer people are now expected to obtain health insurance coverage from their employer or in insurance exchanges; more are now expected to obtain coverage from Medicaid or CHIP or from nongroup or other sources. More are expected to be uninsured."

The implementation of the ACA will be financed by a combination of health care savings resulting from programs that improve efficiency and accountability; incentivize quality and cost-effective care; and reduce waste, fraud, and inefficiencies. Phil Galewitz indicates in "Consumers Guide to Health Reform" (April 13, 2010, http://www.kaiserhealthnews.org/stories/2010/march/22/consumers-guide-health-reform.aspx) that revenues will be generated via taxes on the wealthiest Americans. Beginning in 2013 individuals who earn more than $200,000 per year and couples who earn more than $250,000 per year will pay a Medicare payroll tax of 2.3%. The wealthiest Americans will also pay a 3.8% tax on unearned income such as dividends. Furthermore, in 2018 there will be a 40% excise tax on employers who offer so-called Cadillac insurance plans that cost $10,200 per year for individuals and $27,500 per year for families.

CHAPTER 7

INTERNATIONAL COMPARISONS OF HEALTH CARE

International comparisons are often difficult to interpret because the definitions of terms, the reliability of data, the cultures, and the values differ. What is important in one society may be unimportant or even nonexistent in another. A political or human right that is important in one nation may be meaningless in a neighboring nation. Evaluating the quality of health care systems is an example of the difficulties involved in comparing one culture to another.

Even within the United States there are cultural and regional variations in health care delivery. A visit to a busy urban urgent care center might begin with the patient completing a brief medical history, followed by five or 10 minutes with a nurse who measures and records the patient's vital signs (pulse, respiration, and temperature), and conclude with a 15-minute visit with a physician, who diagnoses the problem and prescribes treatment. In contrast, on the islands of Hawaii a visit with a healer may last several hours and culminate with a prayer, a song, or an embrace. Hawaiian healers, called kahunas, are unhurried and offer an array of herbal remedies, bodywork (massage, touch, and manipulative therapies), and talk therapies (counseling and guidance), because they believe that the healing quality of the encounter, independent of any treatment offered, improves health and well-being.

Even though comparing the performance of health care systems and health outcomes (how people fare as a result of receiving health care services) is of benefit to health care planners, administrators, and policy makers, the subjective nature of such assessments should be duly considered.

A COMPARISON OF HEALTH CARE SPENDING, RESOURCES, AND UTILIZATION

The Organisation for Economic Co-operation and Development (OECD) provides information about 34 member countries that are governed democratically and participate in the global market economy. It collects and publishes data about a wide range of economic and social issues including health and health care policy. The OECD member nations are generally considered to be the wealthier, more developed nations in the world. The OECD (2012, http://www.oecd.org/pages/0,3417,en_36734052 _36761800_1_1_1_1_1,00.html) indicates that its member countries are Australia, Austria, Belgium, Canada, Chile, the Czech Republic, Denmark, Estonia, Finland, France, Germany, Greece, Hungary, Iceland, Ireland, Israel, Italy, Japan, Luxembourg, Mexico, the Netherlands, New Zealand, Norway, Poland, Portugal, the Slovak Republic, Slovenia, South Korea, Spain, Sweden, Switzerland, Turkey, the United Kingdom, and the United States.

Percentage of Gross Domestic Product Spent on Health Care

Even though health has always been a concern for Americans, the growth in the health care industry since the mid-1970s has made it a major factor in the U.S. economy. For many years the United States has spent a larger proportion of its gross domestic product (GDP; the total market value of final goods and services produced within an economy in a given year) on health care than have other nations with similar economic development. In *Health, United States, 2011: With Special Feature on Socioeconomic Status and Health* (May 2012, http://www.cdc.gov/nchs/data/hus/hus11.pdf), the National Center for Health Statistics notes that in 2009 U.S. health expenditures were 17.4% of the GDP, the highest rate in the OECD. (See Table 7.1.) Other nations that spent large percentages of GDP on health care in 2009 included the Netherlands (12%), France (11.8%), Germany (11.6%), Denmark (11.5%), Canada (11.4%), Switzerland (11.4%), Austria (11%), and Belgium (10.9%). Of the member nations that reported health care expenditure data in 2009, Mexico (6.4%), Estonia (7%), Hungary (7.4%), and Poland (7.4%) spent the least in the OECD.

TABLE 7.1

Health expenditure as a share of the gross domestic product (GDP), selected countries and years 1960–2009

Country	1960	1970	1980	1990	1995	2000	2005	2006	2007	2008	2009
					Health expenditures as a percentage of gross domestic product						
Australia	3.6	—	6.1	6.7	7.2	8.0	8.4	8.5	8.5	8.7	—
Austria	4.3	5.2	7.4	†8.3	9.5	9.9	10.4	10.3	10.3	10.4	11.0
Belgium	—	3.9	6.3	7.2	††7.6	††8.1	††10.1	††9.6	††9.7	††10.1	††10.9
Canada	5.4	6.9	7.0	8.9	†9.0	8.8	9.8	10.0	10.0	10.3	11.4
Chile	—	—	—	—	5.3	6.6	6.9	6.6	6.9	7.5	8.4
Czech Republic	—	—	—	4.7	†7.0	†6.5	7.2	7.0	6.8	7.1	8.2
Estonia	—	—	—	—	—	5.3	5.0	5.0	5.2	6.1	7.0
Denmark	—	—	8.9	8.3	8.1	8.7	9.8	9.9	10.0	10.3	11.5
Finland	3.8	5.5	6.3	7.7	†7.9	7.2	8.4	8.4	8.1	8.4	9.2
France	3.8	5.4	7.0	8.4	†10.4	10.1	11.1	11.0	11.0	11.1	11.8
Germany	—	6.0	8.4	8.3	10.1	10.3	10.7	10.6	10.5	10.7	11.6
Greece	—	5.4	5.9	6.6	8.6	7.9	9.6	9.6	9.6	—	—
Hungary	—	—	—	—	7.3	7.0	8.3	8.1	7.5	7.2	7.4
Iceland	3.0	4.7	6.3	7.8	8.2	9.5	9.4	9.1	9.1	9.1	9.7
Ireland	3.7	5.1	8.2	6.1	6.6	6.1	7.6	7.5	7.7	8.8	9.5
Israel[a]	—	—	7.7	7.1	7.6	7.5	7.8	7.6	7.6	7.7	7.9
Italy	—	—	—	7.7	7.3	8.1	8.9	9.0	8.7	9.0	9.5
Japan	3.0	4.5	6.4	5.9	6.9	7.7	8.2	8.2	8.2	8.5	—
Luxembourg	—	3.1	5.2	5.4	5.6	7.5	7.9	7.7	7.1	6.8	7.8
Mexico	—	—	—	4.4	5.2	5.1	5.9	5.7	5.8	5.8	6.4
Netherlands	—	—	7.4	8.0	8.3	8.0	9.8	9.7	9.7	9.9	†§12.0
New Zealand	—	5.2	5.8	6.8	7.1	7.6	8.7	9.1	8.8	9.6	10.3
Norway	2.9	4.4	7.0	7.6	7.9	8.4	9.1	8.6	8.9	§8.6	§9.6
Poland	—	—	—	4.8	5.5	5.5	6.2	6.2	6.4	7.0	7.4
Portugal	—	2.4	5.1	5.7	†7.5	9.3	10.4	10.1	10.0	10.1	—
Republic of Korea	—	—	3.7	4.0	3.8	4.5	5.7	6.0	6.3	6.5	6.9
Slovak Republic	—	—	—	—	—	5.5	7.0	7.3	7.7	8.0	9.1
Slovenia	—	—	—	—	7.5	8.3	8.4	8.3	7.8	8.4	9.3
Spain	1.5	3.5	5.3	6.5	7.4	7.2	8.3	8.4	8.5	9.0	9.5
Sweden	—	6.8	8.9	8.2	8.0	8.2	9.1	8.9	8.9	9.2	10.0
Switzerland	4.9	5.5	7.4	8.2	†9.6	10.2	11.2	10.8	10.6	10.7	11.4
Turkey	—	—	2.4	2.7	2.5	4.9	5.4	5.8	6.0	6.1	—
United Kingdom	3.9	4.5	5.6	5.9	6.8	7.0	8.2	8.5	8.4	8.8	9.8
United States[b]	5.1	7.1	9.0	12.4	13.7	13.7	15.7	15.8	16.0	16.4	17.4
					Per capita health expenditures[c]						
Australia	$90	—	$632	$1,194	$1,607	$2,266	$2,980	$3,164	$3,353	$3,445	—
Austria	77	$196	785	†1,623	2,239	2,862	3,472	3,629	3,792	4,128	$4,289
Belgium	—	149	641	1,353	††1,710	††2,245	††3,23	††3,27	††3,43	††3,71	††3,946
Canada	123	294	777	1,735	†2,056	2,519	3,442	3,665	3,844	4,024	4,363
Chile	—	—	—	—	39	615	843	863	959	1,092	1,186
Czech Republic	—	—	—	558	†897	†981	1,475	1,556	1,661	1,839	2,108
Estonia	—	—	—	—	—	522	831	960	1,113	1,331	1,393
Denmark	—	—	893	1,540	1,86	2,508	3,245	3,577	3,770	4,052	4,348
Finland	63	184	569	1,363	†1,475	1,853	2,589	2,764	2,910	3,158	3,226
France	69	193	666	1,445	†2,100	2,553	3,306	3,493	3,679	3,809	3,978
Germany	—	268	967	1,764	2,26	2,669	3,364	3,565	3,724	3,963	4,218
Greece	—	160	489	844	1,26	1,451	2,352	2,608	2,724	—	—
Hungary	—	—	—	—	65	853	1,411	1,486	1,433	1,495	1,511
Iceland	57	175	752	1,662	1,90	2,740	3,304	3,193	3,320	3,571	3,538
Ireland	43	116	511	788	1,19	1,768	2,959	3,200	3,494	3,784	3,781
Israel[a]	—	—	—	—	1,43	1,766	1,829	1,897	2,012	2,142	2,165
Italy	—	—	—	1,355	1,53	2,064	2,516	2,725	2,771	3,059	3,137
Japan	30	140	541	1,115	1,55	1,974	2,491	2,609	2,750	2,878	—
Luxembourg	—	—	—	—	1,90	3,268	4,152	4,603	4,494	4,451	4,808
Mexico	—	—	—	296	38	508	731	776	842	892	918
Netherlands	—	—	732	1,412	1,79	2,340	3,450	3,613	3,944	4,241	§4,914
New Zealand	—	214	498	983	1,24	1,607	2,197	2,467	2,525	2,784	2,983
Norway	49	143	665	1,366	1,85	3,043	4,301	4,507	4,885	§5,230	§5,352
Poland	—	—	—	289	41	583	857	934	1,078	1,265	1,394
Portugal	—	47	277	628	†1,014	1,654	2,212	2,303	2,419	2,508	—
Republic of Korea	—	—	89	325	48	771	1,291	1,469	1,651	1,736	1,879
Slovak Republic	—	—	—	—	—	604	1,139	1,350	1,619	1,859	2,084
Slovenia	—	—	—	—	98	1,453	1,974	2,106	2,129	2,451	2,579
Spain	16	95	362	870	1,19	1,537	2,269	2,536	2,735	2,971	3,067
Sweden	—	311	942	1,592	1,74	2,286	2,963	3,193	3,432	3,644	3,722
Switzerland	166	344	1,013	2,028	†2,563	3,221	4,015	4,150	4,469	4,930	5,144
Turkey	—	—	70	155	17	433	591	712	798	902	—
United Kingdom	84	159	466	960	1,34	1,828	2,735	3,006	3,051	3,281	3,487
United States[b]	148	355	1,101	2,850	3,78	4,793	6,700	7,073	7,437	7,720	7,960

TABLE 7.1

Health expenditure as a share of the gross domestic product (GDP), selected countries and years 1960–2009 [CONTINUED]

—Data not available.
†Break in series.
††Difference in methodology.
§Data are estimated.
ªThe statistical date for Israel are supplied by and under the responsibility of the relevant Israeli authorities. The use of such data by the Organisation for Economic Co-operation and Development (OECD) is without prejudice to the status of the Golan Heights, East Jerusalem, and Israeli settlements in the West Bank under the terms of international law.
ᵇOECD estimates for the United States differ from the National Health Expenditures estimates because of differences in methodology.
ᶜPer capita health expenditures for each country have been adjusted to U.S. dollars using gross domestic product purchasing power parities for each year.
Notes: These data include revisions in health expenditures and differ from previous editions of *Health, United States*. Trends should be interpreted with caution due to data series breaks and changes in methodology.

SOURCE: "Table 124. Total Health Expenditures As a Percentage of Gross Domestic Product and per Capita Health Expenditures in Dollars, by Selected Countries: Selected Years 1960–2009," in *Health, United States, 2011: With Special Feature on Socioeconomic Status and Health*, U.S. Department of Health and Human Services, Centers for Disease Control and Prevention, National Center for Health Statistics, May 2012, http://www.cdc.gov/nchs/data/hus/hus11.pdf (accessed June 13, 2012). Data from Organisation for Economic Co-operation and Development Health Data.

Per Capita Spending on Health Care

The United States also experienced the highest per capita spending for health care services in 2009, spending an average of $7,960 per citizen. (See Table 7.1.) No other country came close to spending this amount per capita in 2009: Norway spent $5,352 per citizen; Switzerland, $5,144; the Netherlands, $4,914; Luxembourg, $4,808; Canada, $4,363; Denmark, $4,348; Germany, $4,218; France, $3,978; Belgium, $3,946; Ireland, $3,781; Sweden, $3,722; and Iceland, $3,538. In 2009 Mexico ($918) spent the least per capita of any OECD member nation on health care, followed by Chile ($1,186), Estonia ($1,393), and Poland ($1,394).

Who Pays for Health Care?

Public expenditures for health care services as a percentage of GDP vary widely between the OECD member nations. In "OECD Health Data—Frequently Requested Data" (2012, http://www.oecd.org/document/16/0,3746,en_2649_37407_2085200_1_1_1_37407,00.html), the OECD notes that public spending on health accounted for an average of 72.2% of total health spending across OECD member countries in 2010 and that the remaining 27.8% of spending was paid by private sources, mainly private insurance and individuals. In the United States public funding accounted for 48.2% of total health spending. By contrast, public sources in the Netherlands and Norway accounted for 85.7% and 85.5%, respectively, of total health spending. Other nations with above-average contributions of public funding to health expenditures included Denmark (85.1%), Luxembourg (84%), the Czech Republic (83.8%), New Zealand (83.2%), the United Kingdom (83.2%), Sweden (81%), Japan (80.5%), Iceland (80.4%), Italy (79.6%), Estonia (78.9%), France (77%), Germany (76.8%), Austria (76.2%), Belgium (75.6%), Finland (74.5%), Spain (73.6%), Turkey (73%), and Slovenia (72.8%). Public expenditures on health per capita were lowest in Mexico (47.3%), Chile (48.2%), and the United States (48.2%).

In terms of out-of-pocket payments as a share of total health expenditures in 2010, the United States, at 11.8%, was below the OECD average of 20.1%. In France and the United Kingdom out-of-pocket payments as a share of total health expenditures were low, 7.3% and 8.9%, respectively. In contrast, out-of-pocket spending as a share of total health care spending was highest in Mexico (49%) and Greece (38.4%). Out-of-pocket spending as a share of total health care spending was also high in Chile (33.3%), South Korea (32.1%), Israel (27.1%), Hungary (26.2%), Portugal (26%), the Slovak Republic (25.9%), and Switzerland (25.1%).

Private health insurance fills the gap between public expenditures and out-of-pocket costs. Among the OECD member countries declaring private insurance as a percentage of total expenditures for health in 2010, the United States' private insurance expenditure far outstripped all other countries. Because the United States does not currently have a government-funded national health care program that provides coverage for all of its citizens, U.S. private insurance expenditures cover the costs generally assumed by government programs that finance health care delivery in comparable OECD member nations. The Patient Protection and Affordable Care Act and the Health Care and Education Reconciliation Act (which are now commonly known as the ACA) promise not only to provide health insurance coverage for the overwhelming majority of Americans but also to change the ways in which Americans purchase and pay for health care. In 2014, when U.S. citizens will be required to have health care coverage (or pay a penalty), it is anticipated that the mix of payment sources (public, private, and out of pocket) will shift. For example, expanded Medicaid eligibility may increase the share of public expenditures, and the establishment of limits on maximum health plan deductibles may reduce out-of-pocket expenditures.

Spending on Pharmaceutical Drugs

The OECD indicates in "OECD Health Data—Frequently Requested Data" that in 2010 the United

States spent more per capita ($983.1) on pharmaceutical drugs than any other OECD member country. The average pharmaceutical spending was $364.1 per capita. The per capita pharmaceutical spending was also high in Canada ($740.7), Ireland ($686.4), Greece ($676.5), Germany ($640), France ($634.5), and Japan ($630.2). In contrast, Chile spent $134.7, Mexico spent $249.9, Estonia spent $281.8, and New Zealand spent $285.4 per capita on pharmaceuticals.

Hospital Utilization Statistics

The number of hospital beds is a gross measure of resource availability; however, it is important to remember that it does not reflect capacity to provide emergency or outpatient hospital care. In general, it also does not measure the number of beds that are devoted to nonacute or other long-term care, although it is known that in Japan many of the beds designated as acute care are actually used for long-term care. According to the OECD, in "OECD Health Data—Frequently Requested Data," of the OECD member countries reporting acute care hospital beds per 1,000 population, Japan (13.6) and South Korea (8.8) had the highest numbers in 2010. The United States was among the lowest, at 3.1 beds per 1,000 population in 2010, trailed only by the United Kingdom (3), New Zealand (2.7), Sweden (2.7), Turkey (2.5), Chile (2), and Mexico (1.6).

Hospital lengths of stay have consistently declined since 1960, in part because increasing numbers of illnesses can be treated as effectively in outpatient settings and because many countries have reduced inpatient hospital-ization rates and the average length of stay (ALOS) to control health care costs. In 2010 Japan (18.2 days) had the longest acute care ALOS of the OECD member nations, followed by South Korea (14.2 days), Finland (11.6 days), Switzerland (9.6 days), and Germany (9.5 days). The shortest hospital stays in 2010 were in Mexico (3.9 days), Turkey (4.1 days), Israel (4.5 days), Norway (4.5 days), and Denmark (4.6 days). The United States' ALOS was 4.9 days in 2010, which was on par with Australia (5.1 days) and Hungary (5.1 days).

Medical practice, particularly the types and frequency of procedures performed, also varies from one country to another. The OECD looked at rates of cesarean section (delivery of a baby through an incision in the abdomen as opposed to vaginal delivery) per 1,000 births and found both growth in the rates of cesarean section (as a percentage of all births) and considerable variation in the rates for this surgical procedure. In 2010 the highest rates for cesarean sections per 1,000 live births were reported in Mexico (448), Turkey (427), Italy (384), South Korea (352), Portugal (330), the United States (329), Switzerland (328), and Hungary (325). In "Beyond Numbers: The Multiple Cultural Meanings of Rising Cesarean Rates Worldwide" (*American Journal of Bioethics*, vol. 12, no. 7, 2012), Kristina Orfali of Columbia University observes that rates of cesarean sections are at an all-time high. Orfali reports that two-thirds of countries with low rates of maternal and infant deaths have cesarean section rates in excess of the World Health Organization's recommendation of 15%. Figure 7.1 shows the dramatic rise in cesarean sections

FIGURE 7.1

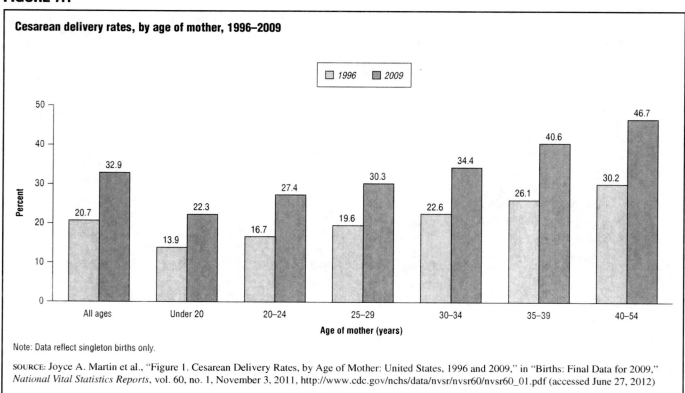

Cesarean delivery rates, by age of mother, 1996–2009

Note: Data reflect singleton births only.

SOURCE: Joyce A. Martin et al., "Figure 1. Cesarean Delivery Rates, by Age of Mother: United States, 1996 and 2009," in "Births: Final Data for 2009," *National Vital Statistics Reports*, vol. 60, no. 1, November 3, 2011, http://www.cdc.gov/nchs/data/nvsr/nvsr60/nvsr60_01.pdf (accessed June 27, 2012)

among mothers of all ages between 1996 and 2009 in the United States. Because cesarean section is performed in the hospital and generally involves at least an overnight stay, the frequency with which it and other surgical procedures are performed contributes to hospitalization rates and expenditures.

Physicians' Numbers Are Increasing

Since 1960 the OECD member nations have all enjoyed growing physician populations. In "OECD Health Data—Frequently Requested Data," the OECD reports that in 2010 Greece and Austria reported the highest ratio of practicing physicians, 6.1 and 4.8 per 1,000 population, respectively, with most countries ranging between 2 and 4 physicians per 1,000 population. The countries that had the fewest practicing physicians were in Chile (1.4 per 1,000 population), Turkey (1.7), Mexico (2), South Korea (2), Japan (2.2), and Poland (2.2). Canada, Slovenia, and the United States each had 2.4 physicians per 1,000 population, below the OECD average of 2.5.

The ratio of physicians to population is a limited measure of health care quality, because many other factors, such as the availability of other health care providers as well as the accessibility and affordability of health care services, also influence the quality of health care systems. Furthermore, during the last 25 years research has shown that more medical care, in terms of numbers and concentration of health care providers, is not necessarily linked to better health status for the population. For example, the Dartmouth Institute for Health Policy and Clinical Practice indicates in "The Physician Workforce" (2012, http://www.dartmouthatlas.org/keyissues/issue.aspx?con=2940) that increasing the physician population will make the U.S. health care system worse rather than better. The institute contends that "first, unfettered growth is likely to exacerbate regional inequities in supply and spending; our research has shown that physicians generally do not choose to practice where the need is greatest. Second, expansion of graduate medical education would most likely further undermine primary care and reinforce trends toward a fragmented, specialist-oriented health care system."

OVERVIEWS OF SELECTED HEALTH CARE SYSTEMS

David Squires of the Commonwealth Fund uses data collected by the OECD and other agencies to compare health care systems and performance in industrialized countries in *Multinational Comparisons of Health Systems Data, 2011* (November 2011, http://www.commonwealthfund.org/) and in *Explaining High Health Care Spending in the United States: An International Comparison of Supply, Utilization, Prices, and Quality* (May 2012, http://www.commonwealthfund.org/).

Squires looks at OECD data for 13 industrialized countries: Australia, Canada, Denmark, France, Germany, Japan, the Netherlands, New Zealand, Norway, Sweden, Switzerland, the United Kingdom, and the United States. He observes that the reasons the United States outspends other industrialized countries are not its aging population, higher income, or greater supply or utilization of health care providers. Instead, Squires attributes excess U.S. health care costs to higher prices for drugs, more office visits and procedures, more readily accessible and expensive technology, and an increased prevalence of obesity. He also notes that the quality of U.S. health care is not significantly superior to other, much less costly health care systems.

Another significant difference between the United States and other OECD countries is the lack of universal health insurance coverage. This gap in coverage explains why Americans go without needed health care more often than people in other OECD countries and why, in comparison to the other industrialized countries, the United States does not fare well in measures of access to care and equity in health care between high- and low-income populations. However, as the provisions of the ACA take effect through 2014, and the overwhelming majority of Americans have health care coverage, these disparities will likely diminish.

Other key findings by the OECD include:

- Spending growth slowed or fell in nearly all OECD member countries in 2010, reversing the trend of escalating health care spending.

- The United States (http://www.oecd.org/newsroom/healththehighcostofdiabetes.htm) reported the second-highest prevalence of diabetes among adults aged 20 to 79 years in 2010, at 10.3%.

- The United States has more diagnostic imaging equipment—magnetic resonance imaging (MRI) and computed tomography scanners—than any other OECD member nation. For example, in 2007, the most recent year for which U.S. data are reported, Australia had 5.1 MRI units per million population, compared with the U.S. rate of 25.9. (See Table 7.2.) The OECD reports in "OECD Health Data—Frequently Requested Data" that in 2010 Australia had 5.6 MRI units per million population, whereas the U.S. rate had climbed to 31.6.

The United States

The U.S. health care financing system is based on the consumer sovereignty, or private insurance, model. Employer-based health insurance is tax subsidized—that is, health insurance premiums are a tax-deductible business expense and are not generally taxed as employee compensation. The premiums for individual policies purchased by self-employed Americans became fully tax deductible in 2003. Benefits, premiums, and provider

TABLE 7.2

Number of magnetic resonance imaging (MRI) units and computed tomography (CT) scanners, selected countries, selected years 1990–2009

Country	1990	1995	2000	2007	2008	2009	1990	1995	2000	2007	2008	2009
	Number of MRI units per million population						Number of CT scanners per million population					
Australia[a]	0.6	2.9	†3.5	5.1	5.6	5.9	13.8	††20.5	††26.1	—	—	††38.7
Austria	—	—	11.0	17.7	18.0	18.4	—	—	26.1	30.0	29.6	29.3
Canada[b]	0.7	1.4	2.5	6.7	—	8.0	7.2	8.0	—	12.7	—	13.9
Czech Republic[c]	—	1.0	1.7	4.4	5.0	5.7	—	6.7	9.6	12.9	13.3	14.1
Denmark	—	—	5.4	—	—	15.4	—	—	11.4	18.5	21.5	23.7
Estonia	—	—	—	5.2	8.2	7.5	—	—	—	11.2	14.9	14.9
Finland	1.8	4.3	9.9	15.3	16.2	16.9	9.8	11.8	13.5	16.5	—	20.4
France	—	—	1.7	5.5	6.1	6.5	—	—	7.0	10.4	10.9	11.1
Greece	—	—	—	17.9	19.6	21.7	—	—	—	29.0	30.6	33.8
Hungary[d]	0.1	1.0	1.8	2.8	2.8	2.8	1.9	4.6	5.7	7.3	7.1	7.2
Iceland	3.9	7.5	10.7	19.3	18.8	21.9	11.8	18.7	21.3	32.1	31.3	34.5
Ireland	—	—	—	8.5	9.0	†11.9	4.3	—	—	14.3	14.5	15.3
Israel[e]	—	0.9	1.4	2.0	2.1	1.9	—	1.6	5.7	8.5	8.8	9.4
Italy[f]	—	—	7.8	18.5	20.1	21.6	—	—	21.1	30.1	30.9	31.7
Japan[g]	6.1	—	—	—	43.1	—	55.2	—	—	—	97.3	—
Luxembourg	2.6	2.5	2.3	10.4	12.4	14.2	5.2	26.9	25.2	27.1	26.9	26.3
Mexico	—	—	—	1.5	1.7	1.9	—	—	—	4.0	4.2	4.3
Netherlands[h]	0.9	3.9	—	7.6	10.4	11.0	7.3	—	—	7.8	10.3	11.3
New Zealand	—	—	—	8.8	9.6	9.7	3.5	—	8.8	12.3	12.4	14.6
Poland	—	—	—	2.7	2.9	3.7	—	—	4.4	9.7	10.9	12.4
Portugal[i]	—	—	—	8.9	—	—	—	—	—	26.0	—	—
Republic of Korea	—	3.9	5.4	16.0	17.6	19.0	—	15.5	28.4	37.1	36.8	37.1
Slovak Republic[j]	—	—	1.1	5.7	6.1	6.1	—	—	—	13.7	13.7	13.3
Slovenia	—	—	—	3.5	4.5	4.5	—	—	—	10.9	12.4	11.9
Switzerland	—	—	—	—	—	—	—	—	—	††31.4	††32.0	††32.8
Turkey	—	—	—	5.4	†7.2	8.9	1.6	—	—	7.7	††10.6	11.6
United Kingdom[k]	—	—	††5.6	—	††5.6	—	—	—	††5.3	—	††7.4	—
United States[l]	—	12.3	—	25.9	—	—	—	—	—	34.3	—	—
	Number of MRI units						Number of CT scanners					
Australia[a]	11	52	†67	108	120	129	235	††370	††500	—	—	†849
Austria	—	—	88	147	150	154	—	—	209	249	247	245
Canada[b]	19	40	76	222	—	266	198	234	—	419	—	464
Czech Republic[c]	—	10	17	45	52	60	—	69	99	133	139	148
Denmark	—	—	29	—	—	85	—	—	61	101	118	131
Estonia	—	—	—	7	11	10	—	—	—	15	20	20
Finland	9	22	51	81	86	90	49	60	70	87	—	109
France	—	—	100	350	389	415	—	—	426	659	696	715
Greece	—	—	—	200	220	245	—	—	—	324	344	381
Hungary[d]	1	10	18	28	28	28	20	47	58	73	71	72
Iceland	1	2	3	6	6	7	3	5	6	10	10	11
Ireland	—	—	—	37	40	†53	15	—	—	62	64	68
Israel[e]	—	5	9	14	15	14	—	9	36	61	64	70
Italy[f]	—	—	442	1,097	1,180	1,272	—	—	1,203	1,785	1,821	1,870
Japan[g]	756	—	—	—	5,503	—	6,821	—	—	—	12,420	—
Luxembourg	1	1	1	5	6	7	2	11	11	13	13	13
Mexico	—	—	—	161	180	209	—	—	—	422	447	467
Netherlands[h]	13	60	—	125	171	181	109	—	—	128	168	186
New Zealand	—	—	—	37	41	42	12	—	34	52	53	63
Poland	—	—	—	103	112	141	—	—	169	368	414	473
Portugal[i]	—	—	—	94	—	—	—	—	—	276	—	—
Republic of Korea	—	174	254	777	855	924	—	699	1,334	1,799	1,788	1,810
Slovak Republic[j]	—	—	6	31	33	33	—	—	—	74	74	72
Slovenia	—	—	—	7	9	9	—	—	—	22	25	24
Switzerland	—	—	—	—	—	—	—	—	—	††237	††245	††254
Turkey	—	—	—	395	517	647	89	—	—	569	†759	838
United Kingdom[k]	—	—	††331	—	††340	—	—	—	††315	—	††449	—
United States[l]	—	3,265	—	7,810	—	—	—	—	—	10,335	—	—

reimbursement methods differ among private insurance plans and among public programs as well.

Most physicians who provide both ambulatory care (hospital outpatient service and office visits) and inpatient hospital care are generally reimbursed on either a fee-for-service or per capita basis (literally, per head, but in managed care frequently per member per month), and payment rates vary among insurers. Increasing numbers of physicians are salaried; they are employees of the government, hospital, and health care delivery systems, universities, and private industry.

The nation's hospitals are paid on the basis of charges, costs, negotiated rates, or diagnosis-related groups, depending on the patient's insurer. There are no overall global

TABLE 7.2

Number of magnetic resonance imaging (MRI) units and computed tomography (CT) scanners, selected countries, selected years 1990–2009 [CONTINUED]

—Data not available.
†Break in series.
††Data are estimated.
aStarting with 2000 data, the number of MRI units includes only those that are approved for billing to Medicare (Australia's national health program). In 1999, approved units represented approximately 60% of total units.
bThe number of units in freestanding imaging facilities was imputed for years prior to 2003 based on data collected in the 2003 National Survey of Selected Medical Imaging Equipment, conducted by the Canadian Institute for Health Information. MRI units in Quebec are not included in 2000.
cPrior to 2000, the data include only equipment of Health Sector establishments.
dEquipment used in military hospitals and the health institutes of Hungarian State Railways are not included.
eThe statistical data for Israel are supplied by and under the responsibility of the relevant Israeli authorities. The use of such data by the Organisation of Economic Co-operation and Development (OECD) is without prejudice to the status of the Golan Heights, East Jerusalem, and Israeli settlements in the West Bank under the terms of international law.
f1990 data include only equipment in public and private hospitals.
gPrior to 2000, the data include only equipment in hospitals.
h2005 data are the number of hospitals reporting having an MRI unit.
iPrior to 2006, numbers are incomplete for the private sector. Starting with 2006, numbers are for equipment installed in both the public and private sectors.
jData include devices in hospitals and do not include equipment in other health care facilities.
kData include devices in public sector establishments only.
lData are from the MRI Census and are comparable with the OECD definition. Devices in U.S. territories are not included.
Notes: Countries use different methods for collecting data. Therefore, estimates may not be directly comparable across countries and comparisons among them should be made with caution. Data for additional years are available.

SOURCE: "Table 123. Number of Magnetic Resonance Imaging (MRI) Units and Computed Tomography (CT) Scanners: Selected Countries, Selected Years 1990–2009," in *Health, United States, 2011: With Special Feature on Socioeconomic Status and Health*, U.S. Department of Health and Human Services, Centers for Disease Control and Prevention, National Center for Health Statistics, May 2012, http://www.cdc.gov/nchs/data/hus/hus11.pdf (accessed June 13, 2012). Data from Organisation for Economic Co-operation and Development Health Data.

budgets or expenditure limits. Nevertheless, managed care (oversight by some group or authority to verify the medical necessity of treatments and to control the cost of health care) has assumed an expanding role. Health maintenance organizations, preferred provider organizations, and other managed care plans and payers (government and private health insurance) now exert greater control over the practices of individual health care providers in an effort to control costs. To the extent that they govern reimbursement, managed care organizations are viewed by many physicians and other industry observers as dictating the methods, terms, and quality of health care delivery.

IS THE UNITED STATES SPENDING MORE AND GETTING LESS? A primary indicator of the quality of health care delivery in any nation is the health status of its people. Many factors can affect the health of individuals and populations: heredity, race and ethnicity, gender, income, education, geography, violent crime, environmental agents, and exposure to infectious diseases, as well as access to and availability of health care services.

Still, in the nation that spends the most on the health of its citizens, it seems reasonable to expect to see tangible benefits of expenditures for health care—that is, measurable gains in health status. This section considers three health outcomes (measures used to assess the health of a population)—life expectancy at birth, infant mortality (death), and health care costs—and selected aspects of health care delivery such as access and quality to determine the extent to which U.S. citizens derive health benefits from record-high outlays for medical care.

Overall, life expectancy at birth consistently increased in all the OECD member countries since 1960; however,

historically, U.S. life expectancy has remained slightly below the OECD average. For example, Table 7.3 shows that in 2009 U.S. life expectancy for women (80.9 years) was surpassed by all OECD member countries except the Czech Republic (80.5 years), Estonia (80.1), Poland (80), the Slovak Republic (78.7 years), Hungary (77.9 years), Mexico (77.6 years), and Turkey (76.1 years). Infant mortality also declined sharply during this period, but the United States fared far worse than most OECD member countries—in 2008 the United States ranked number 27 with an infant mortality rate of 6.6 deaths per 1,000 live births. (See Table 7.4.)

Ida Hellender of Physicians for a National Health Program observes in "The Deepening Crisis in U.S. Health Care: A Review of Data" (*International Journal of Health Services*, vol. 41, no. 3, 2011) that the United States ranks 49th in life expectancy and 42nd globally in deaths among children under the age of five years, trailing every country in western Europe and many other nations. Even though the U.S. child mortality rate has declined by more than 40% since 1990, it remains higher than many other nations.

Hellender also notes that even though the United States spends twice as much per capita on health care as other developed countries, it ranked last in quality, efficiency, and equity when compared with Australia, Canada, Germany, the Netherlands, New Zealand, and the United Kingdom. The United Kingdom was named first in quality and the Netherlands was ranked first in all the other measures. In measures of access, efficiency, equity, premature deaths, infant mortality, and healthy life expectancy among older adults, the United States trailed the other countries, coming in last or next to last. Table 7.5 shows that in 2009 the life expectancy of a man aged 65 was 17.6 years in the United

TABLE 7.3

Life expectancy at birth, OECD countries, selected years 1980–2009

Country	Male					Female				
	1980	1990	2000	2008	2009	1980	1990	2000	2008	2009
At birth					Life expectancy in years					
Australia	71.0	73.9	76.6	79.2	79.3	78.1	80.1	82.0	83.7	83.9
Austria	69.0	72.3	75.2	77.8	77.6	76.1	79.0	81.2	83.3	83.2
Belgium	69 9	72.7	74.6	76.9	77.3	76.7	79.5	81.0	82.6	82.8
Canada	71.7	74.4	76.3	—	—	78.9	80.8	81.7	—	—
Chile	—	69.4	73.7	75.1	75.6[†]	—	76.5	80.0	80.6	80.9[†]
Czech Republic[a]	66.9	67.6	71.7	74.1	74.2	74.0	75.5	78.5	80.5	80.5
Denmark	71.2	72.0	74.5	76.5	76.9	77.3	77.8	79.2	81.0	81.1
Estonia	64.2	64.5	65.1	68.6	69.8	74.2	74.7	76.0	79.2	80.1
Finland	69.3	71.0	74.2	76.5	76.6	78.0	79.0	81.2	83.3	83.5
France	70.2	72.8	75.2	77.6	77.7[†]	78.4	80.9	82.8	84.3	84.4[†]
Germany[b]	69.6	72.0	75.1	77.6	77.8	76.2	78.5	81.2	82.7	82.8
Greece	73.0	74.7	75.5	77.7	77.8	77.5	79.5	80.6	82.3	82.7
Hungary	65.5	65.1	67.4	69.8	70.0	72.7	73.7	75.9	77.8	77.9
Iceland	73.7	75.4	78.4	79.6	79.7	79.7	80.5	81.8	83.0	83.3
Ireland	70.1	72.1	74.0	77.8	77.4	75.6	77.7	79.2	82.4	82.5
Israel[c]	72.1	74.9	76.7	79.0	79.7	75.7	78.4	80.9	83.0	83.5
Italy	70.6	73.8	76.9	79.1	—	77.4	80.3	82.8	84.5	—
Japan	73.3	75.9	77.7	79.3	79.6	78.8	81.9	84.6	86.0	86.4
Luxembourg	70.0	72.4	74.6	78.1	78.1	75.6	78.7	81.3	83.1	83.3
Mexico	64.1	67.7	71.3	72.7	72.9	70.2	73.5	76.5	77.5	77.6
Netherlands	72.5	73.8	75.5	78.3	78.5	79.2	80.1	80.5	82.3	82.7
New Zealand	70.1	72.5	75.9	78.4	78.8	76.2	78.4	80.8	82.4	82.7
Norway	72.4	73.5	76.0	78.4	78.7	79.3	79.9	81.5	83.2	83.2
Poland	66.0	66.2	69.7	71.3	71.5	74.4	75.2	78.0	80.0	80.0
Portugal	67.9	70.6	73.2	76.2	76.5	74.9	77.5	80.2	82.4	82.6
Republic of Korea	61.8	67.3	72.3	76.5	76.8	70.0	75.5	79.6	83.3	83.8
Slovak Republic[a]	66.8	66.6	69.1	70.9	71.3	74.3	75.4	77.4	78.7	78.7
Slovenia	—	69.4	71.9	75.4	75.8	—	77.2	79.1	82.3	82.3
Spain	72.3	73.4	75.8	78.2	78.6	78.5	80.6	82.9	84.5	84.9
Sweden	72.8	74.8	77.4	79.1	79.4	78.8	80.4	82.0	83.2	83.4
Switzerland	72.3	74.0	77.0	79.8	79.9	79.0	80.9	82.8	84.6	84.6
Turkey	55.8	65.4[††]	69.0	71.4	71.5	60.3	69.5[††]	73.1	75.8	76.1
United Kingdom	70.2	72.9	75.5	77.8	78.3	76.2	78.5	80.3	81.9	82.5
United States	70.0	71.8	74.1	75.6	76.0	77.4	78.8	79.3	80.6	80.9

OECD = Organisation for Economic Co-operation and Development.
—Data not available.
[†]Data are estimated.
[††]Break in series.
[a]In 1993, Czechoslovakia was divided into two nations, the Czech Republic and Slovakia. Data for years prior to 1993 are from the Czech and Slovak regions of Czechoslovakia.
[b]Until 1990, estimates refer to the Federal Republic of Germany; from 1995 onwards data refer to Germany after reunification.
[c]The statistical data for Israel are supplied by and under the responsibility of the relevant Israeli authorities. The use of such data by OECD is without prejudice to the status of the Golan Heights, East Jerusalem, and Israeli settlements in the West Bank under the terms of international law.
Notes: Because calculation of life expectancy estimates varies among countries, ranks are not presented; comparisons among countries and their interpretation should be made with caution. Data for additional years are available.

SOURCE: Adapted from "Table 21. Life Expectancy at Birth and at 65 Years of Age, by Sex: Organisation for Economic Co-operation and Development (OECD) Countries, Selected Years 1980–2009," in *Health, United States, 2011: With Special Feature on Socioeconomic Status and Health*, U.S. Department of Health and Human Services, Centers for Disease Control and Prevention, National Center for Health Statistics, May 2012, http://www.cdc.gov/nchs/data/hus/hus11.pdf (accessed June 13, 2012). Data from Organisation for Economic Co-operation and Development Health Data.

States, compared with about 19 years in Australia, Israel, Japan, New Zealand, and Switzerland. For a woman of the same age, the life expectancy in the United States was 20.3 years, compared with between 22 and 24 years in Japan, Spain, and Switzerland.

Likewise, the United States is not a world leader in preventive care. For example, in 2009 only 66.8% of adults aged 65 years and older received a vaccination against influenza in the United States, compared with 88.2% in Mexico, 87.9% in Chile, 74.6% in Australia, 73.3% in the United Kingdom, and 71% in France. (See Table 7.6.) Hellender notes that in the United States, people with chronic conditions were the most likely to

report receipt of the wrong drug or incorrect test results and they experienced the longest delays when awaiting test results. Hellender concludes that "the U.S. system was also the least equitable and least accessible, with 54 percent of people with chronic conditions going without needed care in 2008, compared with 13 percent in Britain and 7 percent in the Netherlands."

Not surprisingly, satisfaction with the U.S. health care system is not high. The Commonwealth Fund indicates in "2010 International Health Policy Survey in Eleven Countries" (2012, http://www.commonwealthfund.org/Topics/International-Health-Policy/Bar.aspx?ind=420) that people were asked about their views of their country's

TABLE 7.4

Infant mortality and international rankings, OECD countries, selected years 1960–2008

Country[b]	1960	1970	1980	1990	2000	2006	2007	2008	International ranking[a] 1960	International ranking[a] 2008
					Infant[c] deaths per 1,000 live births					
Australia	20.2	17.9	10.7	8.2	5.2	4.7	4.2	4.1	6	21
Austria	37.5	25.9	14.3	7.8	4.8	3.6	3.7	3.7	20	13
Belgium	31.4	21.1	12.1	8.0	4.8	4.0	3.9	3.7	18	13
Canada	27.3	18.8	10.4	6.8	5.3	5.0	5.1	—	13	—
Chile	120.3	79.3	33.0	16.0	8.9	7.6	8.3	7.8	28	28
Czech Republic	20.0	20.2	16.9	10.8	4.1	3.3	3.1	2.8	5	7
Denmark	21.5	14.2	8.4	7.5	5.3	3.5	4.0	4.0	9	19
Finland	21.0	13.2	7.6	5.6	3.8	2.8	2.7	2.6	7	3
France	27.7	18.2	10.0	7.3	4.5	3.8	3.8	3.8	14	15
Germany	35.0	22.5	12.4	7.0	4.4	3.8	3.9	3.5	19	11
Greece	40.1	29.6	17.9	9.7	5.9	3.7	3.5	2.7	21	5
Hungary	47.6	35.9	23.2	14.8	9.2	5.7	5.9	5.6	24	24
Iceland	13.0	13.2	7.7	5.9	3.0	1.4	2.0	2.5	1	1
Ireland	29.3	19.5	11.1	8.2	6.2	3.6	3.1	3.8	16	15
Israel[d]	—	22.7	15.6	9.9	5.5	4.0	3.9	3.8	—	15
Italy	43.9	29.6	14.6	8.1	4.3	3.6	3.5	3.3	23	8
Japan	30.7	13.1	7.5	4.6	3.2	2.6	2.6	2.6	17	3
Mexico	92.3	80.9	52.6	39.2	19.4	16.2	15.7	15.2	27	30
Netherlands	16.5	12.7	8.6	7.1	5.1	4.4	4.1	3.8	3	15
New Zealand	22.6	16.7	13.0	8.4	6.3	5.1	4.8	5.0	11	23
Norway	16.0	11.3	8.1	6.9	3.8	3.2	3.1	2.7	2	5
Poland	54.8	36.7	25.5	19.3	8.1	6.0	6.0	5.6	25	24
Portugal	77.5	55.5	24.3	10.9	5.5	3.3	3.4	3.3	26	8
Republic of Korea	—	45.0	—	—	—	4.1	3.6	3.5	—	11
Slovak Republic	28 6	25.7	20.9	12.0	8.6	6.6	6.1	5.9	15	26
Spain	43 7	28.1	12.3	7.6	4.4	3.5	3.5	3.3	22	8
Sweden	16.6	11.0	6.9	6.0	3.4	2.8	2.5	2.5	4	1
Switzerland	21 1	15.1	9.1	6.8	4.9	4.4	3.9	4.0	8	19
Turkey	189.5	145.0	117.5	51.5[†]	31.6	16.9	15.9	14.9	29	29
United Kingdom	22.5	18.5	12.1	7.9	5.6	5.0	4.8	4.7	10	22
United States	26.0	20.0	12.6	9.2	6.9	6.7	6.8	6.6	12	27

OECD = Organisation for Economic Co-operation and Development.
—Data not available.
[†]Break in series.
[a]Rankings are from lowest to highest infant mortality rates (IMR). Countries with the same IMR receive the same rank. The country with the next highest IMR is assigned the rank it would have received had the lower-ranked countries not been tied, i.e., skip a rank. The latest year's international rankings are based on 2008 data because that is the most current data year for which most OECD countries have reported their final data.
[b]Refers to countries, territories, cities, or geographic areas with at least 2.5 million population and with complete counts of live births and infant deaths according to the United Nations Demographic Yearbook.
[c]Under 1 year of age.
[d]The statistical data for Israel are supplied by and under the responsibility of the relevant Israeli authorities. The use of such data by the OECD is without prejudice to the status of the Golan Heights, East Jerusalem, and Israeli settlements in the West Bank under the terms of international law.

SOURCE: "Table 20. Infant Mortality Rates and International Rankings: Organisation for Economic Co-operation and Development (OECD) Countries, Selected Years 1960–2008," in *Health, United States, 2011: With Special Feature on Socioeconomic Status and Health*, U.S. Department of Health and Human Services, Centers for Disease Control and Prevention, National Center for Health Statistics, May 2012, http://www.cdc.gov/nchs/data/hus/hus11.pdf (accessed June 13, 2012). Data from Organisation for Economic Co-operation and Development Health Data.

health care system and were offered three responses: "only minor changes needed," "fundamental changes needed," or "rebuild completely." In the United States 27% of respondents said the health care system should be completely rebuilt and 41% felt it needed fundamental changes. Even though 20% of Australians said their system should be completely rebuilt, less than 15% of the populations of the other countries surveyed thought their health care system required a complete overhaul. For example, just 3% of people in the United Kingdom and 7% of people in the Netherlands wanted to completely rebuild their health care system.

Germany

The German health care system is based on the social insurance model. Statutory sickness funds and private insurance cover the entire population. In "The German Health Care System, 2011" (*International Profiles of Health Care Systems*, November 2011, http://www.commonwealth fund.org/), Reinhard Busse, Miriam Blümel, and Stephanie Stock state that 85% of the population receives health care through the country's statutory health insurance program. Since 2009 health insurance has been mandatory for all citizens and permanent residents. Employees and employers finance these sickness funds through payroll contributions. Nearly all employers, including small businesses and low-wage industries, must participate. The remainder of the population is covered by private health insurance.

During the late 1990s Germany was the second highest among all the OECD member countries in health

TABLE 7.5

Life expectancy at age 65, Organisation for Economic Co-operation and Development (OECD) countries, selected years 1980–2009

Country	Male					Female				
	1980	1990	2000	2008	2009	1980	1990	2000	2008	2009
At 65 years					Life expectancy in years					
Australia	13.7	15.2	16.9	18.6	18.7	17.9	19.0	20.4	21.6	21.8
Austria	12.9	14.4	16.0	17.7	17.7	16.3	18.1	19.6	21.1	21.2
Belgium	12.9	14.3	15.6	17.3	17.5	16.8	18.8	19.7	20.9	21.1
Canada	14.5	15.7	16.5	—	—	18.9	19.9	20.2	—	—
Chile	—	13.7	15.5	17.0	16.8[†]	—	17.2	19.3	20.4	19.9[†]
Czech Republic[a]	11 2	11.7	13.8	15.3	15.2	14.4	15.3	17.3	18.8	18.8
Denmark	13.6	14.0	15.2	16.6	16.8	17.6	17.9	18.3	19.5	19.5
Estonia	—	11.9	12.5	13.6	14.4	—	15.5	16.8	18.6	18.3
Finland	12.6	13.8	15.5	17.5	17.3	17.0	17.8	19.5	21.3	21.5
France	13.6	15.5	16.7	18.2	—	18.2	19.8	21.2	22.5	—
Germany[b]	12.8	14.0	15.8	17.5	17.6	16.3	17.7	19.6	20.7	20.8
Greece	15.2	15.7	16.1	17.8	18.1	17.0	18.0	18.4	19.8	20.2
Hungary	11 6	12.0	12.7	13.6	13.7	14.6	15.3	16.5	17.5	17.6
Iceland	15.8	16.2	18.1	18.2	18.3	19.1	19.5	19.7	20.5	20.6
Ireland	12.6	13.3	14.6	16.8	17.2	15.7	17.0	18.0	20.3	20.6
Israel[3]	—	15.7	17.0	18.5	18.9	—	17.8	19.0	20.7	21.2
Italy	13.3	15.2	16.7	18.2	—	17.1	18.9	20.7	22.0	—
Japan	14.6	16.2	17.5	18.6	18.9	17.7	20.0	22.4	23.6	24.0
Luxembourg	12.6	14.3	15.5	17.4	17.6	16.5	18.5	20.1	21.0	21.4
Mexico	15.4	16.0	16.5	16.8	16.8	17.0	17.8	18.1	18.3	18.3
Netherlands	13.7	14.4	15.3	17.3	17.4	18.0	18.9	19.2	20.5	20.8
New Zealand	13.2	14.6	16.5	18.3	18.6	17.0	18.3	19.8	20.8	21.1
Norway	14.3	14.6	16.1	17.6	18.0	18.2	18.7	19.9	21.0	21.1
Poland	12.0	12.4	13.6	14.7	14.7	15.5	16.1	17.5	19.0	19.1
Portugal	13.1	14.0	15.4	16.9	17.1	16.1	17.1	18.9	20.3	20.5
Republic of Korea	10.5	12.4	14.3	16.6	17.1	15.1	16.3	18.2	21.0	21.5
Slovak Republic[c]	12.3	12.2	12.9	13.8	13.9	15.4	15.7	16.5	17.5	17.6
Slovenia	—	13.2	14.1	16.3	16.3	—	16.7	17.9	20.2	20.1
Spain	14.6	15.5	16.7	18.1	18.3	17.8	19.3	20.8	22.1	22.4
Sweden	14.3	15.3	16.7	17.9	18.2	17.9	19.0	20.0	20.8	21.0
Switzerland	14.3	15.3	17.0	18.9	19.0	18.2	19.7	20.9	22.3	22.2
Turkey	11.7	12.8[††]	13.4	14.0	14.0	12.8	14.3[††]	15.1	15.8	15.9
United Kingdom	12.6	14.0	15.8	17.7	18.1	16.6	17.9	19.0	20.3	20.8
United States	14.1	15.1	16.0	17.3	17.6	18.3	18.9	19.0	20.0	20.3

—Data not available.
[†]Data are estimated.
[†]Break in series.
[a]In 1993, Czechoslovakia was divided into two nations, the Czech Republic and Slovakia. Data for years prior to 1993 are from the Czech and Slovak regions of Czechoslovakia.
[b]Until 1990, estimates refer to the Federal Republic of Germany; from 1995 onwards data refer to Germany after reunification.
[c]The statistical data for Israel are supplied by and under the responsibility of the relevant Israeli authorities. The use of such data by OECD is without prejudice to the status of the Golan Heights, East Jerusalem, and Israeli settlements in the West Bank under the terms of international law.
Notes: Because calculation of life expectancy estimates varies among countries, ranks are not presented; comparisons among countries and their interpretation should be made with caution.

SOURCE: Adapted from "Table 21. Life Expectancy at Birth and at 65 Years of Age, by Sex: Organisation for Economic Co-operation and Development (OECD) Countries, Selected Years 1980–2009," in *Health, United States, 2011: With Special Feature on Socioeconomic Status and Health*, U.S. Department of Health and Human Services, Centers for Disease Control and Prevention, National Center for Health Statistics, May 2012, http://www.cdc.gov/nchs/data/hus/hus11 .pdf (accessed June 13, 2012). Data from Organisation for Economic Co-operation and Development Health Data.

expenditures per capita, but the OECD notes in "OECD Health Data—Frequently Requested Data" that by 2010 Germany ranked ninth in health expenditures per capita. Public funds, a combination of social insurance and general government funds, paid for more than three-quarters (76.8%) of total expenditures for health care, which was higher than the OECD average of 72.2%.

Ambulatory (outpatient) and inpatient care operate in completely separate spheres in the German health care system. German hospitals are public and private, operate for profit and not for profit, and generally do not have outpatient departments. Ambulatory care physicians are paid on the basis of fee schedules that are negotiated

between the organizations of sickness funds and the organizations of physicians. A separate fee schedule for private patients uses a similar scale.

In 1993 Germany's Health Care Reform Law went into effect. Among its many provisions, the law tied increases in physician, dental, and hospital expenditures to the income growth rate of members of the sickness funds. It also limited the licensing of new ambulatory care physicians (based on the number of physicians already in an area) and set a cap for overall pharmaceutical outlays. Still, in 2010 Germany boasted 3.7 practicing physicians per 1,000 population, a ratio that was higher than the OECD member countries' average of 3.1. The 1993

TABLE 7.6

Flu vaccination among adults aged 65 and older, OECD countries, 1998–2009

Country	1998	1999	2000	2003	2004	2005	2006	2007	2008	2009
					Percent receiving influenza vaccination during past 12 months					
Australia	—	69.0	74.0	76.9	79.1	—	77.5	—	—	74.6
Austria	—	23.7	—	—	—	—	36.1	—	—	—
Belgium	—	—	—	—	64.0	—	—	—	66.0	—
Canada	—	—	63.0	67.2	—	70.9	—	69.0	66.6	66.5
Chile	—	—	—	80.3	79.4	73.4	82.0	84.5	78.1	87.9
Czech Republic	—	—	—	—	—	—	—	—	22.1	—
Denmark	—	—	—	19.9	30.6	34.0	33.4	39.3	51.0	48.5
Estonia	—	—	—	—	—	—	—	—	1.1	1.4
Finland	—	—	—	45.0	46.0	52.0	46.0	48.4	51.0	43.0
France	61.0	58.0	65.0	65.0	68.0	68.0	68.0	69.0	70.0	71.0
Germany[a]	—	44.6	—	48.0	—	63.0	60.0	56.0	61.1	—
Hungary	—	—	—	38.9	37.9	37.1	34.0	34.2	37.8	31.6
Ireland	—	—	—	62.2	61.4	63.0	60.6	61.7	70.1	53.8
Israel[b]	—	—	44.7	—	—	—	—	56.0	56.8	56.7
Italy	—	40.7	50.7	63.4	66.6	68.3	66.6	64.9	66.2	66.3
Japan	—	—	—	43.0	48.0	49.0	48.0	53.0	56.0	50.0
Luxembourg	—	—	—	49.1	51.0	55.4	52.0	54.1	53.1	54.7
Mexico	—	—	—	—	—	—	51.1	34.6	76.1	88.2
Netherlands	72.0	72.0	76.0	77.0	73.0	77.0	75.0	78.0	77.0	—
New Zealand	—	—	—	63.1	58.0†	60.6	63.6	63.7	63.7	66.4
Portugal	31.3	39.0	—	46.9	39.0	41.6	50.4	51.0	53.3	52.2
Republic of Korea	—	—	—	—	75.7	77.2	—	70.2	73.6	—
Slovak Republic	—	—	20.7	37.9	22.9	29.3	25.7	33.4	35.5	30.5
Slovenia	—	—	35.0	33.0	30.0	35.0	28.0	26.0	26.0	22.0
Spain	63.5	59.8	61.5	68.0	68.6	70.1	67.6	62.3	65.4	65.7
Sweden	—	—	—	—	—	—	—	57.0	64.0	—
Switzerland	41.0	46.0	51.0	58.0	57.0	59.0	61.0	56.0	—	—
United Kingdom	—	—	65.0	71.0	71.0	75.0	75.1	73.5	75.1	73.3
United States	63.3	65.7	64.4	65.5	64.6	59.7	64.3	66.7	67.2	66.8

OECD = Organisation for Economic Co-operation and Development.
—Data not available.
†Break in series.
[a]1998 data for Germany are for adults 69 years of age and over. Starting with 1999 data, data are for adults 60 years of age and over.
[b]The statistical data for Israel are supplied by and under the responsibility of the relevant Israeli authorities. The use of such data by OECD is without prejudice to the status of the Golan Heights, East Jerusalem, and Israeli settlements in the West Bank under the terms of international law.
Notes: Data are for adults 65 years of age and over. Countries estimate influenza vaccination coverage using different adult age delimitation methods (i.e., 59 or 60 years instead of 65 years of age). Therefore, estimates may not be directly comparable across countries and comparisons among them should be made with caution.

SOURCE: "Table 84. Influenza Vaccination among Adults 65 Years of Age and over: Selected Organisation for Economic Co-operation and Development (OECD) Countries, 1998–2009," in *Health, United States, 2011: With Special Feature on Socioeconomic Status and Health*, U.S. Department of Health and Human Services, Centers for Disease Control and Prevention, National Center for Health Statistics, May 2012, http://www.cdc.gov/nchs/data/hus/hus11.pdf (accessed June 13, 2012). Data from Organisation for Economic Co-operation and Development Health Data.

legislation also changed the hospital compensation system from per diem (per day) payments to specific fees for individual procedures and conditions.

Other German health care reform measures instituted during the 1990s also served to stimulate competition between sickness funds and improved coordination of inpatient and ambulatory care. During the mid-1990s the government also attempted to control health care costs by reducing health benefits, such as limiting how often patients could visit health spas to recuperate.

The health care reforms were not, however, successful at containing health care costs. Growth in health care spending was attributed to the comparatively high level of health care activity and resources, along with rising pharmaceutical expenditures and efforts to meet the health care needs of an aging population. According to Ulrike Siewert et al., in "Health Care Consequences of

Demographic Changes in Mecklenburg-West Pomerania: Projected Case Numbers for Age-Related Diseases up to the Year 2020, Based on the Study of Health in Pomerania (SHIP)" (*Deutsches Ärzteblatt International*, vol. 107, no. 18, May 2010), the German health care system is not adequately prepared to meet the challenges of providing medical care for an aging population. The researchers also observe that decreasing numbers of physicians in rural areas may exacerbate the challenge of delivering needed services.

Canada

The Canadian system is characterized as a provincial government health insurance model, in which each of the 10 provinces operates its own health system under general federal rules and with a fixed federal contribution. All provinces are required to offer insurance coverage for all medically necessary services, including hospital care and physician services. However, additional services and benefits may be offered at the discretion of each province. Most provinces cover preventive services, routine dental care for children, and outpatient drugs for older adults (with a co-payment) and the poor. No restrictions are placed on a patient's choice of physicians.

Canadian citizens have equal access to medical care, regardless of their ability to pay. Entitlement to benefits is linked to residency, and the system is financed through general taxation. Private insurance is prohibited from covering the same benefits that are covered by the public system, yet a majority of Canadians are covered by private supplemental insurance policies. These policies generally cover services such as adult dental care, cosmetic surgery, and private or semiprivate hospital rooms. The OECD notes in "Country Statistical Profile: Canada" (2012, http://www.oecd-ilibrary.org/economics/country-statistical-profile-canada_20752288-table-can) that in 2010 public health expenditures accounted for 8% of the GDP and private expenditures for health were just 3.3% of the country's GDP.

The delivery system consists mostly of community hospitals and self-employed physicians. Nearly all of Canadian hospital beds are public; private hospitals do not participate in the public insurance program. Most hospitals are not for profit and are funded on the basis of global institution-specific or regional budgets. (A global institution-specific budget allocates a lump sum of money to a large department or area; then all the groups in that department or area must negotiate to see how much of the total money each group receives.) Physicians in both inpatient and outpatient settings are paid on a negotiated, fee-for-service basis. Sara Allin and Diane Watson of the Commonwealth Fund report in "The Canadian Health Care System, 2011" (*International Profiles of Health Care Systems*, November 2011, http://www.commonwealthfund.org/) that in 2007–08, 24% of payments to physicians were made through these types of arrangements, up from 21% in 2003–04. The compensation systems vary somewhat from province to province, and certain provinces, such as Quebec, have also established global budgets for physician services. Some provinces, including Alberta, British Columbia, and Ontario, require health care premiums for services; however, the Canada Health Act prohibits denial of health services on the basis of inability to pay premiums.

According to Allin and Watson, 71% of total health expenditures were publicly funded in 2009, and 30% of total health expenditures were from private sources (private insurance and out-of-pocket payments). About two-thirds of Canadians have supplementary private insurance coverage, which many obtain through their employers. These supplemental plans cover services such as vision and dental care, prescription drugs, rehabilitation services, home care, and private rooms in hospitals.

CONTROLLING COSTS. In "Soaring Costs Force Canada to Reassess Health Model" (Reuters, May 31, 2010), Claire Sibonney reports that the combination of an aging population and the need to reduce budget deficits has prompted the Canadian provinces to take measures to control health care costs, which have been rising about 6% per year. The consensus is that no one wants to disassemble what has become Canada's most popular social program, but most agree that change is inevitable. Sibonney notes in "Factbox: Canada's Universal Healthcare System" (Reuters, May 31, 2010) that according to a 2009 poll, 86% of Canadians support "public solutions to make our public healthcare stronger." Given the popularity of the Canadian health care system, the provincial governments have endeavored to cut costs in several ways, such as:

- Ontario has taken steps to reduce the costs of pharmaceutical drugs

- British Columbia has moved to reimburse hospitals using a fee-for-service model rather than block grants

- Quebec has instituted a health tax and proposed a fee, not unlike the co-payments many U.S. health plans use, for each visit to a health care practitioner

- Ontario has proposed tying hospital executives' compensation to the quality of care delivered by hospitals and plans to increase the number of salaried physicians

Allin and Watson suggest that cost containment is achieved through single-payer purchasing power and that increases in health care expenditures generally occur in response to government investment decisions. Actions to control costs include "mandatory annual global budgets for hospitals/health regions, negotiated fee schedules for health care providers, drug formularies, and reviews of the diffusion of technology." The federal Patented Medicine Prices Review Board, an independent body, regulates the prices of newly patented prescription medications. It ensures that drug prices are not "excessive" on the basis of their "degree of innovation" and compares the prices of existing prescription drugs in Canada with the prices of these drugs in seven countries, including the United States.

According to the Canadian Institute for Health Information, in the press release "Health Spending to Reach $200 Billion in 2011" (November 3, 2011, http://www.cihi.ca/cihi-ext-portal/internet/en/document/spending+and+health+workforce/spending/release_03nov11), growth in total health care spending in Canada has slowed from annual increases of 7.4% per year between 1998 and 2008 to just 4% in 2011. Even though health care spending continues to outpace inflation and population growth, it is expected to grow more slowly than the overall economy. In 2011 health care spending topped $200.5 billion and was

11.6% of Canada's GDP. In *Canada's Medicare Bubble: Is Government Health Spending Sustainable without User-Based Funding?* (April 2011, http://www.fraserinstitute.org/), Brett J. Skinner and Mark Rovere of the Fraser Institute examine the public costs of Canada's health care system and conclude that "Canada's health system produces rates of growth in health spending that are not sustainable solely through redistributive public financing. Supplementary user-based, private financing would off-load public cost pressures, encourage economic efficiency, and offer a sustainable source of additional resources."

Europe

Since 2008 nearly every state in the European Union (EU) has suffered an economic downturn or financial crisis marked by increasing deficits, unemployment, and/or public debt. In *The Crisis, Hospitals and Healthcare* (April 2011, http://www.hope.be/05eventsandpublications/docpublications/86_crisis/86_HOPE-The_Crisis_Hospitals_Healthcare_April_2011.pdf), HOPE–European Hospital and Healthcare Federation details the impact of these economic realities on EU health care systems. HOPE observes that throughout the EU health care reforms were instituted in response to the economic downturn and some planned or existing reforms were accelerated to slow health care spending.

Many countries implemented measures that were comparable to those under way in the United States. Some countries established ceilings to restrain health care budget increases. Others instituted strategies to reduce the costs of delivering health services, decrease provider compensation, or ease spending for pharmaceuticals. Still other countries embarked on comprehensive interventions that were aimed at increasing productivity, promoting excellence, leveraging group purchasing, and intensifying coordination of inpatient and outpatient care and services. Because the costs of care, especially hospitalization, have increased, out-of-pocket payments from patients have been instituted or increased.

THE UNITED KINGDOM. The United Kingdom employs the National Health Service (NHS), or Beveridge, model to finance and deliver health care. The entire population is covered under a system that is financed primarily from general taxation. There is minimal cost sharing. In 2009, 84% of all health spending was from public funds. Anthony Harrison et al. note in "The English Health Care System, 2011" (*International Profiles of Health Care Systems*, November 2011, http://www.commonwealthfund.org/) that the NHS "provides or pays for: preventive services, including screening and immunization and vaccination programs; inpatient and outpatient (ambulatory) hospital (specialist) care; physician (general practitioner) services; inpatient and outpatient drugs;

dental care; some eye care; mental health care, including care for those with learning disabilities; palliative care; some long-term care; and rehabilitation." In addition, approximately 89% of prescription drugs are provided free-of-charge.

The United Kingdom's hospital beds are public and generally owned by the NHS. The OECD reports in "OECD Health Data—Frequently Requested Data" that in 2010 there were 3 beds per 1,000 population, which was comparable to the United States (3.1 beds), but fewer than other European nations, such as France (6.4) and Germany (8.3).

Parliament and the Department of Health share the responsibility for health legislation and policy matters. Health services are organized and managed by regional and local public authorities. General practitioners serve as primary care physicians and are reimbursed on the basis of a combination of capitation payments (payments for each person served), fee for service, and other allowances. Hospitals receive overall budget allotments from district health authorities, and hospital-based physicians are salaried. Harrison et al. note that acute hospitals are paid using a system known as "payment by results," which rewards improvement in efficiency. Private insurance reimburses both physicians and hospitals on a fee-for-service basis. Approximately 12% of the population had private health insurance in 2010.

Most general practitioners, who are the frontline of health care delivery, are either self-employed or salaried hospital-based physicians. According to Harrison et al., in 2010 there were 8,324 general practices and each practice saw an average of 6,610 patients. Each general practitioner saw an average of 1,567 patients in 2010.

Michael Ybarra notes in "Healthcare around the World" (*American Academy of Emergency Medicine*, vol. 16, no. 6, 2009) that the NHS pioneered many cost-containment measures that are currently used by the United States and other countries seeking to slow escalating health care expenditures. These approaches to evaluating and managing health care costs include:

- Cost-effective analysis: calculated as a ratio, and often expressed as the cost per year per life saved, the cost-effectiveness analysis of a drug or procedure relates the cost of the drug or procedure to the health benefits it produces. This analysis enables delivery of clinically efficient, cost-effective care.

- Cost-minimization analysis: primarily applied to the pharmaceutical industry, this technique identifies the lowest cost among pharmaceutical alternatives that provide clinically comparable health outcomes.

- Cost-utility analysis: this measures the costs of therapy or treatment. Economists use the term *utility* to describe the amount of satisfaction a consumer receives from a given product or service. This analysis measures outcomes in terms of patient preference and is generally expressed as quality-adjusted life years. For example, an analysis of cancer chemotherapy drugs considers the various adverse side effects of these drugs because some patients may prefer a shorter duration of symptom-free survival rather than a longer life span marked by pain, suffering, and dependence on others for care.

HOPE observes in *Crisis, Hospitals and Healthcare* that "the financial sustainability of the United Kingdom was aggravated by the fact that the country was already in a situation of deficit in the period leading up to the crisis," which only served to worsen the country's situation. To combat a growing government deficit, the United Kingdom is focusing on increasing provider productivity, decreasing administrative and procurement expenses, and improving the efficiency and integration of health services.

FRANCE. The French health care system is based on the social insurance, or Bismarck, model. Virtually the entire population is covered by a legislated, compulsory health insurance plan that is financed through the social security system. Three major programs, and several smaller ones, are quasi-autonomous, nongovernmental bodies. Ybarra explains that the system is financed through employee and employer payroll tax contributions and that individuals pay 5.3% of their income toward the health care system. In "OECD Health Data—Frequently Requested Data," the OECD notes that the total expenditure for health in France was 11.6% in 2010.

The OECD reports that the public share of total health spending in 2010 was 77%, and 7.3% of expenditures represented direct, out-of-pocket payments. Physicians practicing in municipal health centers and in public hospitals are salaried, but physicians in private hospitals and in ambulatory care settings are typically paid on a negotiated, fee-for-service basis. The government establishes the reimbursement schedule for physicians and for other health care goods and services including pharmaceutical drugs. Public hospitals are granted lump-sum budgets, and private hospitals are paid on the basis of negotiated per diem payment rates. According to Ybarra, many employers offer their workers supplemental insurance as a benefit, and individuals can purchase private supplemental insurance to pay for pharmaceutical drugs, prostheses, dental care, and health care at private for-profit hospitals. The OECD reports that the number of hospital beds per 1,000 population declined from 8 in 2000 to 6.4 in 2010.

In April 1996 the French government announced major reforms aimed at containing rising costs in the national health care system. The new system monitored each patient's total health costs and penalized physicians if they overran their budgets for specific types of care and prescriptions. In addition, French citizens were required to consult general practitioners before going to specialists. Initially, physicians—specialists, in particular—denounced the reforms and warned that they could lead to rationing and compromise the quality of health care. Over time, however, these cost-containment efforts met with less resistance from physicians and consumers. By 2010 physicians and hospitals were generally accepting of moderate fee schedules, cost-sharing arrangements, and global budgeting to control costs.

In *Crisis, Hospitals and Healthcare*, HOPE describes the major challenges to the viability of the French health care system as instituting labor market reforms and competition and reducing the public deficit. In 2011 spending cuts were instituted to generate savings on health insurance and providers and efforts were under way to improve the efficiency of the health care system. For example, one strategy to reduce spending and incentivize delivery of quality care is a policy change that does not reimburse hospitals for emergency readmissions that occur within 30 days after hospital discharge.

Japan

Japan's health care financing is also based on the social insurance model and, in particular, on the German health care system. According to the OECD, in "OECD Health Data—Frequently Requested Data," 80.5% of health expenditures were from public funds in 2009. Three general programs cover the entire population: Employee Health Insurance, Community Health Insurance, and Health and Medical Services for the Aged. David Squires of the Commonwealth Fund indicates in "The Japanese Health Care System, 2011" (*International Profiles of Health Care Systems*, November 2011, http://www.commonwealthfund.org/) that 60% of the population obtains coverage through 3,500 insurers. Small businesses, the self-employed, and farmers are covered through Community Health Insurance, which is administered by a conglomeration of local governmental and private bodies. Older adults are covered by a separate plan that largely pools funds from the other plans. The Japanese health expenditure is below the expected level for a country with Japan's standard of living, and its emphasis is on the government, as opposed to business, bearing the major financial burden for the nation's health care.

The OECD indicates that the health care system, which cost 9.5% of Japan's GDP in 2009, is financed through employer and employee income-related premiums. There are different levels of public subsidization of the three general programs. Limited private insurance exists for supplemental coverage and is purchased by about one-third of the population. In 2009 out-of-pocket expenses accounted for 16% of health expenditures.

Physicians and hospitals are paid on the basis of national, negotiated fee schedules. Japan manages with fewer physicians per capita than most OECD member countries—just 2.2 physicians per 1,000 population in 2010. Physicians practicing in public hospitals are salaried, whereas those practicing in physician-owned clinics and private hospitals are reimbursed on a fee-for-service basis. The amount paid for each medical procedure is rigidly controlled. Physicians not only diagnose, treat, and manage illnesses but also prescribe and dispense pharmaceuticals, and a considerable portion of a physician's income is derived from dispensing prescription drugs.

A close physician-patient relationship is unusual in Japan; the typical physician tries to see as many patients as possible in a day to earn a living. A patient going to a clinic for treatment may have to wait many hours in a crowded facility. As a result, health care is rarely a joint physician-patient effort. Instead, physicians tend to dictate treatment without fully informing patients about their conditions or the tests, pharmaceutical drugs, and therapies that have been ordered or prescribed. Squires notes that in 2009 Japan boasted the highest number of physician contacts per person out of all the OECD member countries, at 13.9.

According to Squires, about 55% of Japan's hospitals are not-for-profit and privately operated. Hospitals are paid according to a uniform fee schedule, and for-profit hospitals are prohibited. Even though hospital admissions are less frequent, hospital stays in Japan are typically far longer than in the United States or in any other OECD member nation, allowing hospitals and physicians to overcome the limitations of the fee schedules.

The health status of the Japanese is one of the best in the world. Japanese men and women are among the longest living in all of the OECD member countries. In 2010 life expectancy was 83 years. The Japanese infant mortality rate in 2010, at 2.3 deaths per 1,000 live births, was bested only by Iceland (2.2). These two statistics are usually considered to be reliable indicators of a successful health care system. However, it should be noted that Japan does not have a large impoverished class, as the United States does, and its diet is considered to be among the healthiest in the world.

Squires explains that the disasters that beset Japan in 2011—the destructive earthquake, tsunami, and nuclear emergency—acted to generate a health crisis and devastated a substantial portion of the health care infrastructure, particularly in the regions that were hardest hit. The country is working to rebuild and restore needed services, and Squires observes that "these activities may offer an opportunity to improve upon the previous system, e.g., with improved health information technology infrastructure."

CHAPTER 8
CHANGE, CHALLENGES, AND INNOVATION IN HEALTH CARE DELIVERY

Since the 1970s the U.S. health care system has experienced rapid and unprecedented change. The sites where health care is delivered have shifted from acute inpatient hospitals to outpatient settings, such as ambulatory care and surgical centers, clinics, physicians' offices, and long-term care and rehabilitation facilities. Patterns of disease have changed from acute infectious diseases that require episodic care to chronic conditions that require ongoing care. Even threats to U.S. public health have changed—for example, epidemics of infectious diseases have largely been replaced by epidemics of chronic conditions such as obesity, diabetes, and mental illness. At the end of 2001 the threat of bioterrorism became an urgent concern of health care planners, providers, policy makers, and the American public; between 2009 and 2010 the nation was mobilized to mitigate the effects of the H1N1 pandemic influenza; and in 2010 the government took historic action by passing the Patient Protection and Affordable Care Act and the Health Care and Education Reconciliation Act (which are now commonly known as the ACA), which aim to provide health care coverage to nearly all of the nation's people.

There are new health care providers—midlevel practitioners (advanced practice nurses, certified nurse midwives, physician assistants, and medical technologists)—and new modes of diagnosis such as genetic testing. Furthermore, the rise of managed care, the explosion of biotechnology, and the availability of information on the Internet have dramatically changed how health care is delivered.

The ACA emphasizes the use of health information technology (IT), especially the adoption of electronic health records (EHRs). The act promotes the use of EHRs and other IT not only to help achieve the objectives of health care reform, including intensifying efforts to assess, monitor, and improve patient safety and quality of service delivery, but also to simplify the administration of health services, ensure cost-effective health service delivery, and reduce the growth of health care expenditures.

According to Chad Mather, Carolyn Hettrich, and Ryan Nunley, in "Penalties Coming under PPACA, PQRI" (*AAOS*, vol. 5, no. 1, January 2011), the ACA contains financial incentives and penalties that are aimed at improving the quality and coordination of care and reducing health care costs. It also requires regular and ongoing quality measurement and reporting.

Some health care industry observers suggest the speed at which these changes have occurred has further harmed an already complicated and uncoordinated health care system. There is concern that the present health care system cannot keep pace with scientific and technological advances. Many worry that the health care system is already unable to deliver quality care to all Americans and that it is so disorganized that it will be unable to meet the needs of the growing population of older Americans and the estimated 30 million Americans who will have health care coverage by 2014, or to respond to the threat of another pandemic or an act of bioterrorism.

This chapter considers several of the most pressing challenges and opportunities faced by the U.S. health care system. These include:

- Safety: ensuring safety by protecting patients from harm or injury inflicted by the health care system (e.g., preventing medical errors, reducing hospital-acquired infections, and safeguarding consumers from medical fraud). Besides actions to reduce problems caused by the health care system, safety and quality may be ensured by providers' use of clinical practice guidelines (e.g., standardized plans for diagnosis and treatment of disease and the effective application of technology to information and communication systems).

- Information management: IT, including the Internet, can provide health care providers and consumers with timely access to medical data, patient information, and the clinical expertise of specialists. For example, in *Using Electronic Health Records to Improve Quality and Efficiency: The Experiences of Leading Hospitals* (July 2, 2012, http://www.commonwealthfund.org/), Sharon Silow-Carroll, Jennifer N. Edwards, and Diana Rodin examine nine hospitals that instituted comprehensive EHR systems and find that these hospitals were able to improve patient safety and quality of care. The researchers conclude that "faster, more accurate communication and streamlined processes have led to improved patient flow, fewer duplicative tests, faster responses to patient inquiries, redeployment of transcription and claims staff, more complete capture of charges, and federal incentive payments." Furthermore, EHR systems are credited with improving the timeliness and accuracy of communication and coordination among providers and with patients, creating shorter lengths of stay, reducing numbers of readmissions, and restructuring the peer review processes that make it easier to pinpoint the causes of errors and take action to prevent them.

SAFETY

Patient safety is a critical component of health care quality. Even though the United States is generally viewed as providing quality health care services to its citizens, the Institute of Medicine (IOM) estimates in the landmark report *To Err Is Human: Building a Safer Health System* (1999, http://www.nap.edu/books/0309068371/html/) that as many as 98,000 American deaths per year are the result of preventable medical errors. More than 7,000 of these deaths are estimated to be due to preventable medication errors.

In 2012 HealthGrades, Inc., an independent health care quality research organization that grades hospitals based on a range of criteria and provides hospital ratings to health plans and other payers, issued its ninth update of the 1999 IOM report. In *Patient Safety and Satisfaction: The State of American Hospitals* (May 2012, https://www.cpmhealthgrades.com/CPM/assets/File/HealthGrades PatientSafetySatisfactionReport2012.pdf), HealthGrades finds that hospitals that received the highest patient ratings in physician and nursing communications had fewer patient safety issues as well as higher levels of patient satisfaction.

HealthGrades analyzed Medicare patient records and hospital survey data obtained from the Centers for Medicare and Medicaid Services (CMS) that included approximately 40 million Medicare hospitalizations in 5,000 hospitals to assess the mortality (death) and economic impact of medical errors and injuries that occurred during hospital admissions nationwide between April 2010 to March 2011. The analysis was performed using a method developed by the Agency for Healthcare Research and Quality (AHRQ) to calculate event rates (the rate at which an event occurs in a defined population over time) for indicators of patient safety.

The most significant patient safety findings from the HealthGrades report are:

- Between 2008 and 2010 a total of 254,200 potentially preventable patient safety events affecting hospitalized Medicare beneficiaries were identified. A total of 56,367 deaths occurred among Medicare patients experiencing one or more safety events.

- Patients at Patient Safety Excellence Award hospitals (the top 5% of hospitals) were nearly 48% less likely to experience a patient safety event, compared with hospitals in the bottom 5% in terms of the patient safety indicators.

AHRQ Patient Safety Indicators

The AHRQ has identified qualities and characteristics of organizational culture that contribute to or detract from patient safety in hospitals, clinics, and medical offices. Table 8.1 lists and defines the 10 composites (which include 38 individual indicators) that are used to assess the patient safety culture in medical offices. In *Medical Office Survey on Patient Safety Culture: 2012 User Comparative Database Report* (2012, http://www.ahrq.gov/qual/mosurvey12/mosurvey12pt1.pdf), Joann Sorra et al. report the results of a survey of 934 medical offices with a total of 23,679 medical office providers and staff respondents that was conducted between November 2009 and October 2011.

The key findings of the survey were (see Figure 8.1):

- Teamwork—84% of respondents said their practice engaged in teamwork

- Patient care tracking/follow-up—82% of respondents said their practice tracked and followed up with patients

- Quality and patient safety—76% of respondents said their practice was focused on quality and patient safety

- Work pressure and pace—46% of respondents answered positively about the pressure and pace of their practice

The AHRQ also surveys hospitals to assess selected aspects of hospital culture that are associated with patient safety. Figure 8.2 average percent of positive responses for each of 12 overall aspects of hospital patient safety that contain a total of 42 indicators measured in the 2012 hospital survey. The composite scores, which give each hospital equal weight rather than favoring larger hospitals with more survey respondents, show how hospitals fared on these indicators in 2012. The survey items with the highest average percent positive response (86%) were from the patient safety culture characteristic Teamwork within

TABLE 8.1

Indicators of patient safety in medical offices, 2012

Patient safety culture composite	Definition: The extent to which....
1. Communication about error	Staff are willing to report mistakes they observe and do not feel like their mistakes are held against them, and providers and staff talk openly about office problems and how to prevent errors from happening.
2. Communication openness	Providers in the office are open to staff ideas about how to improve office processes, and staff are encouraged to express alternative viewpoints and do not find it difficult to voice disagreement.
3. Office processes and standardization	The office is organized, has an effective workflow, has standardized processes for completing tasks, and has good procedures for checking the accuracy of work performed.
4. Organizational learning	The office has a learning culture that facilitates making changes in office processes to improve the quality of patient care and evaluates changes for effectiveness.
5. Overall perceptions of patient safety and quality	The quality of patient care is more important than getting more work done, office processes are good at preventing mistakes, and mistakes do not happen more than they should.
6. Owner/managing partner/leadership support for patient safety	Office leadership actively supports quality and patient safety, places a high priority on improving patient care processes, does not overlook mistakes, and makes decisions based on what is best for patients.
7. Patient care tracking/follow-up	The office reminds patients about appointments, documents how well patients follow treatment plans, follows up with patients who need monitoring, and follows up when reports from an outside provider are not received.
8. Staff training	The office provides staff with effective on-the-job training, trains staff on new processes, and does not assign staff tasks they have not been trained to perform.
9. Teamwork	The office has a culture of teamwork, mutual respect, and close working relationships among staff and providers.
10. Work pressure and pace	There are enough staff and providers to handle the patient load, and the office work pace is not hectic.

SOURCE: J. Sorra et al., "Table 1-1. Patient Safety Culture Composites and Definitions," in *Medical Office Survey on Patient Safety Culture: 2012 User Comparative Database Report*, Agency for Healthcare Research and Quality, 2012, http://www.ahrq.gov/qual/mosurvey12/mosurvey12pt1.pdf (accessed June 28, 2012)

FIGURE 8.1

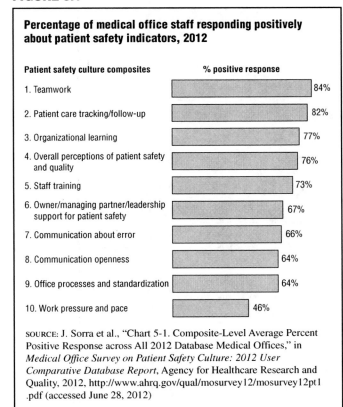

Percentage of medical office staff responding positively about patient safety indicators, 2012

Patient safety culture composites	% positive response
1. Teamwork	84%
2. Patient care tracking/follow-up	82%
3. Organizational learning	77%
4. Overall perceptions of patient safety and quality	76%
5. Staff training	73%
6. Owner/managing partner/leadership support for patient safety	67%
7. Communication about error	66%
8. Communication openness	64%
9. Office processes and standardization	64%
10. Work pressure and pace	46%

SOURCE: J. Sorra et al., "Chart 5-1. Composite-Level Average Percent Positive Response across All 2012 Database Medical Offices," in *Medical Office Survey on Patient Safety Culture: 2012 User Comparative Database Report*, Agency for Healthcare Research and Quality, 2012, http://www.ahrq.gov/qual/mosurvey12/mosurvey12pt1.pdf (accessed June 28, 2012)

Units: "People support one another in this unit" and "When a lot of work needs to be done quickly, we work together as a team to get the work done." The item with the lowest average percent positive response (35%) was from the patient safety culture characteristic Nonpunitive Response to Error: "Staff worry that mistakes they make are kept in their personnel file."

Figure 8.3 shows how survey respondents view their hospital work area or unit in terms of its overall patient safety. On average, most respondents were positive, with three-quarters awarding their work area or unit a patient safety grade of A (30%) or B (45%). Table 8.1 shows the measures used by the AHRQ to assess staff opinions about patient safety and medical errors and reporting safety problems, issues, and concerns. According to Sorra et al., more than half (55%) of the survey respondents had not reported any events in the past 12 months. The frequency of patient safety event reporting was deemed an area for improvement for most hospitals because underreporting of events suggests that potential patient safety problems may go undetected and, as a result, may not be addressed.

Strengthening Safety Measures

In response to a request from the U.S. Department of Health and Human Services (HHS), the IOM's Committee on Data Standards for Patient Safety created a detailed plan to develop standards for the collection, coding, and classification of patient safety information. The 550-page plan, *Patient Safety: Achieving a New Standard for Care* (2004), called on the HHS to assume the lead in establishing a national health information infrastructure that would provide immediate access to complete patient information and decision support tools, such as clinical practice guidelines, and capture patient safety data for use in designing constantly improving and safer health care delivery systems.

FIGURE 8.2

Hospital characteristics associated with patient safety, 2012

Survey item
% positive response

1. Team work within units

1. People support one another in this unit. — 86%

2. When a lot of work needs to be done quickly, we work together as a team to get the work done. — 86%

3. In this unit, people treat each other with respect. — 78%

4. When one area in this unit gets really busy, others help out. — 69%

2. Supv/mgr expectations & actions promoting patient safety

1. My supv/mgr says a good word when he/she sees a job done according to established patient safety procedures. — 73%

2. My supv/mgr seriously considers staff suggestions for improving patient safety. — 76%

3. Whenever pressure builds up, my supv/mgr wants us to work faster, even if it means taking shortcuts. — 74%

4. My supv/mgr overlooks patient safety problems that happen over and over. — 76%

3. Organizational learning—continuous improvement

1. We are actively doing things to improve patient safety. — 84%

2. Mistakes have led to positive changes here. — 64%

3. After we make changes to improve patient safety, we evaluate their effectiveness. — 69%

4. Management support for patient safety

1. Hospital management provides a work climate that promotes patient safety. — 81%

2. The actions of hospital management show that patient safety is a top priority. — 75%

3. Hospital management seems interested in patient safety only after an adverse event happens. — 61%

5. Overall perceptions of patient safety

1. It is just by chance that more serious mistakes don't happen around here. — 62%

2. Patient safety is never sacrificed to get more work done. — 64%

3. We have patient safety problems in this unit. — 64%

4. Our procedures and systems are good at preventing errors from happening. — 72%

6. Feedback & communication about error

1. We are given feedback about changes put into place based on event reports. — 56%

2. We are informed about errors that happen in this unit. — 65%

3. In this unit, we discuss ways to prevent errors from happening again. — 72%

7. Frequency of events reported

1. When a mistake is made, but is caught and corrected before affecting the patient, how often is this reported? — 57%

2. When a mistake is made, but has no potential to harm the patient, how often is this reported? — 59%

3. When a mistake is made that could harm the patient, but does not, how often is this reported? — 74%

FIGURE 8.2

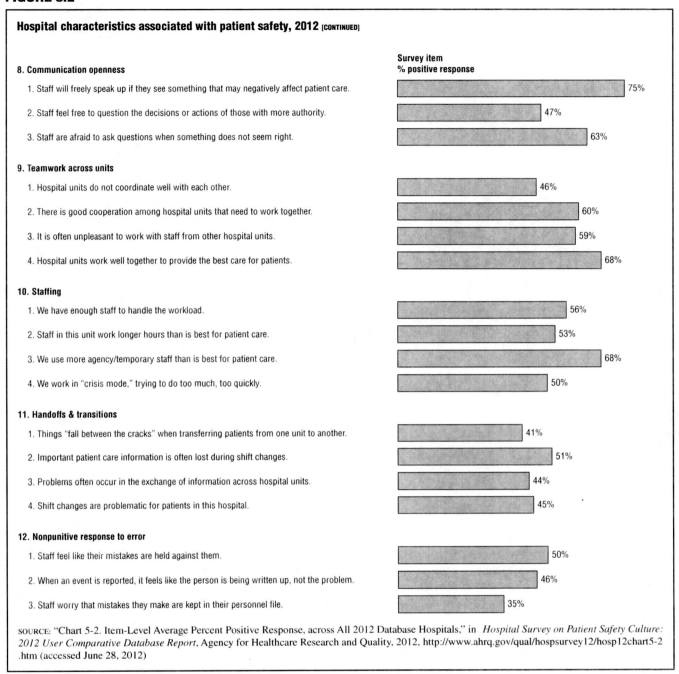

Hospital characteristics associated with patient safety, 2012 [CONTINUED]

Survey item
% positive response

8. Communication openness

1. Staff will freely speak up if they see something that may negatively affect patient care. — 75%

2. Staff feel free to question the decisions or actions of those with more authority. — 47%

3. Staff are afraid to ask questions when something does not seem right. — 63%

9. Teamwork across units

1. Hospital units do not coordinate well with each other. — 46%

2. There is good cooperation among hospital units that need to work together. — 60%

3. It is often unpleasant to work with staff from other hospital units. — 59%

4. Hospital units work well together to provide the best care for patients. — 68%

10. Staffing

1. We have enough staff to handle the workload. — 56%

2. Staff in this unit work longer hours than is best for patient care. — 53%

3. We use more agency/temporary staff than is best for patient care. — 68%

4. We work in "crisis mode," trying to do too much, too quickly. — 50%

11. Handoffs & transitions

1. Things "fall between the cracks" when transferring patients from one unit to another. — 41%

2. Important patient care information is often lost during shift changes. — 51%

3. Problems often occur in the exchange of information across hospital units. — 44%

4. Shift changes are problematic for patients in this hospital. — 45%

12. Nonpunitive response to error

1. Staff feel like their mistakes are held against them. — 50%

2. When an event is reported, it feels like the person is being written up, not the problem. — 46%

3. Staff worry that mistakes they make are kept in their personnel file. — 35%

SOURCE: "Chart 5-2. Item-Level Average Percent Positive Response, across All 2012 Database Hospitals," in *Hospital Survey on Patient Safety Culture: 2012 User Comparative Database Report*, Agency for Healthcare Research and Quality, 2012, http://www.ahrq.gov/qual/hospsurvey12/hosp12chart5-2 .htm (accessed June 28, 2012)

The IOM plan exhorted all health care settings to develop and implement comprehensive patient safety programs and recommended that the federal government launch patient safety research initiatives aimed at increasing knowledge, developing tools, and disseminating results to maximize the effectiveness of patient safety systems. The plan also advised the designation of a standardized format and terminology for identifying and reporting data related to medical errors.

In July 2005 President George W. Bush (1946–) signed into law the Patient Safety and Quality Improvement (PSQI) Act. Angela S. Mattie and Rosalyn Ben-Chitrit surmise in "Patient Safety Legislation: A Look at Health Policy Development" (*Policy, Politics, and Nursing Practice*, vol. 8, no. 4, November 2007) that the IOM call for action to improve patient safety in *To Err Is Human* is credited with heightening awareness of this issue and prompting Congress to pass legislation.

In "No Mention of Patient-Safety Legislation" (*Health Affairs*, vol. 29, no. 2, February 2010), William Riley of the University of Minnesota, Minneapolis, observes that the PSQI Act created a voluntary error reporting system. This

FIGURE 8.3

Hospital workers patient safety grades for their work areas, 2012

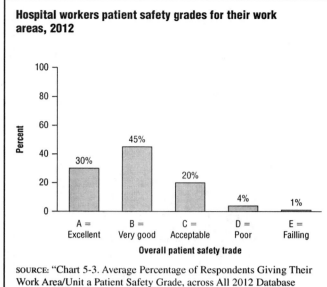

SOURCE: "Chart 5-3. Average Percentage of Respondents Giving Their Work Area/Unit a Patient Safety Grade, across All 2012 Database Hospitals," in *Hospital Survey on Patient Safety Culture: 2012 User Comparative Database Report*, Agency for Healthcare Research and Quality, 2012, http://www.ahrq.gov/qual/hospsurvey12/hosp12chart5-3 .htm (accessed June 28, 2012)

system, called a patient safety organization network, offers the opportunity to "prospectively prevent injury through analysis of mistakes and close calls that have been voluntarily reported by providers." It also protects providers from legal recourse when they report lapses in safety or instances of errors.

How Will the ACA Improve Patient Safety?

Barry R. Furrow of Drexel University states in "Regulating Patient Safety: The Patient Protection and Affordable Care Act" (*University of Pennsylvania Law Review*, vol. 159, May 10, 2011) that "ten years after the IOM report, the level of adverse events in hospitals has not improved in any major way." He explains that the ACA has a range of provisions that are aimed at improving the quality of the health care system by reducing errors and promoting patient safety. The act mandates and funds continuous, data-driven testing of the performance of health care professionals and facilities. It also funds demonstration projects of novel health care delivery systems and requires that their performance be measured and analyzed to determine whether they merit wider adoption. Furrow concludes that the ACA "offers a strong regulatory push toward the goal of 'flawless execution,' the health care equivalent of zero defects in industrial production."

The ACA also aims to improve health care quality and safety by supporting patient safety organizations (PSOs). The AHRQ explains in "Patient Safety Organization Information" (2012, http://www.pso.ahrq.gov/ psos/over view.htm) that "by providing both privilege and confidentiality, PSOs create a secure environment where clinicians and health care organizations can collect, aggregate, and analyze data, thereby improving quality by identifying and reducing the risks and hazards associated with patient care."

Who Is Responsible for Patient Safety?

Many federal, state, and private-sector organizations work together to reduce medical errors and improve patient safety. The Centers for Disease Control and Prevention (CDC) and the U.S. Food and Drug Administration (FDA) are the leading federal agencies that conduct surveillance and collect information about adverse events resulting from treatment or the use of medical devices, drugs, or other products. Mohammed Nabhan et al. observe in "What Is Preventable Harm in Healthcare? A Systematic Review of Definitions" (*BMC Health Services Research*, vol. 12, no. 128, May 25, 2012) that "reducing the risk of harm associated with the delivery of healthcare is a policy priority." In April 2011 the HHS formed the Partnership with Patients initiative. Funded by the ACA, this public-private partnership's goal is to reduce preventable harm by 40%.

The CMS acts to reduce medical errors for Medicare, Medicaid, and Children's Health Insurance Program beneficiaries through its peer review organizations. Peer review organizations concentrate on preventing delays in diagnosis and treatment that have adverse effects on health. The HHS explains in "Partnership for Patients: A Common Commitment" (2012, http://www.healthcare .gov/compare/partnership-for-patients/about/index.html) that in 2011 the CMS formed the Innovation Center, which has $500 million in funding to test models of safer care delivery and promote implementation of best practices in patient safety.

The U.S. Departments of Defense and Veterans Affairs (VA), which is responsible for health care services for U.S. military personnel, their families, and veterans, have instituted computerized systems that have reduced medical errors. The VA established the Centers of Inquiry for Patient Safety, and its hospitals also use bar-code technology and computerized medical records to prevent medical errors.

Safe medical care is also a top priority of the states and the private sector. In 2000 some of the nation's largest corporations, including General Motors and General Electric, joined together to address health care safety and efficacy (the ability of an intervention to produce the intended diagnostic or therapeutic effect in optimal circumstances) and to help direct their workers to health care providers (hospitals and physicians) with the best performance records. Called the Leapfrog Group (http:// www.leapfroggroup.org/), this business coalition was founded by the Business Roundtable, a national association of Fortune 500 chief executive officers, to leverage employer purchasing power that initiates innovation and improves the safety of health care.

The Leapfrog Group publishes hospital quality and safety data to assist consumers in making informed hospital choices. Hospitals provide information to the Leapfrog Group through a voluntary survey that requests information about hospital performance across four quality and safety practices with the potential to reduce preventable medical mistakes and improve health care quality. In "How Safe Is Your Hospital?" (June 6, 2012, http://www.leapfroggroup.org/policy_leadership/leapfrog _news/4894464), the Leapfrog Group notes that it issued safety scores to 2,652 general hospitals. Of the hospitals evaluated, 729 earned an A, 679 earned a B, and 1,243 earned a C or lower. Hospital safety scores are available to the public online at http://hospitalsafetyscore.org/. Website visitors can search for hospital scores for free; the site also offers information on how patients can protect themselves during a hospital stay.

PREVENTING MEDICAL ERRORS AND IMPROVING PATIENT SAFETY. In November 2007 the AHRQ and the Department of Defense launched TeamSTEPPS (http:// teamstepps.ahrq.gov/abouttoolsmaterials.htm), a program that aims to optimize patient outcomes by improving communication and other teamwork skills among health care professionals. TeamSTEPPS applies team training principles that were developed in military aviation and in private industry to health care delivery. Figure 8.4 shows the four competency areas that lead to improved team performance, attitude, and knowledge. TeamSTEPPS helps improve team performance by teaching:

- Leadership—how to direct, coordinate, assign tasks, motivate team members, and facilitate optimal performance

- Situation monitoring—how to develop common understandings of team environment, apply strategies to monitor teammate performance, and maintain a shared mental model

- Mutual support—how to anticipate other team members' needs through accurate knowledge and shift workload to achieve balance during periods of high workload or stress

- Communication—how to effectively exchange information among team members, regardless of how it is communicated

Professional societies are also concerned with patient safety. Over half of all the Joint Commission on Accreditation of Healthcare Organizations' (JCAHO) hospital standards pertain to patient safety. Since 2002 hospitals seeking accreditation from the JCAHO have been required to adhere to stringent patient safety standards

FIGURE 8.4

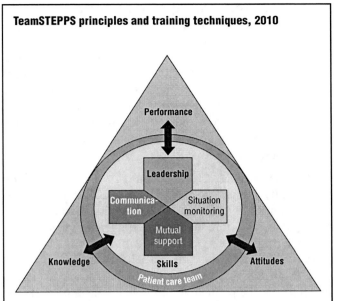

TeamSTEPPS principles and training techniques, 2010

SOURCE: "What Will Our Teams Learn?" in *TeamSTEPPS Leadership Briefing Slides*, Agency for Healthcare Research and Quality, 2010, http://teamstepps.ahrq.gov/abouttoolsmaterials.htm (accessed June 28, 2012)

to prevent medical errors. The JCAHO standards also require hospitals and individual health care providers to inform patients when they have been harmed in the course of treatment. The goal of these standards is to prevent medical errors by identifying actions and systems that are likely to produce problems before they occur. An example of this type of preventive measure, which is called prospective review, is close scrutiny of hospital pharmacies to be certain that the ordering, preparation, and dispensing of medications is accurate. Similar standards have been developed for JCAHO-accredited nursing homes, outpatient clinics, laboratories, and managed care organizations.

On January 1, 2004, the JCAHO began surveying and evaluating health care organizations using new medication management standards. The new standards revise and consolidate existing standards and place even greater emphasis on medication safety. The revised standards increase the role of pharmacists in managing appropriate and safe medication use and strengthen their authority to implement organization-wide improvements in medication safety.

In "Proposed National Patient Safety Goal (NPSG)" (November 14, 2011, http://www.jointcommission.org/ assets/1/6/HAP_NPSG_Overuse_Rpt_2011-11-14.pdf), the JCAHO states its national patient safety goal for 2013: to prevent the misuse and overuse of tests and treatments. The JCAHO instituted a program intended to help achieve this goal by identifying medical procedures that, when used improperly, may harm patients.

Examples of such tests and procedures are early elective induction of labor (inducing deliveries for pregnancies of 39 weeks gestation or less in patients with no known medical conditions that warrant early delivery) and insertion of tubes in the ears of children with middle ear infections for less than 60 days with no other symptoms. By naming inappropriate indications for specific tests, treatments, and procedures and initiating effective performance improvement methods to prevent these health services from being performed inappropriately, patient safety should be improved.

HOSPITALS DESIGNED FOR SAFETY. In "Innovations and Quality Tools" (September 12, 2012, http://www .innovations.ahrq.gov/innovations_qualitytools.aspx), the AHRQ describes initiatives and strategies that hospitals and other health service providers can implement to improve patient safety. Service delivery innovations that were evaluated and presented in 2012 include a set of guidelines to help prevent the development of pressure ulcers, a "strategic nap program" to help health care workers avoid making medical errors caused by sleep deprivation, and a program combining physician-led, multidisciplinary rounds and practice guidelines to reduce the rate of nosocomial (acquired or occurring in the hospital) infections in intensive care units.

In "Effect of Bar-Code Technology on the Safety of Medication Administration" (*New England Journal of Medicine*, vol. 362, no. 18, May 6, 2010), Eric G. Poon et al. look at the frequency of medication errors before and after the implementation of bar-code technology to verify a patient's identity and the medication to be administered. The researchers find that the bar-code technology significantly reduced the rate of medication errors—errors in administering medication were reduced by 41% and there was a 51% reduction in potential adverse effects resulting from these errors. Poon et al. conclude that because the hospital where they conducted the study administers about 5.9 million doses of medication per year, the use of bar-code technology is anticipated to prevent 95,000 potential adverse drug events.

CLINICAL PRACTICE GUIDELINES

Clinical practice guidelines (CPGs) are evidence-based protocols—documents that advise health care providers about how to diagnose and treat specific medical conditions and diseases. CPGs offer physicians, nurses, other health care practitioners, health plans, and institutions objective, detailed, and condition- or disease-specific action plans.

Widespread dissemination and use of CPGs began during the 1990s in an effort to improve the quality of health care delivery by giving health care professionals access to current scientific information on which to base clinical decisions. The use of guidelines also aimed to enhance quality by standardizing care and treatment throughout a health care delivery system such as a managed care plan or hospital and throughout the nation.

Early attempts to encourage physicians and other health professionals to use CPGs was met with resistance, because many physicians rejected CPGs as formulaic "cookbook medicine" and believed they interfered with physician-patient relationships. Over time, however, physicians were educated about the quality problems that resulted from variations in medical practice, and opinions about CPGs gradually changed. Physician willingness to use CPGs also increased when they learned that adherence to CPGs offered some protection from medical malpractice and other liability. Nurses and other health professionals more readily adopted CPGs, presumably because their training and practice was oriented more toward following instructions than physicians' practices had been.

The National Guideline Clearinghouse (http:// www.guideline.gov/) is a database of CPGs that have been produced by the AHRQ in conjunction with the American Medical Association and the American Association of Health Plans. The clearinghouse offers guideline summaries and comparisons of guidelines covering the same disease or condition prepared by different sources and serves as a resource for the exchange of guidelines between practitioners and health care organizations.

CPGs vary depending on their source. All recovery and treatment plans, however, are intended to generate the most favorable health outcomes. Federal agencies such as the U.S. Public Health Service and the CDC, as well as professional societies, managed care plans, hospitals, academic medical centers, and health care consulting firms, have produced their own versions of CPGs.

Practically all guidelines assume that treatment and healing will occur without complications. Because CPGs represent an optimistic approach to treatment, they are not used as the sole resource for development or evaluation of treatment plans for specific patients. CPGs are intended for use in conjunction with evaluation by qualified health professionals able to determine the applicability of a specific CPG to the specific circumstances involved. Modification of the CPGs is often required and advisable to meet specific, organizational objectives of health care providers and payers.

It is unrealistic to expect that all patients will obtain ideal health outcomes as a result of health care providers' use of CPGs. Guidelines may have greater utility as quality indicators. Evaluating health care delivery against CPGs enables providers, payers, and policy makers to identify and evaluate care that deviates from CPGs as part of a concerted program of continuous improvement of health care quality.

COMMUNICATION AND INFORMATION MANAGEMENT TECHNOLOGIES

The explosion of communication and information management technologies has already revolutionized health care delivery and holds great promise for the future. Health care data can be easily and securely collected, shared, stored, and used to promote research and development over great geographic distances and across traditionally isolated industries. Online distance learning programs for health professionals and the widespread availability of reliable consumer health information on the Internet have increased understanding and awareness of the causes and treatment of illness. This section describes several recent applications of technology to the health care system.

Telemedicine

The term *telemedicine* describes a variety of interactions that occur by way of telephone lines. Telemedicine may be as simple and commonplace as a conversation between a patient and a health professional in the same town or as sophisticated as surgery directed via satellite and video technology from one continent to another.

Anita Majerowicz and Susan Tracy describe in "Bridging Gaps in Healthcare Delivery" (*Journal of the American Health Information Management Association*, vol. 81, no. 5, May 2010) the benefits of telemedicine, including:

- Reduced healthcare costs

- Increased patient access to providers, especially in medically underserved areas

- Improved quality and continuity of care

- Faster and more convenient treatment resulting in reduction of lost work time and travel costs for patients

In "The Doctor Will See You Now. Please Log On" (*New York Times*, May 29, 2010), Milt Freudenheim reports that in North America the interactive telemedicine market has grown about 10% each year; in 2010 alone it generated an estimated $500 million in revenue. An example of interactive telemedicine is Internet or telephone-enabled video-teleconferencing, which creates a meeting between a patient and primary care physician in one location and a physician specialist elsewhere when a face-to-face consultation is not feasible because of time or distance. Peripheral equipment even enables the physician specialist to perform a virtual physical examination and hear the patient's heart sounds through a stethoscope. The availability of desktop videoconferencing has expanded this form of telemedicine from a novelty found exclusively in urban, university teaching hospitals to a valuable tool for patients and physicians in rural areas who were previously underserved and unable to access specialists readily.

Another application of telemedicine is transtelephonic pacemaker monitoring. (Cardiac pacemakers are battery-operated implanted devices that maintain normal heart rhythm.) Cardiac technicians at the device monitoring company are able to check the implanted cardiac pacemaker's functions, including the status of its battery. Transtelephonic pacemaker monitoring is able to identify early signs of possible pacemaker failure and detect potential pacemaker system abnormalities, thereby reducing the number of emergency replacements. It can also send an electrocardiogram rhythm strip to the patient's cardiologist (physician specialist in heart diseases).

Freudenheim notes that the entire telemedicine market, which includes health care applications for smart phones and in-home monitoring devices that relay patient data using telephone lines, is about $3.9 billion. Medicare and Medicaid reimburse physicians and hospitals that provide remote care to patients in rural, underserved regions, and some private insurers offer coverage of interactive video technologies. Because the ACA allocates about $1 billion annually for research into telemedicine and other health care innovations, industry observers predict continuing growth in the development and utilization of this technology.

Despite the promise and growing popularity of telemedicine, Freudenheim observes that several groups, including state regulators at the Texas Medical Board, caution that physicians who conduct remote consultations might miss subtle medical indicators. The American Academy of Family Physicians is not opposed to telemedicine; however, the professional society encourages patients to maintain a direct relationship with a physician who can monitor their health and treatment.

Telemedicine appears to improve patient outcomes. For example, Kate Johnson reports in "Telemedicine Improves Diabetes Management in Rural Areas" (*Medscape Medical News*, May 24, 2012) the results of a study that was presented at the annual meeting of the American Association of Clinical Endocrinologists in May 2012. The study indicated that in rural areas where patients may travel hundreds of miles to see a physician specialist and wait months for an appointment, telemedicine is a promising way to deliver needed care. The study consisted of 66 patients with multiple endocrine and metabolic disorders including diabetes, dyslipidemia (abnormal amounts of lipids such as cholesterol and triglycerides in the blood), and thyroid disease. The researchers found that patients who were interviewed and examined via video conferencing were comfortable with this approach to medical care and showed significant improvement in their diabetes management.

Telemedicine has been used in schools to improve access to care, treat middle ear infections, and increase appropriate referral to specialists. It has also proven beneficial in helping manage asthma in school-aged children. David A. Bergman et al. note in "The Use of Telemedicine Access to Schools to Facilitate Expert Assessment of Children with Asthma" (*International Journal of Telemedicine and Applications*, 2008) that asthma care was improved through a telemedicine link between an asthma specialist and a school-based asthma program, which involved real-time video and audio conferencing between the patient and school nurse on site at the school and the asthma specialist at San Francisco General Hospital. The researchers find that the program produced significant improvements in health status outcomes and note that the use of telemedicine ensured that children identified with asthma received comprehensive assessments, action plans, and asthma education. Bergman et al. conclude that telemedicine "allowed for a more efficient use of the asthma subspecialist's time when contrasted with hospital-based asthma clinics."

In "Effect of Telephone-Administered vs Face-to-Face Cognitive Behavioral Therapy on Adherence to Therapy and Depression Outcomes among Primary Care Patients: A Randomized Trial" (*Journal of the American Medical Association*, vol. 307, no. 21, June 6, 2012), David C. Mohr et al. report the results of a study comparing cognitive behavioral therapy (CBT; a type of psychotherapy that attempts to help patients replace negative thoughts and feelings with more positive, optimistic approaches and actions) delivered face to face or transtelephonically. The researchers find that CBT by telephone is as effective as administering it face to face. The benefits of CBT by telephone include the fact it appears to overcome barriers to access, such as travel time, especially for people living in remote or rural locations. It also has a higher patient retention rate.

Telemedicine has also proven to be a cost-effective alternative to psychiatric hospitalization. Caroline Cassels reports in "Telemental Health Dramatically Cuts Psychiatric Hospitalization Rates" (*Medscape Medical News*, May 9, 2012) the results of a study that was presented at the American Psychiatric Association's 2012 annual meeting. The large-scale study, which analyzed four years of data on 98,609 mental health patients between 2006 and 2010, showed that delivering telemental health services via high-definition video transmission to patients in rural areas dramatically reduced psychiatric hospitalization rates.

Telemedicine may lower costs by reducing hospitalization, but other research reports improved patient outcomes using telehealth (the remote exchange of data between the patient and the clinician as part of health care management) with only modest cost savings. In "Effect of Telehealth on Use of Secondary Care and Mortality: Findings from the Whole System Demonstrator Cluster Randomised Trial" (*BMJ*, vol. 344, no. 3874,

June 21, 2012), Adam Steventon et al. analyzed the records of 3,230 patients with chronic health conditions (diabetes, chronic obstructive pulmonary disease, and heart failure), some of whom received telehealth services and some of whom did not. The researchers find that patients who received telehealth services had lower mortality rates and fewer emergency hospital admissions than those who did not receive telehealth care. The modest cost savings observed were attributed to lower utilization of hospital services.

Online Patient-Physician Consultations

Saurage Marketing Research conducted a survey in November and December 2011 and reported the results in "Online Access to Doctors" (2012, http://saurageresearch.com/key-findings-november-december-2011/#5). The research firm finds that nearly three-quarters (73%) of Americans said they want to access their physicians' offices online. The majority (81%) want to schedule appointments online, 68% want to go online to refill prescriptions, 62% want to see lab results online, 59% want to complete medical forms online, and 53% want to be able to view and pay bills online.

Physicians appear to be eager to respond to their patients' wishes for online communication. Chris Gullo reports in "Half of Doctors to Use Medical Apps in 2012" (*MobiHealthNews*, November 16, 2012) on CompTIA's "Third Annual Healthcare IT Insights and Opportunities," a physician survey that was conducted in 2011. Gullo notes that 61% of physicians use telemedicine for continuing medical education, 44% use it for specialist referrals, and 37% use it for general patient consultations. Ten percent of the physicians surveyed said they plan to use video conferencing with patients in the coming year.

Crystale Purvis Cooper et al. surveyed primary care physicians to find out which ones are using e-mail to communicate with patients and frequenting social networking sites and reported their findings in "Physicians Who Use Social Media and Other Internet-Based Communication Technologies" (*Journal of the American Informatics Association*, May 25, 2012). The researchers find that even though the majority (80.6%) of physicians use a portable device to access the Internet, just 12.9% write a blog. More than half (59%) use social networking sites, 49% correspond with patients via e-mail, 41% listen to podcasts, 22% use widgets, and 19% use Really Simple Syndication feeds (delivery of news or other information directly using a web format rather than via e-mail).

In "How to Get Paid for Online Consults" (*American Medical News*, March 22, 2010), Pamela Lewis Dolan reports that "a growing number of insurers are paying for online communication between physicians and patients. And when insurers don't cover it, many patients are willing to pay out of pocket for the convenience." Dolan explains that e-mail exchanges between patients and their physicians are considered to be billable when they address "a specific problem not associated with a prior visit, online or in-office, within the previous seven days." E-mail that is sent as follow-up to a visit that occurred within the past seven days, such as an e-mail that details laboratory test results or requests a prescription refill, cannot be billed separately.

One important advantage of electronic encounters (e-encounters) over telephone conversations is the patient's ability to communicate home monitoring results such as blood pressure or blood glucose levels in a format that is easily included as documentation in the patient's permanent (paper or electronic) medical record. Another advantage is that less time devoted to telephone calls improves the efficiency of the physician's office, thereby boosting productivity and potentially reducing practice expenses.

Concerns about e-encounters center on privacy and security of patient information exchanged and physician reimbursement for the time spent in electronic correspondence with patients. Besides legal and privacy issues, some industry observers suggest that guidelines should be developed for e-encounters to ensure that they are clinically appropriate and are not used as substitutes for needed, but more costly, face-to-face office visits.

Despite promising research findings about the benefits of e-mail correspondence between patients and physicians and increasing consumer demand for e-mail, instant messaging, and texting, industry observers caution that the shift toward e-encounters could create additional expectations for physicians. For example, in "The Future of Your Medical Data" (*Scientific American*, April 12, 2010), Katherine Harmon asserts that physicians could face liability challenges if they fail to address certain information that is contained in an e-mail. Experts also note that e-encounters could raise new reimbursement issues and introduce time pressures that interrupt physicians' already busy work schedules.

Richard J. Baron of Greenhouse Internists in Philadelphia, Pennsylvania, asserts in "What's Keeping Us So Busy in Primary Care? A Snapshot from One Practice" (*New England Journal of Medicine*, vol. 362, no. 17, April 29, 2010) that he and his colleagues respond to an average of 16.8 e-mails per day. Baron states that "59.3% were for the interpretation of test results, 21.7% were for response to patients (either initiated by patients through the practice's interactive Web site or as part of an e-mail dialogue with patients), 9.3% were for administrative problems, 5.0% were for acute problems, 2.8% were for proactive outreach to patients, and 1.9% were for discussions with consultants."

TECHNOLOGY MAY HELP EDUCATE MORE NURSES. One key factor limiting the supply of nurses is a shortage of nursing faculty, which restricts class size and ultimately the numbers of nurses graduating each year. According to the American Association of Colleges of Nursing, in "Nursing Faculty Shortage" (April 2, 2012, http://www.aacn.nche.edu/media-relations/fact-sheets/nursing-faculty-shortage/), in 2009 there were more than 10,000 nursing faculty position vacancies and in 2011–12 approximately 75,587 qualified applicants were turned away from nursing schools because of a lack of faculty. One way to remedy this situation may be to offer some nursing courses online. In "Transforming a RN to BSN Program to an On-line Delivery Format" (*Kentucky Nurse*, vol. 60, no. 1, 2012), Cathy H. Abell, Deborah Williams, and M. Susan Jones of Western Kentucky University describe the transformation of a registered nurse (RN) program that uses a combination of traditional classes and online learning to a bachelor of science in nursing (BSN) program that is completely online. They deem the transformation a success and conclude, "The RN to BSN faculty perceive the on-line program as essential for the seamless transition toward a higher academic degree. They are committed to offering this program as a means for nurses who are place bound to achieve the BSN."

Patricia Allen, Yvonne VanDyke, and Myrna L. Armstrong describe in "'Growing Your Own' Nursing Staff with a Collaborative Accelerated Second-Degree, Web-Based Program" (*Journal of Continuing Education in Nursing*, vol. 41, no. 3, March 2010) the success of an online accelerated degree program that is designed to produce new baccalaureate-prepared nurses. The researchers report that graduates of the program feel well prepared and have excellent career prospects following graduation.

MORE STAFF, RATHER THAN TECHNOLOGY, IS KEY TO IMPROVING PATIENT SAFETY AND QUALITY OF CARE. Despite rapid advances in technology, many industry observers feel that it is not sufficient to solve the nursing shortage that the U.S. Bureau of Labor Statistics projects in "The 30 Occupations with the Largest Projected Number of Total Job Openings Due to Growth and Replacements, 2010–20" (February 1, 2012, http://www.bls.gov/news.release/ecopro.t10.htm) will require over 1.1 million replacement nurses by 2020. In "The Recent Surge in Nurse Employment: Causes and Implications" (*Health Affairs*, vol. 28, no. 4, July–August 2009), Peter I. Buerhaus, David I. Auerbach, and Douglas O. Staiger observe that even though the nursing shortage slowed as a result of the economic recession, it is still forecast to reach 260,000 registered nurses by 2025—twice as large as any U.S. nursing shortage since the mid-1960s. The researchers identify the retirement of older nurses as the key contributor to the anticipated shortfall.

According to Annette Richardson and Julie Storr, in "Patient Safety: A Literature Review on the Impact of Nursing Empowerment, Leadership, and Collaboration"

(*International Nursing Review*, vol. 57, no. 1, March 2010), because of their proximity to patients, nurses are in an ideal position to drive safety and quality initiatives. The researchers conducted a comprehensive review of the relevant literature and conclude that nursing leadership, collaboration, and empowerment can exert a demonstrable impact on patient safety.

Promise of Robotics

One technological advance that promises to reduce hospital operating costs and enable hospital workers to spend more time caring for patients is the use of robots. Once relegated to the realm of science fiction, automated machines such as self-guided robots to perform many routine hospital functions have seen a resurgence in the 21st century.

In "Hospital Robots of the Future" (Hospitalmanagement.net, April 29, 2010), Chris Lo describes several novel uses of robotics in hospitals: self-guiding robots that deliver and dispense medication; robots that enable physicians to perform remote, real-time consultations and communicate with patients at a distance; and robots that monitor critically ill patients in the intensive care unit. According to Kawanza Newson, in "Robot Now Makes Tracks through Hospital" (*Milwaukee [Wisconsin] Journal Sentinel*, March 31, 2008), the Children's Hospital of Wisconsin uses a robotic cart that looks like a train. The robot warns onlookers to "pardon my caboose" when it backs up and makes deliveries of oxygen monitors and feeding pumps. Newson quotes Sarah Currie, a patient care manager, who explains that "people are such a precious resource, so any time you have a chance to outsource and keep the people in contact with patients, it's a good thing. Having [the robot] has improved the waiting time for getting patients to tests quicker."

Some robots are involved in more than simply routine, menial tasks. Barnaby J. Feder notes in "Prepping Robots to Perform Surgery" (*New York Times*, May 4, 2008) that a growing number of surgeons delegate much of their work to medical robots controlled from computer consoles. The robotic system allows a cardiovascular surgeon to perform heart surgery without touching the patient, or a urologist to ensure precise, tremor-free incisions to prevent damage to delicate nerves during prostate surgery. Seated at a console with a computer and video monitor, the surgeon uses handgrips and foot pedals to manipulate robotic arms that hold scalpels, sutures, and other surgical instruments to perform the operation. These robotic systems have been approved for use by the FDA, and in 2008 they represented a $1 billion segment of the medical device industry.

Newer surgical robots are miniature versions that can be inserted through a laparoscope. Bhavin C. Shah et al. describe in "Miniature in Vivo Robotics and Novel Robotic Surgical Platforms" (*Urology Clinics of North America*, vol. 36, no. 2, May 2009) miniature robots that are equipped with cameras and guided by a joystick. These miniature robots can be inserted into the abdominal cavity or peritoneal cavity to perform diagnostic imaging and assist with surgical tasks. They can also be inserted through small orifices or swallowed and can remain implanted for months to perform specific tasks. Shah et al. explain that "small fully implantable robots can be manipulated from the outside with much less force and trauma to the tissues, allowing for more precision and delicate handling of surgical fields."

Some skeptics feel that the effectiveness of robotic surgery has not yet been rigorously evaluated nor has it been compared with other surgical techniques. For example, in "Surgical Robots: Worth the Investment?" (*Hospitals & Health Networks*, vol. 86, no. 4, April 2012), Geri Aston observes that increasing the use of robotic surgery raises concerns about health care spending, the comparative effectiveness of various treatment options, and the pace at which new technology is adopted. Aston reports that more than 1,200 hospitals have invested as much as $2 million in a specific robotic system, but notes that there is considerable controversy among surgeons about the benefits of robotic procedures versus traditional approaches. Advocates assert that the presence of this technology permits more minimally invasive surgeries, attracts surgeons who want to use it, and increases a hospital's market share because the hospital has technology that is popular among physicians and patients alike. Skeptics worry that robots have been rapidly integrated into clinical practice, with only minimal research supporting their effectiveness. Jason D. Wright, an assistant professor of women's health, calls for additional research to resolve this question, "This is an expensive, new and unproven technology, so it is an ideal situation for doing comparative effectiveness studies."

INNOVATION SUPPORTS QUALITY HEALTH CARE DELIVERY

The health care industry is awash in wave after wave of new technologies, models of service delivery, reimbursement formulae, legislative and regulatory changes, and increasingly specialized personnel ranks. Creating change in hospitals and in other health care organizations requires an understanding of diffusion—the process and channels by which new ideas are communicated, spread, and adopted throughout institutions and organizations. Diffusion of technology involves all the stakeholders in the health care system: policy makers and regulatory agencies establish safety and efficacy, government and private payers determine reimbursement, vendors of the technology are compared and one is selected, hospitals and health professionals adopt the technology and are trained in its use, and consumers are informed about the benefits of the new technology.

The decision to adopt new technology involves a five-stage process beginning with knowledge about the innovation. The second stage is persuasion, the period when decision makers form opinions based on experience and knowledge. Decision is the third phase, when commitment is made to a trial or pilot program, and is followed by implementation, the stage during which the new technology is put in place. The process concludes with the confirmation stage, the period during which the decision makers seek reinforcement for their decision to adopt and implement the new technology.

Communicating Quality

As the provisions of the ACA take effect, industry observers hope that consumers armed with data about comparative costs and quality will be better able to make informed health care purchases—choosing providers that offer quality care and competitive fees. In "An Experiment Shows That a Well-Designed Report on Costs and Quality Can Help Consumers Choose High-Value Health Care" (*Health Affairs*, vol. 31, no. 3, March 2012), Judith H. Hibbard et al. examine how employees choose health care providers. The researchers find that health care consumers generally equate quality with cost and mistakenly believe that higher cost providers deliver better care. Regardless, consumers are more concerned about the quality of care than its cost, so when they are provided with cost data along with easy-to-interpret quality information that highlights high-value (optimal combinations of quality and cost) options, the consumers are more likely to choose the high-value options. Hibbard et al. conclude that presenting cost and quality data in a user-friendly format "will help consumers understand that a doctor who provides higher-quality care than other doctors does not necessarily cost more."

In "Evidence That Consumers Are Skeptical about Evidence-Based Health Care" (*Health Affairs*, vol. 29, no. 7, July 2010), Kristin L. Carman et al. considered how consumers define and characterize quality care. The researchers were especially interested in finding out the extent to which consumers understand and appreciate evidence-based health care, which encompasses a range of actions including use of evidence-based practice guidelines, shared decision making, comparative effectiveness research, and transparency of cost and quality information. Consumer attitudes and beliefs about evidence-based health care are of increasing importance because the ACA emphasizes its use. Carman et al. assert that if consumers do not understand evidence-based care or do not view it as a useful way to inform their decisions about providers and treatments, the move to incorporate it in the emerging health care delivery system will not be successful.

Carman et al. report that consumers' beliefs, values, and knowledge were not consistent with what policy makers prescribe as evidence-based health care. There was little understanding and considerable confusion about the meaning of terms such as *medical evidence* and *quality guidelines*. Most consumers continued to believe that when it comes to health care, more care, more costly care, and newer treatments are always better. These gaps in knowledge and misconceptions about the characteristics of quality care may mean that considerable consumer education will be required before consumers can become fully engaged in evidence-based decision making.

In response to these findings, Carman et al. developed a communication toolkit that aims to "enable employers and unions to communicate with consumers about evidence-based health care and help them become active participants in their care through customizable materials that translate these concepts into clear, simple, and relevant language." The researchers report that the toolkit was favorably received by employers and other health care purchasers, health plans, and provider organizations and that in 2010 efforts were under way to help bridge "the gap between the need for evidence-based health care and the consumers' current perceptions of it."

MAKING THE GRADE: HEALTH CARE REPORT CARDS. The publication of medical outcomes report cards and disease- and procedure-specific morbidity rates (the degree of disability caused by disease) and mortality rates (the number of deaths caused by disease) has attracted widespread media attention and sparked controversy. Advocates for the public release of clinical outcomes and other performance measures contend that despite some essential limitations, these studies offer consumers, employers, and payers the means for comparing health care providers.

Some skeptics question the clinical credibility of scales such as surgical mortality, which they claim are incomplete indicators of quality. Others cite problems with data collection or speculate that data are readily manipulated by providers to enhance marketing opportunities sufficient to compromise the utility and validity of published reports. Long term, the effects of published comparative evaluation of health care providers on network establishment, contracting, and exclusion from existing health plans are uncertain and in many instances may be punitive (damaging). Hospitals and medical groups may be forced to compete for network inclusion on the basis of standardized performance measures.

The number of websites that rate physicians and hospitals continues to grow, with Angie's List and Vitals .com joining more established sites such as Health.org and HealthGrades.com. The sites describe physicians' training, experience, certification, and any disciplinary actions taken against them, as well as patient ratings. They also encourage physicians to respond to patient comments. Some industry observers contend that the sites, especially those that use anonymous ratings, have the potential to further erode patient-physician relationships by prompting physicians to behave defensively. Guodong Gordon Gao et al. find in "A Changing Landscape of Physician Quality Reporting: Analysis of Patients' Online Ratings of Their Physicians over a 5-Year Period" (*Journal of Medical Internet Research*, vol. 14, no. 1, February 24, 2012) that despite the proliferation of these websites, and increasing consumer use of them, both to consult and to post comments and reviews, little is known about the characteristics that influence physician ratings or how these ratings relate to quality. The researchers scrutinized more than 386,000 physician ratings between 2005 and 2010 and find that younger physicians, who had graduated from medical school after 2000, received more favorable ratings than older physicians. Board-certified physicians and those who had graduated from one of the top 50 U.S. medical schools received higher ratings than those who were not board certified.

Interestingly, Gao et al. note that consumers were quite positive in their assessments of their physicians and more critical in their ratings of staff and punctuality. The researchers report that even though physicians are concerned that online ratings are simply a venue for disgruntled patients to vent their complaints, their findings indicate that this is not the case—nearly half the rated physicians received perfect scores. Gao et al. conclude that "online ratings appear to be driven by patients who are delighted with their physicians."

Despite legitimate concern about the objectivity, reliability, validity, and potential for manipulating data, there is consensus that scrutiny and dissemination of quality data will escalate. Business groups and employers continue to request physician, hospital, and health plan data to design their health benefit programs. When choosing between health plans involving the same group of participating hospitals and physicians, employers request plan-specific information to guide their decisions. Companies and employer-driven health care coalitions seeking to assemble their own provider networks rely on physician- and hospital-specific data, such as the quality data provided by HealthGrades, during the selection process.

The most beneficial use of the data is not to be punitive, but to be inspiring to improve health care delivery systematically. When evidence of quality problems is identified, health plans and providers must be prepared to launch a variety of interventions to address and promptly resolve problems.

CHAPTER 9

PUBLIC OPINION ABOUT THE HEALTH CARE SYSTEM

As with many other social issues, public opinion about health care systems, providers, plans, coverage, and benefits varies in response to a variety of personal, political, and economic forces. Personal experience and the experience of friends, family, and community opinion leaders (trusted sources of information such as members of the clergy, prominent physicians, and local business and civic leaders) exert powerful influences on public opinion. Health care marketing executives have known for years that the most potent advertising any hospital, medical group, or managed care plan can have is not a full-page newspaper advertisement or prime-time television ad campaign. It is positive word-of-mouth publicity.

The influence of the news media, advertising, and other attempts to sway health care consumers' attitudes and purchasing behaviors cannot be overlooked. A single story about a miraculous medical breakthrough or life-saving procedure can reflect favorably on an entire hospital or health care delivery system. Similarly, a lone mistake, an adverse reaction to a drug, or a misstep by a single health care practitioner can impugn (attack as lacking integrity) a hospital, managed care plan, or pharmaceutical company for months or even years, prompting intense media scrutiny of every action taken by the practitioner, facility, or organization.

Political events, the economy, and pending legislation can focus public attention on a particular health care concern, supplant one health-related issue with another, or eclipse health care from public view altogether. For example, in 2009 and 2010 federal, state, and local government officials implemented successful plans to contain the H1N1 influenza pandemic in the United States. During the same period there was heated debate about the scope and provisions of health care reform legislation, which did not subside even after the March 2010 passage of the Patient Protection and Affordable Care Act and the

Health Care and Education Reconciliation Act (which are now commonly known as the ACA).

In fact, opposition to the ACA mounted with questions about the constitutionality of many of its provisions, such as requiring individuals to obtain health insurance coverage (called the individual mandate) and officials from 26 states filed a lawsuit against the ACA. The plaintiffs argued that the individual mandate violated the U.S. Constitution's commerce clause, which empowers Congress to regulate interstate commerce. They conceded that health care is a form of interstate commerce but questioned whether Congress could compel individuals to engage in it—that is, force them to buy health insurance coverage. They perceived the individual mandate as an assault on personal liberty.

Even though a federal district court in Florida and a federal appeals court in Georgia agreed with the plaintiffs, other lower federal courts that ruled on similar challenges concurred with the Obama administration's position, that people without health insurance coverage could still participate in the health care marketplace because they will one day require medical care. An individual's decision to forgo coverage harms the public because the cost of the free or subsidized care he or she might receive is borne by others in the form of higher insurance premiums. Furthermore, when healthy Americans decide to go without or drop their health insurance, the balance of the pool of insured Americans grows smaller and sicker, which also serves to increase insurance premiums.

The case eventually went before the U.S. Supreme Court and was argued in March 2012. Some industry observers speculated that the court would strike the individual mandate but uphold the rest of the law. Others thought the court would strike down the expansion of Medicaid or even the entire health care reform law. In a decision that surprised many observers, on June 28, 2012, the Supreme

Court ruled in *National Federation of Independent Business v. Sebelius, Secretary of Health and Human Services* (No. 11-393) that the ACA is constitutional. Chief Justice John G. Roberts (1955–) joined the majority in affirming the ACA. Roberts ruled that the individual mandate, which would impose a fine on Americans opting to forgo health insurance coverage, was a tax that the government had the authority to impose and that the mandate was not unconstitutional. The court did, however, significantly restrict the expansion of Medicaid by affording the states some leeway: They could choose not to expand their Medicaid programs without incurring the financial penalties the ACA would have imposed.

Besides government funding of entitlement programs and other public policy issues that are frequently divisive, some industry observers believe health care providers, policy makers, biomedical technology and research firms, and academic medical centers have fanned the flames of consumer dissatisfaction with the U.S. health care system by overselling the promise and the progress of modern medicine. They fear that the overzealous promotion of every scientific discovery with a potential clinical application has created unrealistic expectations of modern medicine. Health care consumers who believe there should be "one pill for every ill" or feel all technology should be made widely available even before its efficacy (the ability of an intervention to produce the intended diagnostic or therapeutic effect in optimal circumstances) has been demonstrated are more likely to be dissatisfied with the present health care system.

AMERICANS' CHANGING VIEWS ABOUT HEALTH CARE REFORM

In *Gallup Editors: Americans' Views on the Healthcare Law* (June 22, 2012, http://www.gallup.com/poll/155300/Gallup-Editors-Americans-Views-Healthcare-Law.aspx), Frank Newport, Jeffrey M. Jones, and Lydia Saad of the Gallup Organization observe that Americans' support for the ACA did not increase after the law was passed—in fact, their views were relatively unchanged or were more negative than they were before the law passed. The Gallup editors explain that Americans oppose the ACA because they do not want government involvement in health care. Even though the ACA relies heavily on private insurance coverage, it allows the government to dictate who will be covered and which services must be covered. Table 9.1 shows that in November 2011 most Americans preferred a health care system based on private insurance (56%). It also shows that support for a government-run system increased by five percentage points between November 2010 and November 2011.

Interestingly, Americans' belief that it is the federal government's responsibility to provide health care coverage to all of its citizens declined from a high of 69% in

TABLE 9.1

Public opinion on preference for a government-run or private health care system, November 2010 and November 2011

	Government-run system	System based on private insurance	No opinion
	%	%	%
2011 Nov 3–6	39	56	6
2010 Nov 4–7	34	61	5

SOURCE: Frank Newport, Jeffrey M. Jones, and Lydia Saad, "Which of the Following Approaches for Providing Healthcare in the United States Would You Prefer—[ROTATED: A Government Run Healthcare System, (or) a System Based Mostly on Private Health Insurance?" in *Gallup Editors: Americans' Views on the Healthcare Law*, The Gallup Organization, June 22, 2012, http://www.gallup.com/poll/155300/Gallup-Editors-Americans-Views-Healthcare-Law.aspx (accessed July 5, 2012). Copyright © 2012 Gallup, Inc. All rights reserved. The content is used with permission; however, Gallup retains all rights of republication.

2006 to a low of 50% in 2011. (See Figure 9.1.) Views about federal government responsibility for health care coverage fall predictably along political party lines. In November 2011 just one-fifth (20%) of Republicans felt it is the responsibility of the federal government to provide coverage, whereas seven out of 10 (71%) Democrats felt it is the government's responsibility. (See Figure 9.2.)

In November 2011 Americans were divided about the ACA, and many favored repealing it. Frank Newport of the Gallup Organization reports in *Americans Tilt toward Favoring Repeal of Healthcare Law* (November 16, 2011, http://www.gallup.com/poll/150773/Americans-Tilt-Toward-Favoring-Repeal-Healthcare-Law.aspx) that 47% favored repealing the ACA and 42% supported its enactment. (See Table 9.2.) Support for the ACA was largely from Democrats, whereas Republicans favored its repeal.

Jeffrey M. Jones of the Gallup Organization indicates in *Confidence in U.S. Medical System up since Health Law Passed* (June 28, 2012, http://www.gallup.com/poll/155381/Confidence-Medical-System-Health-Law-Passed.aspx) that after the ACA was signed into law, Americans' confidence in the U.S. health care system increased. In 2009, 36% of respondents said they have a "great deal/quite a lot" of confidence in the health care system, whereas in 2012, 41% shared this sentiment. (See Figure 9.3.) Historically, Republicans have expressed greater confidence in the U.S. health care system, and this trend persisted in 2012. Nearly half (49%) of Republicans said they have a "great deal/quite a lot" of confidence in the health care system, compared with 44% of Independents and 34% of Democrats. (See Figure 9.4.)

Even confidence in health maintenance organizations (HMOs), which has historically been low, has increased. In 2012 nearly one-fifth (19%) of Americans said they have a "great deal/quite a lot" of confidence in HMOs.

FIGURE 9.1

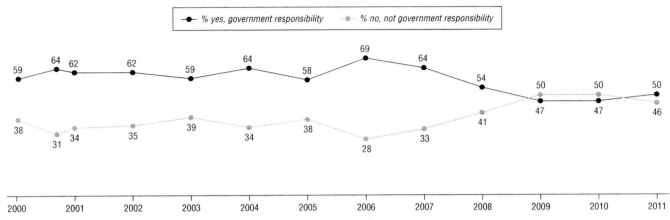

Public opinion on whether federal government should ensure that all Americans have health coverage, 2000–11

DO YOU THINK IT IS THE RESPONSIBILITY OF THE FEDERAL GOVERNMENT TO MAKE SURE ALL AMERICANS HAVE HEALTHCARE COVERAGE, OR IS THAT NOT THE RESPONSIBILITY OF THE FEDERAL GOVRNMENT?

SOURCE: Frank Newport, Jeffrey M. Jones, and Lydia Saad, "Do You Think It Is the Responsibility of the Federal Government to Make Sure All Americans Have Healthcare Coverage, or Is That Not the Responsibility of the Federal Government?" in *Gallup Editors: Americans' Views on the Healthcare Law*, The Gallup Organization, June 22, 2012, http://www.gallup.com/poll/155300/Gallup-Editors-Americans-Views-Healthcare-Law.aspx (accessed July 5, 2012). Copyright © 2012 Gallup, Inc. All rights reserved. The content is used with permission; however, Gallup retains all rights of republication.

FIGURE 9.2

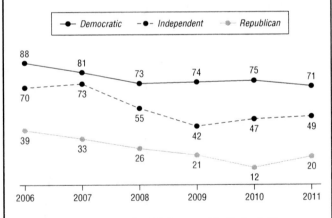

Public opinion on whether federal government should ensure that all Americans have health coverage, by political party afiliation, 2006–11

SOURCE: Frank Newport, Jeffrey M. Jones, and Lydia Saad, "Percentage Saying Federal Government Should Have Responsibility for Making Sure All Americans Have Healthcare Coverage," in *Gallup Editors: Americans' Views on the Healthcare Law*, The Gallup Organization, June 22, 2012, http://www.gallup.com/poll/155300/Gallup-Editors-Americans-Views-Healthcare-Law.aspx (accessed July 5, 2012). Copyright © 2012 Gallup, Inc. All rights reserved. The content is used with permission; however, Gallup retains all rights of republication.

(See Figure 9.5.) Simultaneously, the percentage of Americans that had "very little" or no confidence in HMOs declined from 47% in 2002 to 32% in 2012.

TABLE 9.2

Public opinion on whether the health reform legislation should be repealed or left in place, November 2011

NOW THINKING ABOUT THE HEALTHCARE OVERHAUL BILL PASSED BY CONGRESS AND SIGNED INTO LAW BY PRESIDENT OBAMA LAST YEAR: IF YOU HAD TO CHOOSE, DO YOU THINK THE HEALTHCARE LAW [ROTATED: SHOULD BE KEPT IN PLACE OR SHOULD BE REPEALED]?

	Kept in place	Repealed	No opinion
	%	%	%
National adults	42	47	11
Republicans	10	80	9
Independents	43	48	9
Democrats	64	21	15

Nov. 3–6, 2011

SOURCE: Frank Newport, "Now Thinking about the Healthcare Overhaul Bill Passed by Congress and Signed into Law by President Obama Last Year: If You Had to Choose, Do You Think the Healthcare Law [ROTATED: Should Be Kept in Place or Should Be Repealed]?" in *Americans Tilt Toward Favoring Repeal of Healthcare Law*, The Gallup Organization, November 16, 2011, http://www.gallup.com/poll/150773/Americans-Tilt-Toward-Favoring-Repeal-Healthcare-Law.aspx (accessed July 5, 2012). Copyright © 2011 Gallup, Inc. All rights reserved. The content is used with permission; however, Gallup retains all rights of republication.

AMERICANS ARE CONCERNED ABOUT THE ECONOMIC IMPACT OF THE ACA

In view of the fact that health care spending accounts for nearly one-fifth of the U.S. gross domestic product (the total market value of final goods and services produced within an economy in a given year) and that health care costs and out-of-pocket expenses are escalating, it is understandable that Americans are extremely concerned

FIGURE 9.3

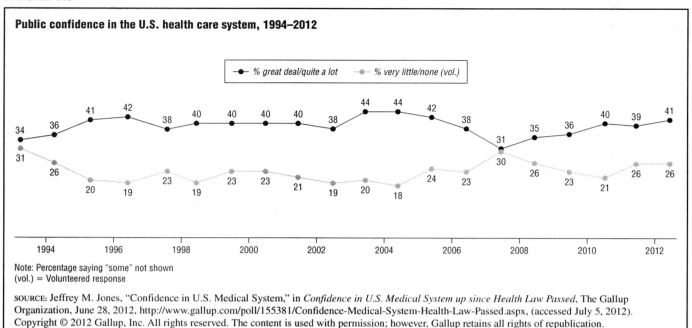

Public confidence in the U.S. health care system, 1994–2012

Note: Percentage saying "some" not shown
(vol.) = Volunteered response

SOURCE: Jeffrey M. Jones, "Confidence in U.S. Medical System," in *Confidence in U.S. Medical System up since Health Law Passed*, The Gallup Organization, June 28, 2012, http://www.gallup.com/poll/155381/Confidence-Medical-System-Health-Law-Passed.aspx, (accessed July 5, 2012). Copyright © 2012 Gallup, Inc. All rights reserved. The content is used with permission; however, Gallup retains all rights of republication.

FIGURE 9.4

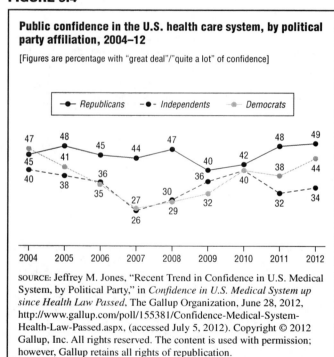

Public confidence in the U.S. health care system, by political party affiliation, 2004–12

[Figures are percentage with "great deal"/"quite a lot" of confidence]

SOURCE: Jeffrey M. Jones, "Recent Trend in Confidence in U.S. Medical System, by Political Party," in *Confidence in U.S. Medical System up since Health Law Passed*, The Gallup Organization, June 28, 2012, http://www.gallup.com/poll/155381/Confidence-Medical-System-Health-Law-Passed.aspx, (accessed July 5, 2012). Copyright © 2012 Gallup, Inc. All rights reserved. The content is used with permission; however, Gallup retains all rights of republication.

about health care costs. Gallup surveys have repeatedly found that health care costs, which continue to rise much faster than inflation, top the list of health problems Americans believe beset the nation and are perceived as more urgent than threats of specific diseases.

The Gallup Organization notes that in July 2012, just days after the Supreme Court ruling on the ACA's con-stitutionality, Americans were worried about the act's economic consequences. Nearly half (46%) of those surveyed felt the ACA will hurt the U.S. economy, compared with 37% who believed it will help the economy. (See Table 9.3.) Feelings about the economic impact of the ACA were highly partisan; Democrats were more likely to say the ACA will help the U.S. economy (62%), whereas Republicans were more likely to say it will harm the economy (78%). (See Table 9.4.) Independents were more likely to say it will hurt (47%) rather than help (34%) the economy.

Another poll gauging public opinion about the ACA following the Supreme Court decision found that the ruling did little to change overall views on the ACA, which have been roughly stable since its passage. The Kaiser Family Foundation conducted a poll at the end of June 2012 and published the results in "Kaiser Poll: Early Reaction to Supreme Court Decision on ACA" (July 2, 2012, http://healthreform.kff.org/en/scan/2012/july/kaiser-poll-early-reaction-to-supreme-court-decision-on-aca.aspx). The foundation notes that equal percentages of Americans (41%) viewed the ACA as favorable and unfavorable. Democrats viewed the law more favorably than they had prior to the Supreme Court ruling—47% were "'very favorable' toward the law," compared with 31% just one month before the ruling. The majority (56%) of Americans said "they would like to see the law's detractors stop their efforts to block its implementation and move on to other national problems." The overwhelming majority (82%) of Democrats said "opponents should move on to other issues," as did half (51%) of Independents. In contrast, the majority (69%) of Republicans said they want to pursue efforts "to stop the law."

FIGURE 9.5

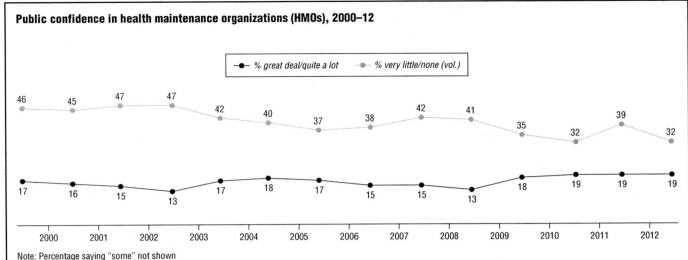

Public confidence in health maintenance organizations (HMOs), 2000–12

Note: Percentage saying "some" not shown
(vol.) = Volunteered response

SOURCE: Jeffrey M. Jones, "Confidence in Health Maintenance Organizations," in *Confidence in U.S. Medical System up since Health Law Passed*, The Gallup Organization, June 28, 2012, http://www.gallup.com/poll/155381/Confidence-Medical-System-Health-Law-Passed.aspx, (accessed July 5, 2012). Copyright © 2012 Gallup, Inc. All rights reserved. The content is used with permission; however, Gallup retains all rights of republication.

TABLE 9.3

Public opinion on whether health care reform law will help or hurt the U.S. economy, July 2012

ALL IN ALL, DO YOU THINK THE 2010 HEALTHCARE LAW UPHELD BY THE SUPREME COURT LAST WEEK WILL HELP OR HURT THE NATIONAL ECONOMY?

National adults

	Help	Hurt	No effect (vol.)	No opinion
Jul 2–3, 2012	37%	46%	1%	17%

(vol.) = Volunteered response

SOURCE: Frank Newport, "All in All, Do You Think the 2010 Healthcare Law Upheld by the Supreme Court Last Week Will Help or Hurt the National Economy?" in *Americans See More Economic Harm Than Good in Health Law*, The Gallup Organization, July 5, 2012, http://www.gallup.com/poll/155513/Americans-Economic-Harm-Good-Health-Law.aspx, (accessed July 6, 2012). Copyright © 2012 Gallup, Inc. All rights reserved. The content is used with permission; however, Gallup retains all rights of republication.

TABLE 9.4

Public opinion on whether health care reform law will help or hurt the U.S. economy by political party affiliation, July 2012

ALL IN ALL, DO YOU THINK THE 2010 HEALTHCARE LAW UPHELD BY THE SUPREME COURT LAST WEEK WILL HELP OR HURT THE NATIONAL ECONOMY?

July 2–3, 2012

	Help	Hurt	No effect (vol.)	No opinion
	%	%	%	%
Republicans	13	78	1	8
Independents	34	47	1	19
Democrats	62	20	*	18

*Less than 0.5%
(vol.) = Volunteered response

SOURCE: Frank Newport, "All in All, Do You Think the 2010 Healthcare Law Upheld by the Supreme Court Last Week Will Help or Hurt the National Economy?" in *Americans See More Economic Harm Than Good in Health Law*, The Gallup Organization, July 5, 2012, http://www.gallup.com/poll/155513/Americans-Economic-Harm-Good-Health-Law.aspx, (accessed July 6, 2012). Copyright © 2012 Gallup, Inc. All rights reserved. The content is used with permission; however, Gallup retains all rights of republication.

Even though the Supreme Court decision was eagerly awaited and hotly contested, Frank Newport observes in *Americans Don't Often Name Healthcare as Top U.S. Problem* (June 29, 2012, http://www.gallup.com/poll/155414/Americans-Dont-Often-Name-Healthcare-Top-Problem.aspx) that in 2012 few Americans named health care as the most important problem facing the country. In a June 2012 poll a scant 6% identified health care as the top problem facing the nation. (See Figure 9.6.) Newport notes that health care trailed "behind mentions of the economy, jobs, the deficit, and problems in government."

The national economy and the rate of increase of health care costs, especially out-of-pocket expenses, also play important roles in shaping public opinion. Many surveys show a direct relationship between rising out-of-pocket expenses and dissatisfaction with the health care system.

Most U.S. Physicians Favor Health Care Reform

Charles Feng reports in "Doctors' Groups Applaud Health Care Ruling" (ABCNews.com, June 29, 2012) that the majority of physicians' professional organizations—including the American Medical Association (AMA), the National Physicians Alliance, the American Academy of Pediatrics, and the Association of American Medical

FIGURE 9.6

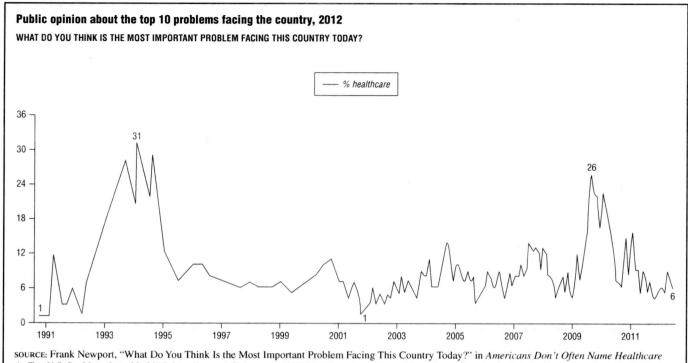

Public opinion about the top 10 problems facing the country, 2012

WHAT DO YOU THINK IS THE MOST IMPORTANT PROBLEM FACING THIS COUNTRY TODAY?

SOURCE: Frank Newport, "What Do You Think Is the Most Important Problem Facing This Country Today?" in *Americans Don't Often Name Healthcare As Top U.S. Problem*, June 29, 2012, http://www.gallup.com/poll/155414/Americans-Dont-Often-Name-Healthcare-Top-Problem.aspx, (accessed July 6, 2012). Copyright © 2012 Gallup, Inc. All rights reserved. The content is used with permission; however, Gallup retains all rights of republication.

Colleges—are pleased with the Supreme Court's ruling that the ACA is constitutional. However, some groups do take issue with specific provisions of the act. For example, the American Association of Orthopedic Surgeons is concerned that administrative requirements of the ACA will compromise the time available to spend with patients. Likewise, the American Urological Association, the American Association of Clinical Urologists, and the Large Urology Group Practice Association opine that some provisions of the ACA will "ultimately, hurt this nation's ability to provide widespread care for its citizens."

Nevertheless, even groups that support the ACA have concerns about its implementation and the nation's capacity to provide care for an additional 30 million people. In "Your Health Care Is Covered, but Who's Going to Treat You?" (CNN.com, June 29, 2012), Jacque Wilson quotes Ardis Hoven, the president-elect of the AMA, who said, "We've expressed some concerns before about whether or not we're going to have enough physicians out there." Hoven suggested that the most severe shortage will be of primary care physicians.

CONSUMER SATISFACTION WITH HEALTH CARE FACILITIES

Despite the problems that continue to plague hospitals, such as shortages of nurses and other key personnel, diminished reimbursement, shorter inpatient lengths of stay, sicker patients, and excessively long waiting times for patients in emergency and other hospital departments, consumer satisfaction with hospital services has remained relatively high. In fact, Press Ganey Associates Inc. reports in *2011 Pulse Report: Perspectives on American Health Care* (November 2011, http://www.pressganey.com/Documents_secure/Pulse%20Reports/2011_Press_Ganey_Pulse_Report.pdf?viewFile), which considers the experiences of more than 3 million patients who were treated at 3,062 hospitals nationwide, that overall patient satisfaction with inpatient hospital care steadily increased between July 2006 and October 2010, rising from 83.9% to 86.1%. Press Ganey finds a wide gap in performance among hospitals that are in the top 10% of performance and those in the bottom 10%. The study also identifies significant variations based on hospital size and geographic location.

Patient satisfaction with hospital care was linked to the hospital's success in communicating and meeting patients' spiritual and emotional needs. This finding, that satisfaction is associated with patient-centered care and intangible qualities of the hospital experience such as sensitivity, attention, and responsiveness to emotional needs, concerns, and complaints, underscores the fact that many health care consumers assess the quality of service they receive in terms of the care and compassion displayed by hospital personnel.

Other patient-related variables and hospital characteristics also influence satisfaction with care. Fewer patients admitted through the emergency department (64%) were satisfied, compared with those who did not have emergency admissions (68.2%). This difference may be attributed to the understandable stress and discomfort surrounding an emergency hospital admission, but it may also reflect dissatisfaction with specific hospital qualities such as long waits for admission.

Abby Swanson Kazley et al. report in "Is Electronic Health Record Use Associated with Patient Satisfaction in Hospitals?" (*Health Care Management Review*, vol. 37, no. 1, January–February 2012) that electronic health record (EHR) use positively and significantly influences patient satisfaction. EHR use is associated with measures of patient satisfaction, such as rating hospitals as a 9 or a 10, and patients' willingness to recommend the hospital. In "Interdisciplinary Teamwork in Hospitals: A Review and Practical Recommendations for Improvement" (*Journal of Hospital Medicine*, vol. 7, no. 1, January 2012), Kevin J. O'Leary et al. indicate that the extent that hospitals use teamwork and collaborative practice is positively associated with higher levels of patient satisfaction as well as with higher nurse retention and lower hospital costs.

Gienna Shaw explains in "Time to Put Patients First" (*HealthLeaders Magazine*, May 12, 2010) some of the origins of patient dissatisfaction. She notes that "Americans can't understand why they must wait months for an appointment with a specialist. They continually hear horror stories about wrong-site surgeries and hospital-acquired infections. They have trouble getting their physicians, specialists, and alternative providers to talk to each other—let alone communicate effectively with them. And then they get a bill for it all that they can't understand." Shaw asserts that hospitals have lost sight of their mission—caring for patients—and lauds efforts to promote patient-centered care, which is defined as "compassionate care delivered with the highest quality and level of patient safety."

Government Website Posts Patient Satisfaction Survey Data

Amid multiple reports of patient dissatisfaction with selected aspects of health care delivery, there are some hopeful signs, such as improving levels of satisfaction with inpatient hospital care. Industry observers attribute some of the improvement in inpatient hospital care satisfaction to the fact that the federal government posts the results of the Hospital Consumer Assessment of Healthcare Providers and Systems survey on the website "Hospital Compare" (http://www.hospitalcompare.hhs.gov/), which enables consumers to compare up to three hospitals. The website is a public-private venture led by organizations that represent the hospital industry, providers, and consumers with coordination and oversight from government agencies.

The website aims to help consumers choose the best hospital for selected surgical procedures by detailing how often hospitals give recommended treatments that are known to get the best results for patients with certain medical conditions. The website includes mortality rates and hospital readmission rates for each hospital as well as other information such as whether the hospital uses EHRs and the waiting times for selected emergency departments. It also provides information about a hospital's quality of care, as measured by patient surveys.

Consumer groups, employers, labor unions, and other government agencies applaud the dissemination of these data, asserting that it helps promote transparency and accountability. Diana Manos reports in "CMS Adds Mortality, Readmission Data to Its Online Hospital Rating Site" (*Healthcare IT News*, July 9, 2009) that the Centers for Medicare and Medicaid Services (CMS) considers the "Hospital Compare" website to be a vital resource for consumers and notes that in 2008 the site had more than 18 million page views. According to Manos, Kathleen Sebelius (1948–), the secretary of health and human services, explained that the government is particularly focused on preventing readmissions: "When we reduce readmissions, we improve the quality of care patients receive and cut health care costs." Manos quotes Barry M. Straube, the chief medical officer and director of the CMS's Office of Clinical Standards and Quality, as saying, "More data gives a clearer picture of the quality of care delivered at different hospitals over time, which ultimately increases the value of our mortality information to hospital patients, health care payers, employers, policymakers, and other health care stakeholders."

A GROWING NUMBER LOOK FOR HEALTH INFORMATION ONLINE

Even though public trust in hospitals and personal physicians remains relatively high, and many people seek and receive health education from physicians, nurses, and other health professionals, a growing number of Americans are seeking health information online.

In "The Prepared Patient: Information Seeking of Online Support Group Members before Their Medical Appointments" (*Journal of Health Communication*, May 10, 2012), Xinyi Hu et al. looked at more than 500 online support group members' use of Internet communities and other online and offline health resources as they prepared for appointments with their doctors. The researchers find that the study subjects were more likely to seek information online when their medical condition caused them distress or when they felt they had some ability to control the symptoms or progress of their illness. Participants who believed that their medical condition was chronic or will persist were also more likely to search for information online.

Hu et al. find that use of the Internet to research medical conditions was not associated with mistrust of physicians. Nearly 70% of the study subjects said they planned to ask their physicians about the information they obtained, and 40% printed information to discuss with their physicians during their upcoming visit. More than half said they planned to make at least one request during their visit in response to information they had obtained on the Internet. Interestingly, Hu et al. find that the Internet did not replace more traditional sources of health information; it was used in addition to traditional sources to confirm or refute information that was obtained from friends, family, magazines, and books.

Is there a relationship between anxiety about health concerns and seeking health information online? Kate Muse et al. examined the relationship between health anxiety and searching for health information online, a phenomenon called *cyberchondria*, and reported their findings in "Cyberchondriasis: Fact or Fiction? A Preliminary Examination of the Relationship between Health Anxiety and Searching for Health Information on the Internet" (*Journal of Anxiety Disorders*, vol. 26, no. 1, January 2012). The researchers indicate that people "with higher levels of health anxiety sought online health information more frequently, spent longer searching, and found searching more distressing and anxiety provoking," and conclude that searching for health information online may intensify health anxiety.

Social media have the potential to serve as an important platform for health education, information, and intervention. In "Health Information Seeking and Social Media Use on the Internet among People with Diabetes" (*Online Journal of Public Health Informatics*, vol. 3, no. 1, 2011), Ryan J. Shaw and Constance M. Johnson of the Duke University School of Nursing examined health information-seeking behaviors of people with diabetes to determine whether they use online social media and verify their willingness to use these sites to discuss health information. The researchers questioned 57 people with diabetes about their Internet use and how they seek and share health information. Shaw and Johnson find that the majority of study subjects read blogs and used the Internet to search for health information. In total, 78.5% said the health information they found online "changed the way they think about health." More than two-thirds (65.4%) of the subjects were "willing to discuss health information online in chat rooms, discussion groups or online support groups." Because Shaw and Johnson recruited study participants from urban, suburban, and rural locations in the United States, they conclude that their findings "may indicate that using these online venues could reach diverse and non-urban populations."

Mina Kim reports in "Consumers Increasingly Turning to Internet, Social Media for Health Care Informa-

tion" (*iHealthBeat*, April 15, 2010) that adults are increasingly looking for health information online. She notes that "in addition to health care Web sites, such as WebMD, consumers are turning to user-generated health content, such as physician and hospital rankings, blogs and chat groups." Robin A. Cohen and Patricia F. Adams of the National Center for Health Statistics confirm in *Use of the Internet for Health Information: United States, 2009* (July 2011, http://www.cdc.gov/nchs/data/data briefs/db66.pdf) that "74% of all U.S. adults use the Internet, and 61% have looked for health or medical information on the Internet."

Cohen and Adams note that among adults aged 18 years and older, women (50.9%) were more likely than men (39.8%) to search for health information online in 2009. (See Figure 9.7.) Non-Hispanic white people (57.3%) were nearly twice as likely as Hispanic people (28.8%) to seek health information on the Internet. (See Figure 9.8.) Adults with higher incomes (63.4%) were more likely to have used the Internet for health information in 2009 than those with lower incomes (28.9%). Figure 9.9 shows that college graduates (73.8%) were more than five times as likely to seek health information online as people with less than a high school education (13.8%). Adults who were employed (53.4%) were more likely than adults who were not in the workforce (42.5%) or unemployed (40.9%) to have used the Internet for health information. (See Figure 9.10.) Figure 9.11 shows that adults with private health insurance (58.7%) were more likely to seek health information online than adults on Medicaid (31.3%), adults who were uninsured (33.3%), or adults with other coverage (42.9%).

According to the Deloitte Center for Health Solutions, in *2011 Survey of Health Care Consumers in the United States: Key Findings, Strategic Implications* (July 2011, https://www.deloitte.com/assets/Dcom-United-States/Local%20Assets/Documents/US_CHS_2011Con sumerSurveyinUS_062111.pdf), less than half (43%) of consumers surveyed said they had looked for health information online in 2011, down from 55% in 2010 and 57% in 2009. The extent to which consumers were going online for health information varied by age. For example, 45% of Generation X (people born between 1965 and 1979) and 39% of Generation Y (people born in 1980 and after) searched online for treatment-related information in 2011, compared with 44% of baby boomers (people born between 1946 and 1964) and 38% of older adults.

The Deloitte survey indicates that younger people were more interested in looking for information about provider quality and cost. In 2011 nearly one-third of Generation Y (34% for quality information and 30% for cost information) sought cost and quality information online, and the percentage of adults seeking this information declined with

FIGURE 9.7

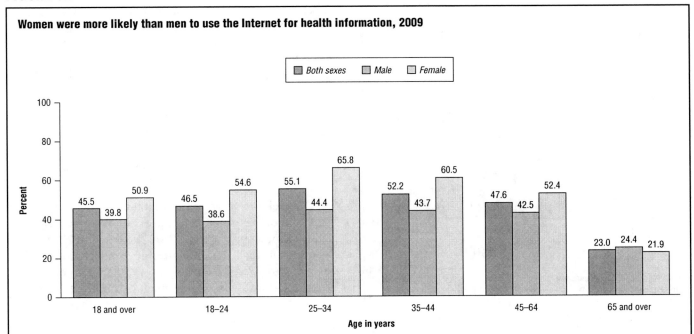

Women were more likely than men to use the Internet for health information, 2009

Notes: Data are based on household interviews of a sample of the civilian noninstitutionalized population.

SOURCE: Robin A. Cohen and Patricia F. Adams, "Figure 1. Percentage of Adults Aged 18 and over Who in the Past 12 Months Looked up Health Information on the Internet, by Sex and Age, United States, 2009," in "Use of the Internet for Health Information: United States, 2009," *NCHS Data Brief*, no. 66, Centers for Disease Control and Prevention, National Center for Health Statistics, July 2011, http://www.cdc.gov/nchs/data/databriefs/db66.pdf (accessed July 9, 2012)

FIGURE 9.8

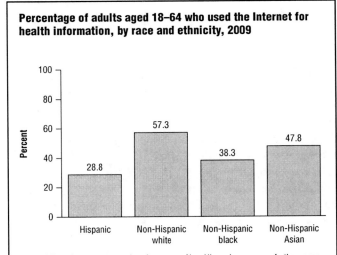

Percentage of adults aged 18–64 who used the Internet for health information, by race and ethnicity, 2009

Notes: Hispanic persons may be of any race. Non-Hispanic persons of other races or of mixed race are not shown. Data are based on household interviews of a sample of the civilian noninstitutionalized population.

SOURCE: Robin A. Cohen and Patricia F. Adams, "Figure 2. Percentage of Adults Aged 18–64 Who in the Past 12 Months Looked up Health Information on the Internet, by Race and Ethnicity, United States, 2009," in "Use of the Internet for Health Information: United States, 2009," *NCHS Data Brief*, no. 66, Centers for Disease Control and Prevention, National Center for Health Statistics, July 2011, http://www.cdc.gov/nchs/data/databriefs/db66.pdf (accessed July 9, 2012)

FIGURE 9.9

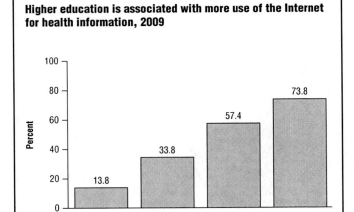

Higher education is associated with more use of the Internet for health information, 2009

Notes: GED is General Educational Development high school equivalency diploma. Data are based on household interviews of a sample of the civilian noninstitutionalized population.

SOURCE: Robin A. Cohen and Patricia F. Adams, "Figure 3. Percentage of Adults Aged 25–64 Who in the Past 12 Months Looked up Health Information on the Internet, by Education Status, United States, 2009," in "Use of the Internet for Health Information: United States, 2009," *NCHS Data Brief*, no. 66, Centers for Disease Control and Prevention, National Center for Health Statistics, July 2011, http://www.cdc.gov/nchs/data/databriefs/db66.pdf (accessed July 9, 2012)

FIGURE 9.10

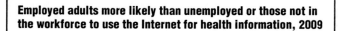

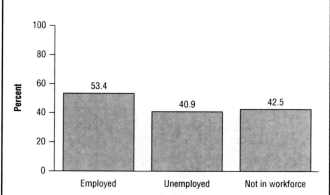

Employed adults more likely than unemployed or those not in the workforce to use the Internet for health information, 2009

Notes: Data are based on household interviews of a sample of the civilian noninstitutionalized population.

SOURCE: Robin A. Cohen and Patricia F. Adams, "Figure 5. Percentage of Adults Aged 18–64 Who in the Past 12 Months Looked up Health Information on the Internet, by Employment Status, United States, 2009," in "Use of the Internet for Health Information: United States, 2009," *NCHS Data Brief*, no. 66, Centers for Disease Control and Prevention, National Center for Health Statistics, July 2011, http://www.cdc.gov/nchs/data/databriefs/db66.pdf (accessed July 9, 2012)

FIGURE 9.11

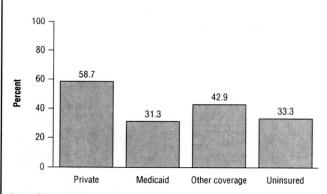

Seeking health information on the Internet is related to health insurance status, 2009

Notes: Data are based on household interviews of a sample of the civilian noninstitutionalized population.

SOURCE: Robin A. Cohen and Patricia F. Adams, "Figure 6. Percentage of Adults Aged 18–64 Who in the Past 12 Months Looked Up Health information on the Internet, by Health Insurance Coverage Status, United States, 2009," in "Use of the Internet for Health Information: United States, 2009," *NCHS Data Brief*, no. 66, Centers for Disease Control and Prevention, National Center for Health Statistics, July 2011, http://www.cdc.gov/nchs/data/databriefs/db66.pdf (accessed July 9, 2012)

advancing age—Generation X (quality, 33%, and cost, 24%), Boomers (quality, 24%, and cost, 13%), and older adults (quality, 19%, and cost, 5%).

Just one out of 10 (11%) adults used a social networking site in 2011 to communicate their experiences with the health care system (6%), and even fewer used social networking sites to learn about prescription drugs (5%), to communicate with their insurance companies (2%), or to communicate with their physicians (2%).

Similarly, blogs are not popular means of seeking or communicating health information. Less than 10% of adults said they used a blog in 2011 to share their experiences with others (8%), to learn about others' health care experiences (5%), or to post comments about a physician (3%) or a hospital (2%).

The Deloitte survey finds that there is limited interest in and use of electronic personal health records (PHRs)—just 11% of consumers in 2011 had their PHRs in an electronic format. People suffering from chronic conditions (14%) were more likely to maintain electronic PHRs than those without chronic conditions (8%). Older adults (17%) had more electronic PHRs than Boomers (12%), Generation X (8%), and Generation Y (11%).

There is considerable interest in using mobile devices to monitor health conditions and access electronic PHRs. More than half (52%) of the survey respondents said they would use a smart phone or personal digital assistant "to monitor their health if they were able to access their medical records and download information about their medical condition and treatments." Not unexpectedly, the youngest survey respondents were the most enthusiastic about using mobile devices to seek and exchange health information, and interest declined with age—from 72% of Generation Y, to 62% of Generation X, to 42% of Boomers, and 26% of older adults.

Reliable public sources of consumer and provider health information on the Internet include the National Institutes of Health, the Centers for Disease Control and Prevention, and MEDLINE, as well as websites that are produced by medical professional organizations such as the AMA, the American Heart Association, and the Cancer Society. Using technology effectively is a health system challenge, especially in terms of protecting patient privacy and confidentiality and ensuring that consumers have access to accurate and reliable health information.

MARKETING PRESCRIPTION DRUGS TO CONSUMERS

Even though health care consumers continue to receive much of their information from physicians, nurses, other health professionals, and the Internet, many also learn about health care services and products from reports in the news media and from advertising. Media advertising (the promotion of hospitals, health insurance, managed care plans, medical groups, and related health services and products) has been a mainstay of health care marketing efforts since the 1970s. During the early 1990s pharmaceutical companies made their first forays into advertising of prescription drugs directly to consumers. Before the 1990s pharmaceutical companies' promotion efforts had focused almost exclusively on physicians, the health professionals who prescribe their products.

Since the mid-1990s spending on prescription drugs has escalated and has become the fastest-growing segment of U.S. health care expenditures. In 1997 the U.S. Food and Drug Administration released guidelines governing direct-to-consumer advertising and seemingly opened a floodgate of print, radio, and television advertisements promoting prescription drugs. Industry observers wondered if this upsurge of direct-to-consumer advertising had resulted in more, and possibly inappropriate, prescribing and higher costs.

Is Direct-to-Consumer Advertising Effective?

It stands to reason that pharmaceutical companies must be receiving significant returns on their direct-to-consumer advertising investments to justify increasing budgets for consumer advertising, but it is difficult to measure the precise impact of consumer advertising on drug sales. In the press release "Real Per Capita Spending on U.S. Medicines Grows 0.5 Percent" (*IMS News*, April 4, 2012), the IMS Institute for Healthcare Informatics reports that despite less prescription drug use by older adults in 2011, prescription drug sales grew by 3.7% to more than $320 billion. In "Direct-to-Consumer Advertising in Pharmaceutical Markets: Effects on Demand and Prices" (*Vox*, June 3, 2010), Dhaval Dave of Bentley University notes that spending on direct-to-consumer prescription drug advertising was responsible for 18% of the total increase in prescription drug sales between 1993 and 2005. Of this 18%, about 12% was attributable to more sales and 6% to higher prices. Dave asserts that media promotion may affect price by increasing demand and/or reducing the price-sensitivity of purchasers (individual consumers and group purchasers), which may raise the price of pharmaceuticals. In addition, spending for media advertising may be passed along to consumers in the form of higher prescription drug prices.

According to Bruce Japsen, in "Drug Makers Dial down TV Advertising" (*New York Times*, February 2, 2012), spending on the television advertising of prescription drugs declined by more than 20% between 2007 and 2011, from $3.1 billion to $2.4 billion. The 2% decline in spending in 2011 marked the fourth consecutive year that pharmaceutical advertising spending fell. Japsen predicts further declines as generic competitors vie for customers of brand-name drugs that are advertised on television. He adds that "pharmacies and health insurance companies offer incentives to patients with drug coverage to choose cheaper generics over brand-name drugs, limiting the power of television advertising."

Is Direct-to-Consumer Advertising of Psychoactive Drugs Helpful or Harmful?

It's difficult to ascertain whether efforts aimed directly at consumers ultimately translate into real sales. A recent marketing study found that fewer than 3 percent of patients mentioned a marketed drug by name and less than 1 percent asked for a prescription.

—Pauline W. Chen, "Have These Symptoms? Buy This Drug"
(*New York Times*, January 26, 2012)

In *The Numbers Count: Mental Disorders in America* (2012, http://www.nimh.nih.gov/health/publications/the-numbers-count-mental-disorders-in-america/index.shtml), the National Institute of Mental Health estimates that 26.2% of Americans aged 18 years and older are affected by a mental disorder and that 6% suffer from a serious mental illness. Other surveys find that as many as 30% of adults in the United States suffer from mental disorders. For example, the Harvard School of Medicine's National Comorbidity Survey (July 2007, http://www.hcp.med.harvard.edu/ncs/) finds that in any given year 32.4% of all Americans meet the criteria for having a mental illness and that the lifetime prevalence of any diagnosable mental disorder is 57.4%.

Even though these studies rely primarily on self-reporting, they do suggest that the United States is in the throes of an epidemic of mental illness. However, some researchers argue that Americans' mental health is no worse than it was in past decades. They contend that the availability and aggressive marketing of psychopharmacological agents (prescription drugs that are used to treat mental health problems such as nervousness, anxiety, panic, and shyness) have prompted the overdiagnosis of mental health problems and conditions motivated primarily by the desire to increase drug sales.

Shirley S. Wang reports in "Psychiatric Drug Use Spreads" (*Wall Street Journal*, November 16, 2011) that psychiatric medications are among the most widely prescribed and best-selling drugs in the United States and that their sales increased 22% during the first decade of the 21st century. Wang observes that in 2010 Americans spent $16.1 billion on antipsychotic drugs, $11.6 billion on antidepressants, and $7.2 billion on drug treatment for attention-deficit hyperactivity disorder.

According to Rosemary J. Avery, Matthew Eisenberg, and Kosali I. Simon, in "The Impact of Direct-to-Consumer Television and Magazine Advertising on Antidepressant Use" (*Journal of Health Economics*, vol. 31, no. 5, September 2012), direct-to-consumer advertising of antidepressant drugs affects the use of these drugs. The researchers estimate that television advertising produces an increase of between 6% and 10% in antidepressant drug use.

Nathan P. Greenslit and Ted J. Kaptchuk explain in "Antidepressants and Advertising: Psychopharmaceuticals in Crisis" (*Yale Journal of Biology and Medicine*, vol. 85, no. 1, March 2012) that "psychopharmaceuticals are currently in crisis [because] the science of depression has become a contest between scientists, pharmaceutical marketing, physicians, professional medical organizations, regulatory agencies, and patients." The mechanisms of action (how the drugs work) and the efficacy of antidepressant drugs have been called into question by rigorous population studies that find them no more effective than placebo (an inactive compound; the placebo effect is a health benefit, such as pain relief, that arises from the patient's expectation that the placebo will provide relief, rather than from the placebo itself). Greenslit and Kaptchuk note that "despite such broad uncertainty over both the scientific explanations and efficacy of antidepressants, [direct-to-consumer] advertising is still a nearly 5 billion dollar per year industry (and practically unique to the United States, as no other country except New Zealand allows it)."

Greenslit and Kaptchuk observe that since 1997, when the Food and Drug Administration approved direct-to-consumer advertising, pharmaceutical companies have been accused of overstating claims of drug efficacy, minimizing the health risks that are associated with antidepressant use, and increasing consumer demand for the drugs by characterizing everyday experiences such as sadness, anxiety, and shyness as symptoms of mental illness. In contrast, advocates contend that direct-to-consumer advertising reduces the stigmas that are associated with mental illness, educates consumers, promotes patient participation in clinical decision making, and improves patient adherence to medication and other treatment. Critics counter that advertising is intended to persuade, not educate, and that it promotes inappropriate use of prescription drugs or diverts consumers from safer, less costly alternatives.

Opponents usually contend that direct-to-consumer advertising is primarily intended to drive sales and that it:

- Increases prescription drug costs

- Does not provide the impartial, objective information that would enable consumers to make informed health choices

- Increases risk because, unlike other consumer goods, prescription drugs, even when administered properly, may cause serious adverse reactions

- Takes unfair advantage of vulnerable people facing difficult treatment choices, especially people who suffer from mental illness

- Aims to increase awareness and utilization of newer products to gain market share and recoup development costs (new drugs are not necessarily safer or more effective but are usually costlier, and often little is known about their long-term risks)

- Does not enhance consumer awareness or public health because there is no evidence that advertising helps patients to make better choices about prescription drug use

- May unduly influence physician-prescribing practices; physicians often rely on manufacturers for information about drugs, rather than on independent sources, and many studies show that the physicians most influenced by pharmaceutical advertising tend to prescribe less judiciously

Dominick L. Frosch et al. contend in "A Decade of Controversy: Balancing Policy with Evidence in the Regulation of Prescription Drug Advertising" (*American Journal of Public Health*, vol. 100, no. 1, January 2010) that such advertising may mislead consumers or prompt them to consider drug treatment for a condition that does not warrant it. The researchers cite the example of advertising campaigns for drugs to treat various anxiety disorders that emphasized feelings of social discomfort with slogans such as "imagine being allergic to people." Similarly, antidepressant print advertisements were found to mislead consumers to believe that their emotional symptoms are best treated with prescription medications. An analysis of advertisements found that direct-to-consumer advertising frequently identifies conditions that may not be recognized by consumers as problems in need of treatment or as treatable. Frosch et al. recommend that "to minimize potential harm and maximize the benefits of [direct-to-consumer advertising] for population health, the quality and quantity of information should be improved to enable consumers to better self-identify whether treatment is indicated, more realistically appraise the benefits, and better attend to the risks associated with prescription drugs."

Regardless, many mental health professionals and consumers favor direct-to-consumer advertising because they believe it informs consumers that there is effective treatment for potentially debilitating mental disorders and helps them to overcome reluctance to seek needed treatment. Nile M. Khanfar, Hyla H. Polen, and Kevin A. Clauson observe in "Influence on Consumer Behavior: The Impact of Direct-to-Consumer Advertising on Medication Requests for Gastroesophageal Reflux Disease and Social Anxiety Disorder" (*Journal of Health Communications*, vol. 14, no. 5, July–August 2009) that 40% of people with a social anxiety disorder reported that direct-to-consumer advertising helped them to initiate conversations with their physicians that led to a change of therapy.

IMPORTANT NAMES
AND ADDRESSES

Accreditation Association for Ambulatory Health Care
5250 Old Orchard Rd., Ste. 200
Skokie, IL 60077
(847) 853-6060
FAX: (847) 853-9028
E-mail: info@aaahc.org
URL: http://www.aaahc.org/

Administration on Aging
One Massachusetts Ave. NW
Washington, DC 20001
(202) 619-0724
FAX: (202) 357-3555
E-mail: aoainfo@aoa.hhs.gov
URL: http://www.aoa.gov/

Agency for Healthcare Research and Quality
Office of Communications and Knowledge Transfer
540 Gaither Rd., Ste. 2000
Rockville, MD 20850
(301) 427-1104
URL: http://www.ahrq.gov/

American Academy of Child and Adolescent Psychiatry
3615 Wisconsin Ave. NW
Washington, DC 20016-3007
(202) 966-7300
FAX: (202) 966-2891
URL: http://www.aacap.org/

American Academy of Family Physicians
11400 Tomahawk Creek Pkwy.
Leawood, KS 66211-2680
(913) 906-6000
1-800-274-2237
FAX: (913) 906-6075
URL: http://www.aafp.org/

American Academy of Physician Assistants
2318 Mill Rd.
Alexandria, VA 22332

(703) 836-2272
FAX: (703) 684-1924
E-mail: aapa@aapa.org
URL: http://www.aapa.org/

American Association for Geriatric Psychiatry
7910 Woodmont Ave., Ste. 1050
Bethesda, MD 20814-3004
(301) 654-7850
FAX: (301) 654-4137
E-mail: main@aagponline.org
URL: http://www.aagponline.org/

American Association for Marriage and Family Therapy
112 S. Alfred St.
Alexandria, VA 22314-3061
(703) 838-9808
FAX: (703) 838-9805
URL: http://www.aamft.org/

American Association of Pastoral Counselors
9504A Lee Hwy.
Fairfax, VA 22031-2303
(703) 385-6967
FAX: (703) 352-7725
E-mail: info@aapc.org
URL: http://www.aapc.org/

American Cancer Society
250 Williams St. NW
Atlanta, GA 30303
(404) 220-2700
1-800-227-2345
URL: http://www.cancer.org/

American Chiropractic Association
1701 Clarendon Blvd.
Arlington, VA 22209
(703) 276-8800
FAX: (703) 243-2593
E-mail: memberinfo@acatoday.org
URL: http://www.acatoday.org/index.cfm

American College of Nurse Practitioners
225 Reinekers Lane, Ste. 525
Alexandria, VA 22314
(703) 740-2529
FAX: (703) 740-2533
E-mail: acnp@acnpweb.org
URL: http://www.acnpweb.org/

American Counseling Association
5999 Stevenson Ave.
Alexandria, VA 22304
1-800-347-6647
FAX: 1-800-473-2329
URL: http://www.counseling.org/

American Dental Association
211 E. Chicago Ave.
Chicago, IL 60611-2678
(312) 440-2500
URL: http://www.ada.org/

American Diabetes Association
1701 N. Beauregard St.
Alexandria, VA 22311
1-800-342-2383
URL: http://www.diabetes.org/

American Geriatrics Society
40 Fulton St., 18th Floor
New York, NY 10038
(212) 308-1414
FAX: (212) 832-8646
E-mail: info.amger@americangeriatrics.org
URL: http://www.americangeriatrics.org/

American Heart Association
7272 Greenville Ave.
Dallas, TX 75231
1-800-242-8721
URL: http://www.americanheart.org/

American Hospital Association
155 N. Wacker Dr.
Chicago, IL 60606
(312) 422-3000
URL: http://www.aha.org/

American Medical Association
515 N. State St.
Chicago, IL 60654
1-800-621-8335
URL: http://www.ama-assn.org/

American Osteopathic Association
142 E. Ontario St.
Chicago, IL 60611
(312) 202-8000
1-800-621-1773
FAX: (312) 202-8200
URL: http://www.osteopathic.org/

American Pharmacists Association
2215 Constitution Ave. NW
Washington, DC 20037
(202) 628-4410
FAX: (202) 783-2351
URL: http://www.aphanet.org/

American Physical Therapy Association
1111 N. Fairfax St.
Alexandria, VA 22314-1488
(703) 684-2782
1-800-999-2782
FAX: (703) 684-7343
URL: http://www.apta.org/

American Psychiatric Association
1000 Wilson Blvd., Ste. 1825
Arlington, VA 22209
(703) 907-7300
E-mail: apa@psych.org
URL: http://www.psych.org/

American Psychiatric Nurses Association
3141 Fairview Park Dr., Ste. 625
Arlington, VA 22042
(571) 533-1919
1-855-863-2762
FAX: 1-855-883-2762
URL: http://www.apna.org/

American Psychological Association
750 First St. NE
Washington, DC 20002-4242
(202) 336-5500
1-800-374-2721
URL: http://www.apa.org/

American Psychological Society
1133 15th St. NW, Ste. 1000
Washington, DC 20005
(202) 293-9300
FAX: (202) 293-9350
URL: http://www.psychologicalscience.org/

Association of American Medical Colleges
2450 North St. NW
Washington, DC 20037-1126
(202) 828-0400
FAX: (202) 828-1125
URL: http://www.aamc.org/

Center for Mental Health Services Substance Abuse and Mental Health Services Administration
(240) 276-1310
FAX: (240) 276-1320
URL: http://www.samhsa.gov/about/cmhs.aspx

Center for Studying Health System Change
1100 First St. NE, 12th Floor
Washington, DC 20002-4221
(202) 484-5261
FAX: (202) 863-1763
URL: http://www.hschange.org/

Centers for Disease Control and Prevention
1600 Clifton Rd.
Atlanta, GA 30333
1-800-232-4636
E-mail: cdcinfo@cdc.gov
URL: http://www.cdc.gov/

Centers for Medicare and Medicaid Services
7500 Security Blvd.
Baltimore, MD 21244
(410) 786-3000
1-877-267-2323
URL: http://www.cms.gov/

Children's Defense Fund
25 E St. NW
Washington, DC 20001
1-800-233-1200
E-mail: cdfinfo@childrensdefense.org
URL: http://www.childrensdefense.org/

Families USA
1201 New York Ave. NW, Ste. 1100
Washington, DC 20005
(202) 628-3030
FAX: (202) 347-2417
E-mail: info@familiesusa.org
URL: http://www.familiesusa.org/

Health Coalition on Liability and Access
PO Box 78096
Washington, DC 20013-8096
URL: http://www.hcla.org/

Health Resources and Services Administration
U.S. Department of Health and Human Services
5600 Fishers Lane
Rockville, MD 20852
(301) 443-2216
1-888-275-4772
E-mail: ask@hrsa.gov
URL: http://www.hrsa.gov/index.html/

Hospice Association of America
228 Seventh St. SE
Washington, DC 20003

(202) 546-4759
FAX: (202) 547-9559
URL: http://www.nahc.org/HAA

Joint Commission on Accreditation of Healthcare Organizations
One Renaissance Blvd.
Oakbrook Terrace, IL 60181
(630) 792-5800
FAX: (630) 792-5005
URL: http://www.jcaho.org/

March of Dimes Birth Defects Foundation
1275 Mamaroneck Ave.
White Plains, NY 10605
(914) 997-4488
URL: http://www.marchofdimes.com/

Medical Group Management Association
104 Inverness Terrace East
Englewood, CO 80112-5306
(303) 799-1111
1-877-275-6462
E-mail: support@mgma.com
URL: http://www.mgma.com/

Mental Health Association
2000 N. Beauregard St., Sixth Floor
Alexandria, VA 22311
(703) 684-7722
1-800-969-6642
FAX: (703) 684-5968
URL: http://www.nmha.org/

National Association of Community Health Centers
7501 Wisconsin Ave., Ste. 1100W
Bethesda, MD 20814
(301) 347-0400
URL: http://www.nachc.com/

National Association of Public Hospitals and Health Systems
1301 Pennsylvania Ave. NW, Ste. 950
Washington, DC 20004
(202) 585-0100
FAX: (202) 585-0101
E-mail: info@naph.org
URL: http://www.naph.org/

National Association of School Psychologists
4340 East West Hwy., Ste. 402
Bethesda, MD 20814
(301) 657-0270
1-866-331-NASP
FAX: (301) 657-0275
URL: http://www.nasponline.org/

National Association of Social Workers
750 First St. NE, Ste. 700
Washington, DC 20002-4241
(202) 408-8600
URL: http://www.socialworkers.org/

National Center for Health Statistics
U.S. Department of Health and Human Services
3311 Toledo Rd.
Hyattsville, MD 20782
1-800-232-4636
URL: http://www.cdc.gov/nchs/

National Committee for Quality Assurance
1100 13th St. NW, Ste. 1000
Washington, DC 20005
(202) 955-3500
1-888-275-7585

FAX: (202) 955-3599
URL: http://www.ncqa.org/

National Institute of Mental Health
Science Writing, Press, and Dissemination Branch
6001 Executive Blvd.
Rm. 8184, MSC 9663
Bethesda, MD 20892-9663
(301) 443-4513
1-866-615-6464
FAX: (301) 443-4279
E-mail: nimhinfo@nih.gov
URL: http://www.nimh.nih.gov/

United Network for Organ Sharing
700 N. Fourth St.
Richmond, VA 23219
(804) 782-4800
1-888-894-6361
FAX: (804) 782-4817
URL: http://www.unos.org/

World Health Organization
Avenue Appia 20
Geneva 27, 1211 Switzerland
(011-41) 22-791-2111
FAX: (011-41) 22-791-3111
URL: http://www.who.int

RESOURCES

Agencies of the U.S. Department of Health and Human Services collect, analyze, and publish a wide variety of health statistics that describe and measure the operation and effectiveness of the U.S. health care system. The Centers for Disease Control and Prevention tracks nationwide health trends and reports its findings in several periodicals, especially its *Advance Data* series, *National Ambulatory Medical Care Survey*, *HIV Surveillance Reports*, and *Morbidity and Mortality Weekly Reports*. The National Center for Health Statistics provides a complete statistical overview of the nation's health in its annual *Health, United States*.

The National Institutes of Health provides definitions, epidemiological data, and research findings about a comprehensive range of medical and public health subjects. The Centers for Medicare and Medicaid Services monitors the nation's health spending. The agency's quarterly *Health Care Financing Review* and annual *Data Compendium* provide complete information on health care spending, particularly on allocations for Medicare and Medicaid. The Administration on Aging provides information about the health, welfare, and services available for older Americans.

The Agency for Healthcare Research and Quality researches and documents access to health care, quality of care, and efforts to control health care costs. It also examines the safety of health care services and ways to prevent medical errors. The Joint Commission on Accreditation of Healthcare Organizations and the National Committee for Quality Assurance are accrediting organizations that focus attention on institutional health care providers including the managed care industry.

The U.S. Census Bureau, in its *Current Population Reports* series, details the status of insurance among selected U.S. households.

Medical, public health, and nursing journals offer a wealth of health care system information and research findings. The studies cited in this edition are drawn from a range of professional publications, including *AAOS, American Journal of Nursing, Annals of Emergency Medicine, BMC Health Services Research, BMJ, Chest, Forum for Health Economics and Policy, Health Affairs, Health Care Management Review, Hospitals and Health Networks, International Journal of Clinical Practice, Journal of the American Medical Association, Journal of Hospital Medicine, New England Journal of Medicine, Policy, Politics, and Nursing Practice*, and *Primary Care: Clinics in Office Practice*.

Gale, Cengage Learning thanks the Gallup Organization for the use of its public opinion research about health care costs, quality, and concerns. It would also like to thank the many professional associations, voluntary medical organizations, and foundations dedicated to research, education, and advocacy about the efforts to reform and improve the health care system that were included in this edition.

INDEX

Balanced Budget Act of 1997
home health care and, 58–59
Medicare+Choice program, 97, 116
Bamezai, Anil, 45
Bar-code technology, 150
Barnes, Patricia M.
on access to health care, 7, 8
on CAM use, 36–37
on regular source of health care, 5
Baron, Richard J., 153
"Basic Head Start Facts" (National Head Start Association), 68
"Becoming a PA" (Commission on Accreditation of Allied Health Education Programs), 28
Beds
hospital beds in France, 140
hospital utilization statistics for OECD countries, 130–131
of mental health organizations, 56, 57t
of nursing homes, 52–53, 53t–54t
of United Kingdom's hospitals, 139
Bell, Derek, 19
Ben-Chitrit, Rosalyn, 147
Benjamin, Regina M., 68
Berenson, Julia, 46
Bergman, David A., 152
"The Best Jobs of 2012" (Graves), 24
"Beyond Numbers: The Multiple Cultural Meanings of Rising Cesarean Rates Worldwide" (Orfali), 130
Biotechnology
cost of health care and, 86, 89
online patient-physician consultations, 152–154
robotics, 154
telemedicine, 151–152
Bioterrorism
HHS and, 66
threat of, 143
Birth
cesarean delivery rates, by age of mother, 130f
cesarean delivery rates for OECD countries, 130
Birth defects, 81
Blogs, 164, 166
Bloom, Barbara
on CAM use, 36–37
on children's access to health care, 8, 10, 12
BLS. See Bureau of Labor Statistics
Blümel, Miriam, 135
"Bogus Arguments for Unproven Treatments" (Ernst), 37
Bok, Derek, 2
Boyle, Brian, 64
Brawley, Otis, 108
Breast cancer, 76

"Bridging Gaps in Healthcare Delivery" (Majerowicz & Tracy), 151
British Columbia, health care system of, 138
Bronchitis, 78
Brox, Denene, 48
Bryant, Natasha, 55
Budget
ACA, budgetary effects of insurance coverage provisions in, 125t
CMS, budgeted net outlays, 67(f4.3)
of HHS agencies, 66, 68
of National Institutes of Health, 73–74
of U.S. Department of Health and Human Services, 65, 66, 66t, 69t–71t
Buerhaus, Peter I., 153
Buettgens, Matthew, 86
Bureau of Labor Statistics (BLS)
on chiropractors, 39
on clinical social workers, 35
on counselors, 35
on dentists, 28, 29
on nursing shortage, 153
on pharmacists, 33
on physical therapists, 31–32
on physician working conditions, 21–22
on psychologists, 34
on registered nurses, 24
Burrage, PacifiCare of Oklahoma, Inc. v., 63
Bush, George W.
Deficit Reduction Act, 99–100
Medicare Prescription Drug, Improvement, and Modernization Act of 2003, 117
MSAs and, 120
Patient Safety and Quality Improvement Act, 147
Business Roundtable, 148–149
Busse, Reinhard, 135
Bynum, Julie P., 108
Byock, Ira, 60

C

California, 63
"California Limits HMO Wait Times" (Helfand), 63
Calmes, Jackie, 98
CAM. See Complementary and alternative medicine
Canada, health care system of, 137–139
Canada Health Act, 138
Canada's Medicare Bubble: Is Government Health Spending Sustainable without User-Based Funding? (Skinner & Rovere), 139
"The Canadian Health Care System, 2011" (Allin & Watson), 138
Canadian Institute for Health Information, 138–139

Cancer
American Cancer Society, 80–81
NIH website about, 76
research milestones, 65
Cancer Society, 166
Cardiac pacemakers, 151
Cardiologist, 19
Cardiovascular disease, 80
The Care of Patients with Severe Chronic Illness: An Online Report on the Medicare Program by the Dartmouth Atlas Project (Wennberg et al.), 108
Carman, Kristin L., 155
Cassel, Christine K., 52
Cassels, Caroline, 152
CBO. See Congressional Budget Office
CDC. See Centers for Disease Control and Prevention
CDC Coordinating Center for Health Information and Service, 71
"CDC Fact Sheet" (Centers for Disease Control and Prevention), 69–70
"CDC Organization" (Centers for Disease Control and Prevention), 70
CDHPs. See Consumer-driven health plans
"Census Bureau Reports World's Older Population: Projected to Triple by 2050" (U.S. Census Bureau), 40
Center for Medicare and Medicaid Innovation, 46
Center for Mental Health Services Substance Abuse and Mental Health Services Administration, 170
Center for Studying Health System Change, 170
Centers for Disease Control and Prevention (CDC)
actions to protect health of nation, 70–71
community health care needs and, 4–5
contact information, 170
on emergency department use, 48
employees of, 69–70
establishment of, 65
health care cost statistics, 83
for health information online, 166
influenza, percentage of visits for, by week, 73f
on nursing home beds, residents, occupancy rates, 52
organization and leadership, 72f
patient safety and, 148
preventive health services, 67
on regular source of health care, 5
responsibilities of, 68
Centers for Medicare and Medicaid Services (CMS)
budgeted net outlays, 67(f4.3)
contact information, 170
establishment of, 66
on health expenditures, rise in, 39
Hospital Compare website, 163

health care workers and wages, 33*t*

industrial-organizational psychologists, 34

Internet for health information, employed adults more likely to use, 166(*f*9.10)

medical specialties, compensation for, 23*t*

of pharmacists, 33

of physical therapists, 31–32

physician working conditions/earnings, 21–23

for physicians/surgeons, change in, 23*f*

of registered nurses, 24, 27, 27(*f*2.3)

registered nurses, supply/demand for, 27(*f*2.4)

searching for health information online by, 164

Employment-based health insurance, 111, 114–115

End-of-life care, 108

Endocrinologists, 24

"The English Health Care System, 2011" (Harrison), 139

Epidemiologists, 69–70

EPOs (exclusive provider organizations), 64

Ernst, Edzard, 37

Errors. *See* Medical errors; Patient safety

Estimates for the Insurance Coverage Provisions of the Affordable Care Act Updated for the Recent Supreme Court Decision (Congressional Budget Office), 13, 86, 109

"Estimates of Funding for Various Research, Condition, and Disease Categories (RCDC)" (National Institutes of Health), 104

European Union (EU)

France's health care system, 140

health care systems in, 139

United Kingdom's health care system, 139–140

Evaluation of the Wellspring Model for Improving Nursing Home Quality (Stone et al.), 55

Eviatar, Daphne, 89

"Evidence That Consumers Are Skeptical about Evidence-Based Health Care" (Carman et al.), 155

Evidence-based health care, 155

Exclusive provider organizations (EPOs), 64

Expenditures

Canadian health expenditures, 138–139

of France's health care system, 140

German health expenditures, 135–137

international comparison of health care expenditures, 127, 129–131

of Japan's health care system, 140–141

OECD countries, spending on pharmaceutical drugs, 129–130

of United Kingdom's health care system, 139–140

of U.S. health care system, 131–135

See also Cost; Spending

"An Experiment Shows That a Well-Designed Report on Costs and Quality Can Help Consumers Choose High-Value Health Care" (Hibbard et al.), 155

"Experts Talk Health-Care Reform Bill Impact" (Seligman), 64

Explaining High Health Care Spending in the United States: An International Comparison of Supply, Utilization, Prices, and Quality (Squires), 131

F

"Factbox: Canada's Universal Healthcare System" (Sibonney), 138

"Facts about ACS" (American Cancer Society), 80

"Facts about the Joint Commission" (JCAHO), 77

"Facts at a Glance" (National Institutes of Health), 73

Families USA Foundation

on consequences of being uninsured, 114

contact information, 170

on health care costs, 104–105

Family

costs of health care, hardships of, 104–106

hospice care and, 59, 60

Family Economics and Nutrition Review, 58

Family practitioner

earnings of, 23

job of, 19

Family therapists, 36

"FAQ about the Entry-Level Master's and Doctoral Degrees for Occupational Therapist" (American Occupational Therapy Association), 32

"Fast Facts on US Hospitals" (American Hospital Association), 43, 44

FDA. *See* U.S. Food and Drug Administration

Feder, Barnaby J., 154

Federal Community Mental Health Centers Act of 1963, 56

Federal government

ACA, impact on health care spending, 94

community mental health centers and, 56

Medicaid, 99–100

Medicare, 96–99

as payer of health care expenses, 84–86

public opinion on ACA, 158–159

public opinion on whether federal government should ensure that all Americans have health coverage, 159(*f*9.1)

public opinion on whether federal government should ensure that all Americans have health coverage, by political party affiliation, 159(*f*9.2)

spending on health care, increased, 93

website for patient satisfaction survey data, 163

"Feds to Put up $1.9B for Oregon Health Overhaul" (Cooper), 107

Fellowship training, 18

Females

cesarean delivery rates, by age of mother, 130*f*

life expectancy for women in U.S., 133

physician office visits by, 23

women's access to health care, 8, 8(*f*1.7)

See also Gender

Feng, Charles, 161–162

"Fight Erupts over Rules Issued for 'Mental Health Parity' Insurance Law" (Pear), 124

Fischer, Staci A., 20

Fisher, Elliott S., 108

Fisher, Peter, 37

Five-Star Quality Rating System, 53

Fleming, Sara A., 37–38

Flower, Joe, 1–2

"Focus and Impact: The AMA's Long-Range Strategic Plan" (Madera), 79

"For the Elderly, Emergency Rooms of their Own" (Hartocollis), 48

"43% Say Cost of Prescription Drugs Will Go up If Health Plan Becomes Law" (Rasmussen Reports), 105–106

France

health care system of, 140

out-of-pocket spending for health care, 129

"Francis Collins: 3 Scientific Breakthroughs Changing Medicine" (Reed), 76

Frappier Estate v. Wishnov, 63

Freeman, Gulnar, 8, 10, 12

Frenk, Julio, 2

"Frequent Users of Emergency Departments: The Myths, the Data, and the Policy Implications" (LaCalle & Rabin), 46, 48

"Frequently Asked Questions" (American Geriatrics Society), 18

Freudenheim, Milt, 151

Frieden, Thomas R., 70

Frieder, Miryam, 64

Frosch, Dominick L., 168

Funding

for cancer research by American Cancer Society, 80

national health expenditures, by source of funds, 88*t*–89*t*

National Institutes of Health total funding, fiscal year 2013, 75*f*

National Institutes of Health total funding, fiscal years 2011–13, 74*t*

personal health expenditures, by source of funds, 92*t*–93*t*

prescription drug expenditures, by source of funds, 95*t*–96*t*

See also Budget; Expenditures

Furrow, Barry R., 148

"The Future of Your Medical Data" (Harmon), 153

G

Galewitz, Phil, 94, 125

Gallup Editors: Americans' Views on the Healthcare Law (Newport, Jones, & Saad), 158

Gallup Organization
public opinion on ACA, 158–159
public opinion on impact of ACA on economy, 160, 161

Gao, Guodong Gordon, 156

Garrett, Bowen, 86

Gastroenterologist, 19

GDP. *See* Gross domestic product

Gebhart, Fred, 105

Gender
access, percentage of persons of all ages who failed to obtain needed medical care due to cost at some time during past 12 months, by age group and sex, 8(*f*1.7)
access, percentage of persons of all ages with usual place to go for medical care, by age, sex, 6(*f*1.3)
dentist visits by, 29
hospital discharge rates by, 48
persons under age 65 without health insurance at time of interview, percentage of, by age group/sex, 113(*f*6.3)
physician office visits by, 23
searching for health information online by, 164, 165(*f*9.7)
uninsured people by, 112
women's access to health care, 8

General Departmental Management, 67

General Electric, 148–149

General Motors, 148–149

Generic drugs, 105

"Generics Continue to Roll up Medication Markets" (Gebhart), 105

Genome sequencing, 75

Genomic medicine, 76

Geographical region
HMO enrollment by, 62
uninsured people by, 112

Geography and the Debate over Medicare Reform (Wennberg, Fisher, & Skinner), 108

Georgia, number of dentists in, 29

Geriatric psychiatry, 34

Geriatricians, 18

Geriatrics, 18

Germany, health care system of, 135–137

"The German Health Care System, 2011" (Busse, Blümel, & Stock), 135

Geropsychologists, 34

Gindi, Renee M.
on emergency department use, 48
on regular source of health care, 5, 7

Goldwyn, Samuel, 43

Goodman, John, 122

Government. *See* Federal government; States

Government health insurance, percentage of Americans covered by, 111

"Government Health Spending Seen Hitting $1.8 Trillion" (Morgan), 93

Government-run health care system, 158*t*

Grants
of HHS, 65
from National Institutes of Health, 74
from SAMHSA Mental Health Block Grant, 104

Graves, Jada A., 24

"The Great Health Care Debate of 1993–94" (Bok), 2

Greece, physicians practicing in, 131

Greenslit, Nathan P., 167–168

"A Grim Diagnosis for Our Ailing Health Care System" (Samuelson), 1

Gross domestic product (GDP)
Canadian health expenditures, 138
health expenditures as share of, selected countries/years, 128*t*–129*t*
increase in, 93
national health expenditures, per capita amounts, average annual percent change, 84*t*
OECD countries, percentage of GDP spent on health care, 127
percent spent on health care, 83

Group model HMO, 62

"'Growing Your Own' Nursing Staff with a Collaborative Accelerated Second-Degree, Web-Based Program" (Allen, VanDyke, & Armstrong), 153

"Growth of Consumer-Directed Health Plans to One-Half of All Employer-Sponsored Insurance Could Save $57 Billion Annually" (Haviland et al.), 93–94

Guidelines, clinical practice, 150

"Guidelines for Human Stem Cell Research" (National Institutes of Health), 75

Gulf Worker Study, 75

Gullo, Chris, 152

Gutknecht, Nancy C., 37–38

H

H1N1 influenza
CDC tracking/reporting of, 71
containment of, 157
NIH trials of vaccine for, 75

Hadley, Jack, 112, 114

Hahnemann, Samuel, 37

"Half of Doctors to Use Medical Apps in 2012" (Gullo), 152

Harmon, Katherine, 153

Harrison, Anthony, 139

Hartocollis, Anemona, 48

Harvard School of Medicine's National Comorbidity Survey, 167

"Have These Symptoms? Buy This Drug" (Chen), 167

Haviland, Amelia M.
on CDHPs, 93–94
on health savings accounts, 122

Hawaii, healers of, 127

Head Start program
administered by ACF, 66
development of, 65
services of, 68

Health, United States, 2007: With Chartbook on Trends in the Health of Americans (National Center for Health Statistics), 62

Health, United States, 2011: With Special Feature on Socioeconomic Status and Health (National Center for Health Statistics)
GDP, percentage spent on health care, 127
on health insurance source for people aged 65 years and older, 116
on hospital discharge rates, 48
on Medicaid enrollment, 118
on mental health organizations, 56
on nursing home beds, residents, occupancy rates, 52

Health and Medical Services for the Aged, of Japan, 140

Health anxiety, 164

Health care
less health care, benefits of, 107–108
quality of, 83

Health care, researching/measuring/monitoring quality of
accreditation of health care providers, 76–79
Centers for Disease Control and Prevention, 68–71
Centers for Disease Control and Prevention organization and leadership, 72*f*
Centers for Medicare and Medicaid Services, budgeted net outlays, 67(*f*4.3)
Health and Human Services budget, by operating division, 69*t*–71*t*
health care research, cycle of, 67(*f*4.1)
health care research pipeline, 67(*f*4.2)
influenza, percentage of visits for, by week, 73*f*
National Institutes of Health, 71, 73–76
National Institutes of Health, views when setting research priorities, 76*f*

"Heart Attack Patients Taken to PCI Hospitals First Treated Faster" (American Heart Association), 80

Heart disease, 75

Heart-Check Meal Certification program, 80

Heineman, Janice, 55

Helfand, Duke, 63

Hellender, Ida, 133–134

Hettrich, Carolyn, 143

HHS. *See* U.S. Department of Health and Human Services

"HHS: What We Do" (U.S. Department of Health and Human Services), 65

Hibbard, Judith H., 155

HIPAA (Health Insurance Portability and Accountability Act), 120

Hispanics
  access to health care for, 7, 14
  children's access to health care, 8
  mental health care access for, 16
  searching for health information online by, 164

"Historical Highlights" (U.S. Department of Health and Human Services), 65

"History of the American Heart Association" (American Heart Association), 80

HIV (human immunodeficiency virus)
  identification of, 65
  research budget for, 104

HMO Act of 1973, 62

HMOs. *See* Health maintenance organizations

Holahan, John, 86

Home health care
  cost of, 100
  growth in, 52
  Medicare enrollees/expenditures by type of service, 60*t*–61*t*
  Medicare limits services, 58–59
  Medicare-certified providers/suppliers, 59*t*
  overview of, 58

"Home Health Care" (*Family Economics and Nutrition Review*), 58

Homelessness
  goals for mental health service delivery, 57, 58
  mentally ill people and, 56

Homeopathic medicine, 37

HOPE–European Hospital and Healthcare Federation, 139, 140

Hospice Association of America, 170

Hospice care
  description of, 59–60
  use of, 61

Hospital Compare website, 163

Hospital Consumer Assessment of Healthcare Providers and Systems survey, 163

"Hospital Performance Trends on National Quality Measures and the Association with Joint Commission Accreditation" (Schmaltz et al.), 78

"Hospital Robots of the Future" (Lo), 154

Hospitalists, 18–19

Hospitalization
  organ transplants, 48, 50–51
  statistics on, 48

Hospitals
  accreditation of, 76–79
  American Hospital Association, 80
  in Canada, 138
  community hospitals, 44–45
  consumer satisfaction with health care facilities, 162–163
  emergency department visits within past 12 months among adults, 49*t*–50*t*
  emergency department visits within past 12 months among children under 18, 47*t*–48*t*
  emergency departments, 46, 48
  general hospitals with psychiatric services, 56
  in Germany, 136, 137
  health care at, 1
  history of, 43
  home health care, incentives for, 58
  hospital insurance with Medicare, 96
  hospital utilization statistics for OECD countries, 130–131
  hospital workers patient safety grades for their work, 148*f*
  hospitalists specialty for, 18–19
  hospitals, beds, and occupancy rates, by type of ownership/size of hospital, 44*t*
  intensivists for intensive care units, 18, 18*f*
  in Japan, 141
  national health expenditures on, 84
  patient safety, hospital characteristics associated with, 146*f*–147*f*
  patient safety, prevention of medical errors, 149–150
  patient safety ratings for, 144–145
  patient safety scores, 149
  psychiatric, 56, 57
  public hospitals, 45–46
  robots for, 154
  safety, hospitals designed for, 150
  teaching hospitals, 45
  types of, 43
  in United Kingdom, 139
  in U.S. health care system, 132–133

"House Gears up to Repeal Obamacare (Again)" (Parkinson), 3

Hoven, Ardis, 162

"How Do Consumer-Directed Health Plans Affect Vulnerable Populations?" (Haviland et al.), 122

"How Does Health Reform Affect the Health Care Workforce?" (Adamson), 41

"How Does the ACA Control Health Care Costs?" (Robert Wood Johnson Foundation), 94

"How Safe Is Your Hospital?" (Leapfrog Group), 149

"How the Affordable Care Act Supports a High-Performance Safety Net" (Riley, Berenson, & Dermody), 46

"How the Health Care Overhaul Could Affect You" (*New York Times*), 100

"How to Get Paid for Online Consults" (Dolan), 152–153

HRSA. *See* Health Resources and Services Administration

HSA. *See* Health savings account

Hu, Xinyi, 163–164

Human Genome Project, 65

Human immunodeficiency virus (HIV)
  identification of, 65
  research budget for, 104

"Human Right to Health" (NESRI), 16

Human rights, 16

I

ICF. *See* Intermediate care facility

ICUs (intensive care units), 18, 18*f*

IHS (Indian Health Service), 67

Imaging study, 4

Immunization
  pharmacists and, 32
  as preventive service, 4

"The Impact of Direct-to-Consumer Television and Magazine Advertising on Antidepressant Use" (Avery, Eisenberg, & Simon), 167

Impact of Health Reform on Women's Access to Coverage and Care (Kaiser Family Foundation), 8

Improving America's Hospitals: The Joint Commission's Annual Report on Quality and Safety (JCAHO), 78

IMS Institute for Healthcare Informatics, 167

"In Health Care Overhaul, Boons for Hospitals and Drug Makers" (Abelson), 105–106

"In Health Law, a Clearer View of Coverage" (Rabin), 123

Income
  access measures for which disparities related to age, race, ethnicity, and income improved, were unchanged, or worsened, 14*f*
  access to health care and, 16
  health care workers and wages, 33*t*
  health insurance for children and, 10
  long-term-care coverage by Medicaid and, 100
  Medicaid for low-income Americans, 99–100

"Mission of the U.S. Public Health Service Commissioned Corps" (Office of the Surgeon General), 68

Mobile devices, for health information, 166

Mohr, David C., 152

Montgomery, Lori, 98

Morbidity and Mortality Weekly Report (Centers for Disease Control and Prevention), 71

Morgan, David, 92–93

Mortality rates
infant mortality and international rankings, OECD countries, 135*t*
infant mortality in U.S., 133
reduction of with health insurance, 114
telemedicine and, 152

Mothers
cesarean delivery rates, by age of mother, 130*f*
cesarean delivery rates for OECD countries, 130

Mount Sinai Hospital, New York City, 48

Moxibustion, 38

MRI. *See* Magnetic resonance imaging

MSAs. *See* Medical savings account

Multinational Comparisons of Health Systems Data, 2011 (Squires), 131

Muñoz, Eric, 89

Murray, Patty, 116

Muse, Kate, 164

Mutual support principle, 149, 149*f*

N

Nabhan, Mohammed, 148

NACHC. *See* National Association of Community Health Centers

Nahin, Richard L., 36–37

Names/addresses, of organizations, 169–171

NAPH. *See* National Association of Public Hospitals and Health Systems

"NAPH Annual Survey Shows Increasingly Important Role of Safety Net Hospitals" (National Association of Public Hospitals and Health Systems), 46

"NAPH Concerned about Health Care Cuts in President's Budget" (Siegel), 46

"National and Surgical Health Care Expenditures, 2005–2025" (Muñoz et al.), 89

National Association of Community Health Centers (NACHC)
contact information, 170
on medically disenfranchised, 7

National Association of Public Hospitals and Health Systems (NAPH)
contact information, 170
on mission of public hospitals, 45–46

National Association of School Psychologists, 170

National Association of Social Workers
contact information, 170
work of, 35

National Bipartisan Commission on the Future of Medicare, 98

National Board for Certified Counselors, 35

National Cancer Act, 65

National Cancer Institute, 73

National Center for Complementary and Alternative Medicine (NCCAM), 36

National Center for Health Statistics (NCHS)
on children's access to health care, 8, 10, 12
contact information, 171
on GDP, percentage spent on health care, 127
on health insurance source for people aged 65 years and older, 116
on HMO enrollment, 62
on hospital discharge rates, 48
on Medicaid enrollment, 118
on mental health organizations, 56
on nursing home beds, residents, occupancy rates, 52
on regular source of health care, 5
on uninsured people, 111
work of, 70

National Center on Minority Health and Health Disparities, 73

National Commission on Fiscal Responsibility and Reform, 98

National Committee for Quality Assurance (NCQA)
accreditation of health care providers, 78
contact information, 171

National Committee on Quality Health Care, 79

National Economic and Social Right Initiative (NESRI), 16

National Federation of Independent Business v. Sebelius, Secretary of Health and Human Services, 3, 158

National Guideline Clearinghouse, 150

National Head Start Association, 68

National Health Care Workforce Commission, 41

National Health Expenditure Projections 2010–2020 (Centers for Medicare and Medicaid Services), 39

National Health Expenditures Projections 2011–2021 (Centers for Medicare and Medicaid Services), 83

National Health Interview Survey (NHIS) (Centers for Disease Control and Prevention), 5

National Health Policy Forum, 101–102

National Health Service, of United Kingdom, 139

National Health Service Corps, 65

National Healthcare Disparities Report 2011 (Agency for Healthcare Research and Quality), 13–14, 16

National Hospice and Palliative Care Organization (NHPCO), 61

National Institute for Occupational Safety and Health, 70

National Institute of Child Health and Human Development, 75

National Institute of Mental Health
on advertising for prescription drugs, 167
contact information, 171

National Institutes of Health (NIH)
achievements of, 75–76
budget of, 73–74
community health care needs and, 4–5
on costs of research, 104
establishment of, 65
for health information online, 166
overview of, 71, 73
preventive health services, 67
research priorities, establishing, 74–75
total funding, fiscal year 2013, 75*f*
total funding, fiscal years 2011–13, 74*t*
views taken into consideration when setting research priorities, 76*f*

National Library of Medicine, 73

National Nursing Home Survey, 52

National Organ Transplant Act, 65

National Physicians Alliance, 161–162

National Quality Forum, 79

"National Spending for Long-Term Services and Supports (LTSS)" (National Health Policy Forum), 101–102

Native Americans and Alaskan Natives, 67, 68

Naturopathic medicine, 37–38

"Naturopathy and the Primary Care Practice" (Fleming & Gutknecht), 37–38

NCCAM (National Center for Complementary and Alternative Medicine), 36

NCHS. *See* National Center for Health Statistics

NCQA. *See* National Committee for Quality Assurance

NESRI (National Economic and Social Right Initiative), 16

Netherlands
health care system ranking, 133
public expenditures for health care, 129

Network model HMO, 62

Neuman, Tricia, 98, 99

Neurologist, 19

Neuropsychologist, 34

"New Rules Promise Better Mental Health Coverage" (Pear), 124

New York Times, 100

Newport, Frank, 158, 161

Newson, Kawanza, 154

nursing home beds, residents, occupancy rates, 53t–54t

patient safety, hospital characteristics associated with, 146f–147f

patient safety indicators, percentage of medical office staff responding positively about, 145f

personal health expenditures, by source of funds, 92t–93t

physician offices, visits to, by age, 24t

physician offices, visits to, by selected characteristics, 25t–26t

prescription drug expenditures, by source of funds, 95t–96t

public confidence in health maintenance organizations, 161f

public confidence in U.S. health care system, 160(f9.3)

public confidence in U.S. health care system, by political party affiliation, 160(f9.4)

public opinion on preference for government-run or private health care system, 158t

public opinion on top 10 problems facing country, 162f

public opinion on whether federal government should ensure that all Americans have health coverage, 159(f9.1)

public opinion on whether federal government should ensure that all Americans have health coverage, by political party affiliation, 159(f9.2)

public opinion on whether health care reform law will help or hurt U.S. economy, 161(t9.3)

public opinion on whether health care reform law will help or hurt U.S. economy, by political party affiliation, 161(t9.4)

public opinion on whether health reform legislation should be repealed or left in place, 159t

registered nurses, supply/demand for, 27(f2.4)

U.S. Department of Health and Human Services budget, fiscal years 2011–13, 66t

usual place of health care for children under age 18, frequency/location of, 9t–10t

"Stemming the Tide of Overtreatment in U.S. Healthcare" (Sherman), 108

Steventon, Adam, 152

Stock, Stephanie, 135

Stone, Robyn, 55

Storr, Julie, 153–154

Straube, Barry M., 163

Stroke, 80

"Study: Fewer Employers Are Offering Health Insurance" (Kliff), 115

Subacute care, 53–54

Substance abuse and behavioral disorder counselors, 36

Substance Abuse and Mental Health Services Administration (SAMHSA)
function of, budget of, 67
mental health spending, 103

Substance abuse treatment
mental health/substance abuse expenditures as a percent of total health care expenditures, 103(f5.1)
spending for, 102–103

Suicide, 57

Summary Health Statistics for U.S. Children: National Health Interview Survey, 2010 (Bloom, Cohen, & Freeman), 8, 10, 12

Summary of New Health Reform Law (Kaiser Family Foundation), 99

Supplemental Medical Insurance (SMI)
with Medicare, 96–97
Medicare reform and, 98–99

Surgeons
earnings of, 23
employment for physicians/surgeons, change in, 23f

Surgery, robots for, 154

Surgical centers, 51

"Surgical Robots: Worth the Investment?" (Aston), 154

T

Tax Equity and Fiscal Responsibility Act of 1982, 97

Taxes
ACA and health care spending, 94
economic impact of ACA, 109
federal budget deficit and, 98
health savings accounts and, 120, 121
Medicare payroll tax, 125
U.S. health care financing system, 131–132

TCM (traditional Chinese medicine), 38

Teaching hospitals
overview of, 45
services of, 43

TeamSTEPPS program, 149, 149f

Teamwork
as patient safety indicator, 144–145
patient satisfaction with hospitals and, 163
TeamSTEPPS program, 149, 149f

Technology
consumer dissatisfaction with health care system and, 158
information management for health care system, 143–144
online patient-physician consultations, 152–154
for quality health care delivery, 154–156
robotics, 154
telemedicine, 151–152

Telemedicine, 151–152

"Telemedicine Improves Diabetes Management in Rural Areas" (Johnson), 151

"Telemental Health Dramatically Cuts Psychiatric Hospitalization Rates" (Cassels), 152

Television advertising, 166–168

"10 Least Expensive Public Medical Schools for In-State Students" (McMullen), 19

"10 Medical Schools That Lead to the Most Debt" (Sheehy), 19

Terminal illness, 59–61

Tertiary hospitals, 43

Testing
MRI units/CT scanners, number of, selected countries/years, 132t–133t
for patient safety, 148
See also Diagnostic tests

"Third Annual Healthcare IT Insights and Opportunities" (CompTIA), 152

"The 30 Occupations with the Largest Projected Number of Total Job Openings Due to Growth and Replacements, 2010–20" (U.S. Bureau of Labor Statistics), 153

"Time to Expand NP Scope of Practice" (Sanchez), 28

"Time to Put Patients First" (Shaw), 163

To Err Is Human: Building a Safer Health System (Institute of Medicine), 144, 147

"Too Little? Too Much? Primary Care Physicians' Views on US Health Care: A Brief Report" (Sirovich, Woloshin, & Schwartz), 2

"Tort Reform Unlikely to Cut Health Care Costs" (Eviatar), 89

"Toward Universal Health Coverage" (De Ferranti & Frenk), 2

Tracking, 144

Tracy, Susan, 151

Traditional Chinese medicine (TCM), 38

Training
of advanced practice nurses, physician assistants, 28
of clinical social workers, 35
costs of, hours involved in, 19–20
of dentists, 29
of occupational therapists, 32
of pharmacists, 33
of physical therapists, 32
of physicians, 17–18
of psychologists, 34
at teaching hospitals, 45
See also Education

"Transforming a RN to BSN Program to an On-line Delivery Format" (Abell, Williams, & Jones), 153

Transplants. *See* Organ transplants

Transtelephonic pacemaker monitoring, 151